THEORY AND APPLICATIONS OF CT IMAGING AND ANALYSIS

Edited by **Noriyasu Homma**

Theory and Applications of CT Imaging and Analysis
Edited by Noriyasu Homma

Published by InTech
Janeza Trdine 9, 51000 Rijeka, Croatia

Publishing Process Manager Katarina Lovrecic

Technical Editor Teodora Smiljanic

Cover Designer InTech Design Team

Additional hard copies can be obtained from orders@intechopen.com

Theory and Applications of CT Imaging and Analysis, Edited by Noriyasu Homma
p. cm.
ISBN 978-953-307-234-0

Meet the editor

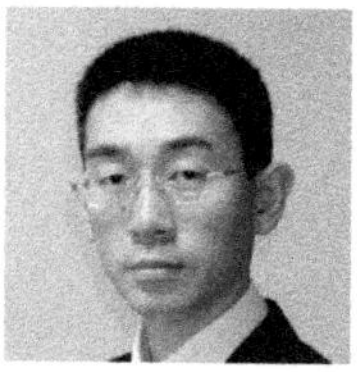

Dr. Noriyasu Homma received a BA, MA, and PhD in electrical and communication engineering from Tohoku University, Japan, in 1990, 1992, and 1995, respectively. From 1995 to 1998, he was a lecturer at the Tohoku University, Japan. He is currently an associate professor of the Cyberscience Center at the Tohoku University. From 2000 to 2001, he was a visiting professor at the Intelligent Systems Research Laboratory, University of Saskatchewan, Canada. His current research interests include neural networks, complex and chaotic systems, soft-computing, cognitive sciences, medical systems and brain sciences. He has published over 100 papers, and co-authored 1 book and 10 chapters in 10 research books in these fields.

Contents

Contents

Preface

The x-ray computed tomography (CT) is well known as a useful imaging method and the invention of several pioneers such as G. Hounsfield and A. M. Cormack in 1970's. This was a brilliant breakthrough as people could not see only fluoroscopic, but tomographic inside shapes of a target without cutting it. Since that time, CT images have continuously been used for many applications, especially in medical fields. This book discloses recent advances and new ideas in theories and applications of CT imaging and its analysis.

The book contains 16 chapters, which are classified by application purposes into the following five parts:

Part 1: CT Image Analysis for Computer-Aided Diagnosis (Chapters 1 to 4)
Part 2: CT Image Analysis for Preoperational Planning (Chapters 5 to 7)
Part 3: CT Image Analysis for Radiotherapy (Chapters 8 and 9)
Part 4: Advanced CT Imaging and Analysis (Chapters 10 to 14)
Part 5: CT Imaging and Analysis for Non-Medical Applications (Chapters 15 and 16)

Parts 1 to 4 are devoted to theories and applications of CT imaging and analysis in medical fields where several image processing techniques such as segmentation, registration, and recognition can be used for observing important pieces of medical information such as positions and shapes of targets to diagnose and treat them accurately. Parts 1, 2, 3, and 4 provide CT imaging and analysis for computer-aided diagnosis (CAD), preoperational (surgery) planning, radiotherapy, and other advanced purposes, respectively. On the other hand, Part 5 is devoted to non-medical CT imaging and analysis such as for forensic and industrial applications.

The 16 chapters selected in this book cover not only the major topics of CT imaging and analysis in medical fields, but also some advanced applications for forensic and industrial purposes. These chapters propose state-of-the-art approaches and cutting-edge research results. I could not thank enough to the contributions of the authors. This book would not have been possible without their support.

February 2011

Noriyasu Homma
Cyberscience Center
Tohoku University
Sendai,
Japan

Part 1

CT Image Analysis for Computer-Aided Diagnosis

1

CT Image Based Computer-Aided Lung Cancer Diagnosis

Noriyasu Homma
Cyberscience Center, Tohoku University
Japan

1. Introduction

An early stage detection of lung cancer is extremely important for survival rate and quality of life (QOL) of patients (Naruke et al., 1988). Although a nationwide periodical group medical examination is conducted in Japan by diagnosing chest X-ray images, such group examination is not often good enough to detect the lung cancer accurately and thus there is a high possibility that the cancer at an early stage cannot be detected by using only the chest X-ray images. To improve the detection rate for the cancer at early stages, X-ray computed tomography (CT) has been used for a group medical examination as well (Iinuma et al., 1992; Yamamoto et al., 1993).

Using the X-ray CT, pulmonary nodules that are typical shadows of pathological changes of the lung cancer (Prokop and Galanski, 2003) can be detected more clearly compared to the chest X-ray examination even if they are at early stages. This is an advantage of the X-ray CT diagnosis. In fact, it has been reported that the survival rate of the later ten years can reach 90% after the detection at early stages using X-ray CT images (I-ECAP, 2006).

On the other hand, compared to the chest X-ray images diagnosis, the X-ray CT diagnosis may exhaust radiologists because the CT generates a large number of images (at least over 30 images per patient) and they must diagnose all of them. The radiologists' exhaustion and physical tiredness might cause a wrong diagnosis especially for a group medical examination where most of CT images are healthy and only very few images involve the pathological changes. Therefore, some computer-aided diagnosis (CAD) systems have been developed to help their diagnosis work (Okumura et al., 1998; Lee et al., 1997; Yamamoto et al., 1994; Miwa et al., 1999). Core techniques of CAD systems can be found in feature extraction and pattern recognition. Because of the fuzziness of the diagnosis target in the medical images, it often requires different methods from those for artificial targets.

Miwa et al. have developed a variable N-quoit filter to detect isolated pulmonary nodules (Miwa et al., 1999) and Homma et al. have further improved the detection accuracy by discriminating between the isolated nodules and blood vessels those are both in a circle-like shape in CT images (Homma et al., 2008). The discrimination was achieved by developing new feature extraction techniques and combining those features extracted by the techniques. These methods, however, aimed at detecting only isolated circle-like shapes with the some morphological features, and thus non-isolated nodules (pathological changes) may not be detected by such methods. Indeed, it has been demonstrated that the conventional methods can detect isolated nodules shown in Fig. 1 (a) (Homma et al., 2008), but cannot or hard to detect a non-isolated nodule shown in Fig. 1 (b). A schematic difference between isolated and non-isolated targets is depicted in Fig. 2.

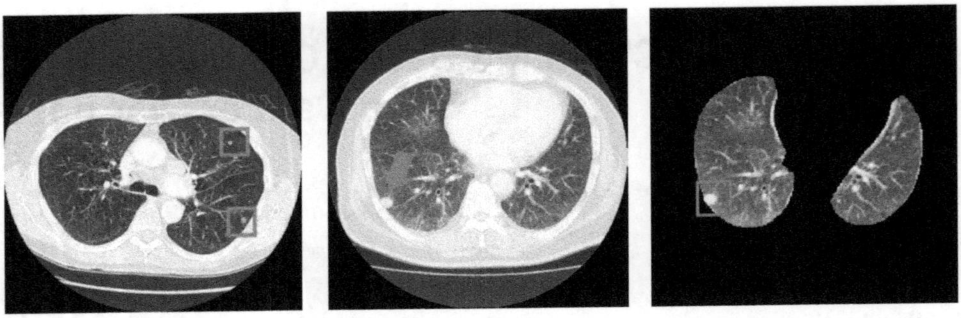

(a) Red squares show locations of isolated-nodules

(b) Red arrow indicates a non-isolated nodule

(c) Red square shows a converted isolated nodule from non-isolated one

Fig. 1. (a) Isolated and (b) non-isolated nodules, and the conversion (c) from non-isolated into isolated one.

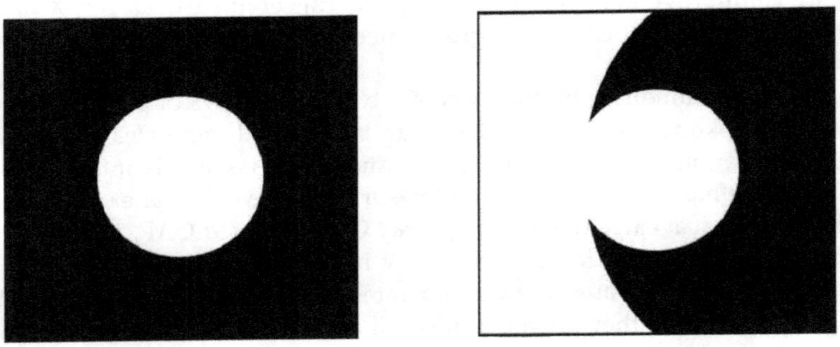

(a) Isolated target

(b) Non-isolated target

Fig. 2. A schematic difference between isolated and non-isolated targets.

Although non-isolated nodules are not very often seen in lung cancer observations, they can be a lung cancer with a high possibility and should not be missed from the viewpoint of the early stages detection of cancers (I-ECAP, 2006).

In this chapter, to improve the detection rate of such non-isolated nodules, we propose a technique transforming the *non-isolated nodules* connected to the walls of the chest into *isolated ones* that can be detected more easily by the conventional CAD systems. The transformation of Fig. 2 (b) into (a) can be achieved by extracting the lung area from the original whole CT image as shown in Fig. 1 (c).

The rest of this chapter consists of as follows. In section 2, a fundamental theory of active contour models (Kass et al., 1998) that can be used for such extraction and its local optimum problem will be introduced. Then, by setting appropriate initial contours for solving the local optimum problem, a novel extraction technique based on the contour model will be developed in section 3. Experimental results using clinical data of X-ray CT images will be discussed to demonstrate the usefulness of the proposed method in section 4. Concluding remarks will be given in section 5.

2. Active contour model

The active contour model proposed by Kass ((Kass et al., 1998) uses a gradient decent-based optimal method. The optimality can be defined by an energy function. The time evolution of the model is controlled by the following partial differential equation.

$$\frac{\partial v}{\partial t} = -\eta \frac{\partial E}{\partial v} \tag{1}$$

where $v(t,x,y)$ is a function of time t and coordinates x and y in the two dimensional space of the original image. η is a positive coefficient. The contour can be defined by a set of coordinates (x,y) satisfying a condition $v = L$ where L is a constant. Obviously, the final contour evolved by (1) is depended on the energy function E.

A well known simple energy function is related to the edge of the original image and can be defined as follows.

$$E = -\iint_{\Omega} \left|\nabla I(x,y)\right|^2 dxdy \tag{2}$$

where $I(x,y)$ is a pixel value at the coordinates (x,y) and $\nabla I(x,y)$ is the spatial gradient of the pixel value. Ω is a domain of the coordinates (x,y) on the contour, i.e, $\Omega = \{(x,y) | v(x,y) = L\}$. By using the energy function E in Eq. (2), the final contour may be on an edge of the original image in which the gradient of the pixel value is the local maximum (i.e., the local minimum for the energy function). Fig. 3 shows an example of the time evolution of the contour given by the active contour model where the energy function was defined by Eq. (2).

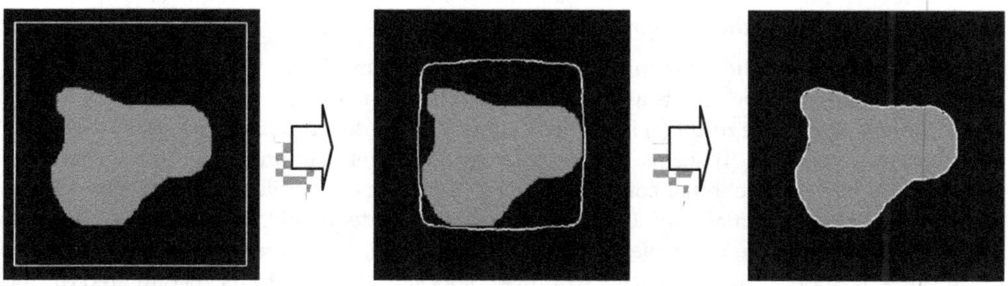

(a) Initial contour (b) Contour in a halfway (c) Final contour

Fig. 3. A sample time evolution of active contour. White lines show contours.

Since the active contour model is controlled by a gradient-decent evolution as mentioned above, the final result is also depended on the initial settings of the contour. In other words, such model can converge to a local optimal solution instead of the global optimal one. Thus, as well as the right design of the energy function, an appropriate setting of the initial contour is required to obtain the desired contour. Fig. 4 shows an example illustrating

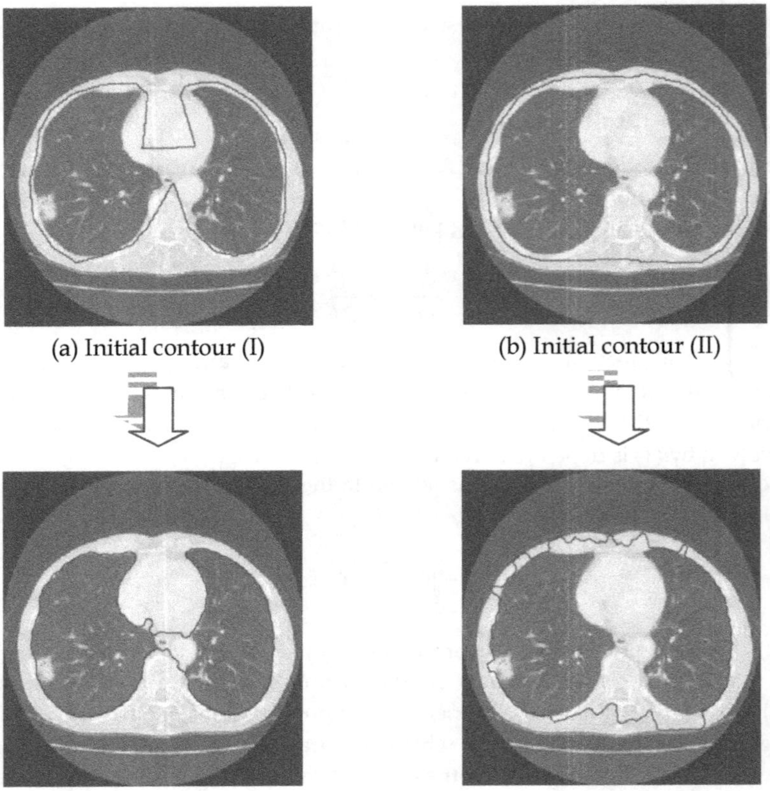

(a) Initial contour (I) (b) Initial contour (II)

(c) Final contour for the initial contour (I) (d) Final contour for the initial contour (II)

Fig. 4. Effect of initial contours on the final results: Examples using the same lung X-ray CT image. Black lines near the walls on the CT images are contours.

results obtained from different initial contours for the same X-ray CT image. In fact, as is clear from this figure, the results are quite different from each other.

In addition, note that the result (I) in Fig. 4 (c) may be more desirable than the result (II) in Fig. 4 (d) because the result (I) seems more similar to the target contour inside the walls of the chest. This is because the initial contour (I) in Fig. 4 (a) is more similar to the target and thus appropriate than the initial contour (II) in Fig. 4 (b). Consequently, if an initial contour as similar as possible to the desirable contour could be given, it may be expected that the final result is the most desirable one since the number of local optimal contours encountered during the time evolution can be the minimum compared to those for the other initial settings.

3. Advanced active contour model for lung cancer diagnosis

As expected in the last paragraph of section 2, the local optimum problem can be avoided by starting from the appropriate initial contours. Note that a lung shape changes smoothly in axial direction as shown in Fig. 5 and recently the interval between X-ray CT slices next to each other is at most 10 [mm] in the direction. Then lung shapes in CT slices (axial tomography) next to each other are almost the same or at least similar as shown in original CT images of Fig. 6. Thus a novel technique proposed here initializes the contour by using such anatomical characteristics of the lung shape. That is, the resulting contour obtained from the active contour model on the CT slice next to a target slice can be an appropriate candidate for the initial contour of the target CT slice. This is a key idea of the proposed initialization. Let us define, in this chapter, a lung area as inside the thorax that includes the center area of heart and aorta, and consider the walls of the chest that does not include the center area.

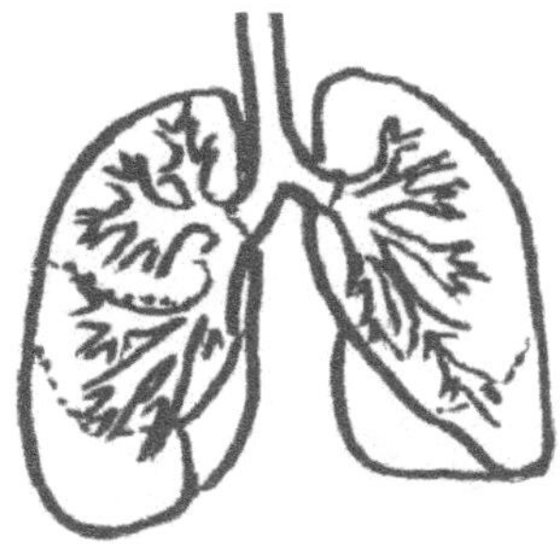

Fig. 5. A schema of a human lung.

A flowchart of the proposed algorithm for extracting the lung area is shown in Fig. 7. In this algorithm, only the first CT slice is needed to be initialized in a specific way and called the *initial slice* of a series of the slices. Because of the specific initialization, steps (i) and (ii) in the flowchart for the initial slice are different from those of the other slices. In the followings, it is assumed, for simplicity, that the algorithm processes the series of CT slices from the head to the legs in the axial direction, but the algorithm is the same for the reverse direction.

(i). Selection of the target slice: If the current target is the initial slice of the series, select a slice without non-isolated nodules connected to the walls of the chest. Otherwise, select the slice below the previous target slice.

(ii). Initialization: There are many local optima during the time evolution of the model due to the edges created by the costae (bones) in the walls of the chest as shown in Fig. 4 (d). The resulting contour of the previous target slice can be a good candidate for the initial contour of the current slice as described above. The initialization except for the initial slice can thus be done easily by setting the candidate.

There is, however, no previous final contour for the initial slice. In this case, to remove such undesirable edges, an equalization of the pixel values that are larger than a threshold is conducted within the walls of the initial slice. The equalization can be given as follows.

$$I'(x,y) = \begin{cases} I_{max}, & (I(x,y) > I_{Th}) \\ I(x,y), & (otherwise) \end{cases} \quad (3)$$

where $I'(x,y)$ denotes a new pixel value after the equalization, I_{Th} is the threshold, and I_{max} is the maximum pixel value that usually represents the white color.

As shown in Fig. 8, lung area of the initial slice can be extracted by using a mask processing. Then, a good result can be obtained from any contour outside the mask

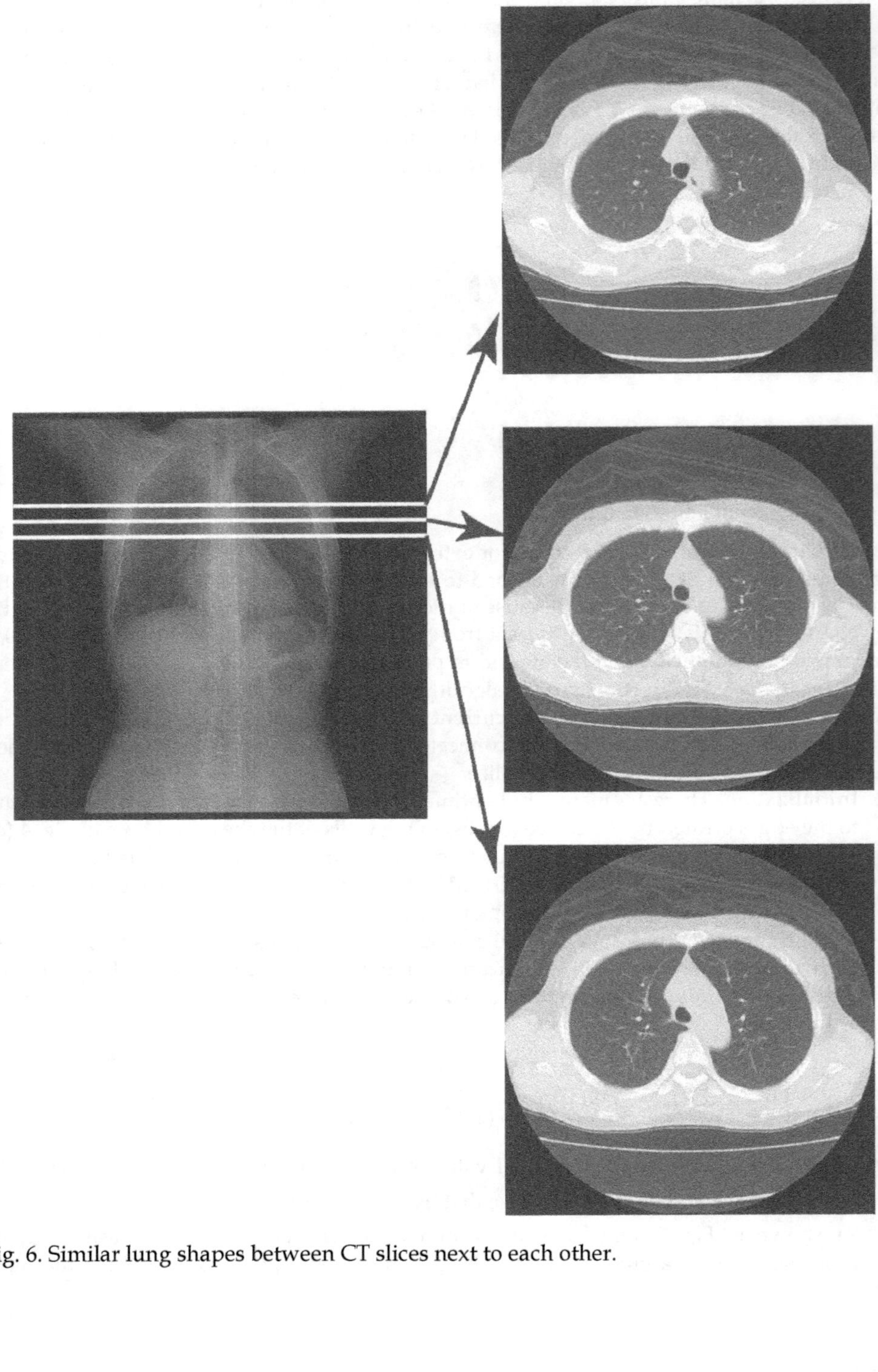

Fig. 6. Similar lung shapes between CT slices next to each other.

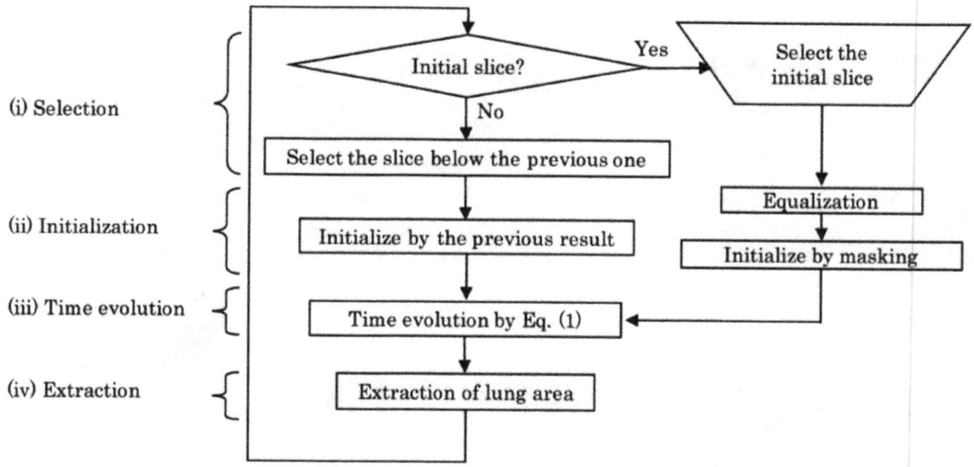

Fig. 7. Flowchart of the proposed method.

area. Note that lung area, however, could not often be extracted correctly if there is a non-isolated nodule connected to the walls of the chest as shown in Fig. 9. In this case, the non-isolated nodule that we want to detect is regarded as outside the lung area and thus cannot be detected by the mask processing. This is only the reason why we need to select the initial slice manually.

(iii). Time evolution: By using Eq. (1), the resulting contour for the current target slice selected in step (i) can be obtained from the contour initialized in step (ii).

(iv). Extraction: The lung area for the current target is extracted as the inside the resulting contour obtained in step (iii).

Steps (i) - (iv) are repeatedly conducted until all lung areas in all CT slices are extracted.

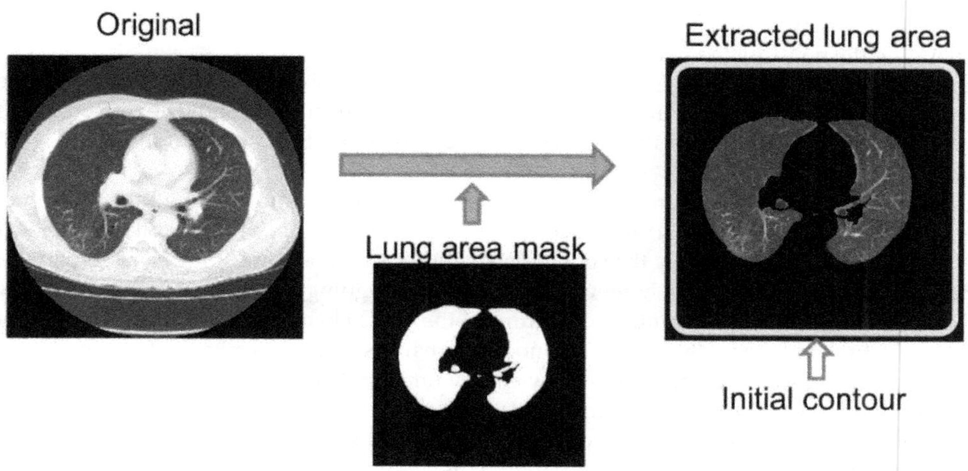

Fig. 8. A mask processing to extract the lung area.

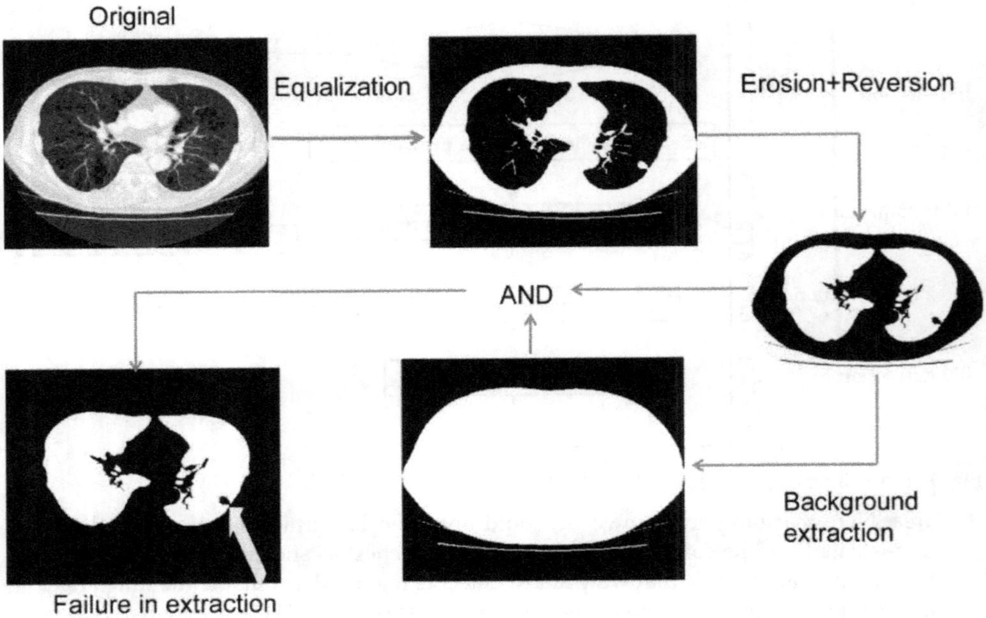

Fig. 9. A failure case of the mask processing for a slice where there is a non-isolated nodule connected to the walls of the chest.

4. Application to lung cancer diagnosis

We have tested the proposed method using an extraction task in which the clinical CT images (https://imaging.nci.nih.gov/ncia/faces/baseDef.tiles) including non-isolated nodules connected to the walls of the chest are used. Examples of the extraction results are shown in Figs. 10 and 11. It is clear that the proposed method can extract the lung area including the non-isolated nodules.

Extracted areas by the initial and the resulting contours for the original slice in Fig. 10 (c) are shown in Fig. 12. Note that the initial contour that is the resulting contour obtained in the previous slice in Fig. 10 (f) is similar enough to the target and thus, the final result in Fig. 10 (g) is good enough.

On the other hand, there are a few examples in which non-isolated nodules were not extracted as the lung area, but regarded as within the walls. In such case, still non-isolated nodules cannot be detected by the conventional CAD systems aiming at the isolated nodules detection. This problem may, however, be solved by designing a further appropriate energy function. For example, the contour curvature of the walls changes smoothly in general, but the curvature involving the connected nodules changes more sharply. Differences in the curvature may be incorporated into a new energy function to discriminate such non-isolated nodules from the walls of the chest.

Furthermore, the active contour model has an ability of making a smooth contour line even if the initial contour has a sharp corner with a high curvature. We can then select the initial slice in an automatic way, i.e., random selection, the first (top), middle, or last (bottom) slice

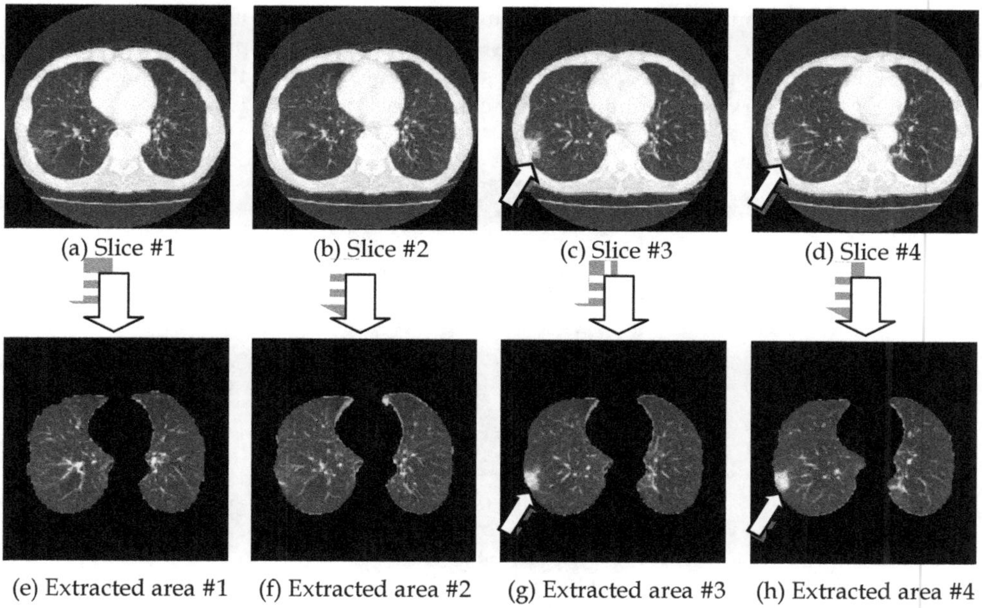

Fig. 10. Extracted results for case 1 by the proposed active contour method. (a) - (d): Original CT images. (e) - (h): Extracted lung areas.

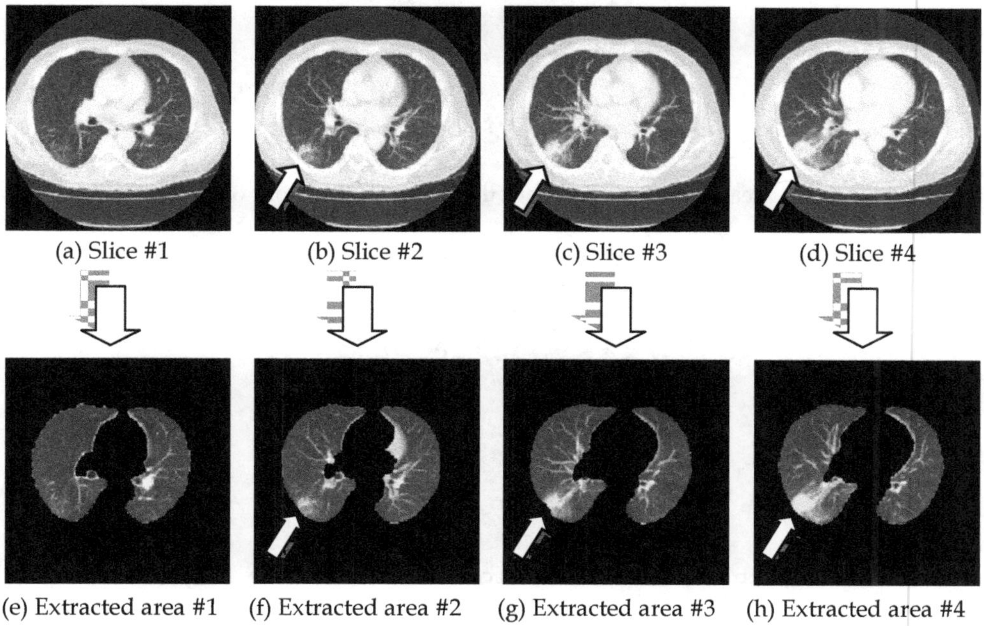

Fig. 11. Extracted results for case 2 by the proposed active contour method. (a) - (d): Original CT images. (e) - (h): Extracted lung areas.

of the series, and so on. The masking problem with the initial slice including non-isolated nodules connected to the walls of the chest can be solved by applying the proposed algorithm with an appropriate parameters setting repeatedly to the same series. This direction of future works can be important for clinical use.

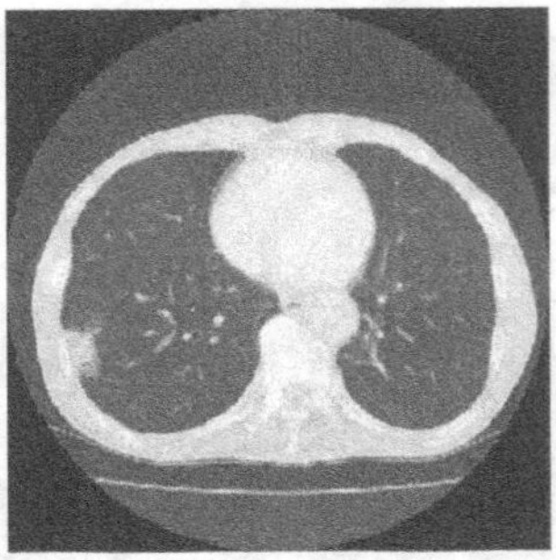

(a) Original CT image (same as in Fig. 10 (c))

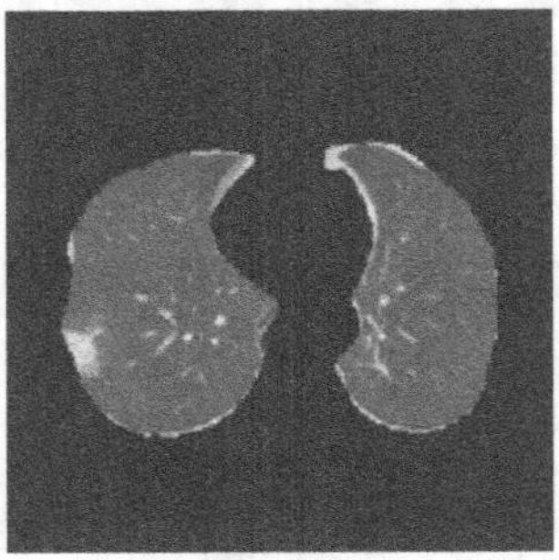

(b) Extracted area by the initial contour that is the final contour of the above slice

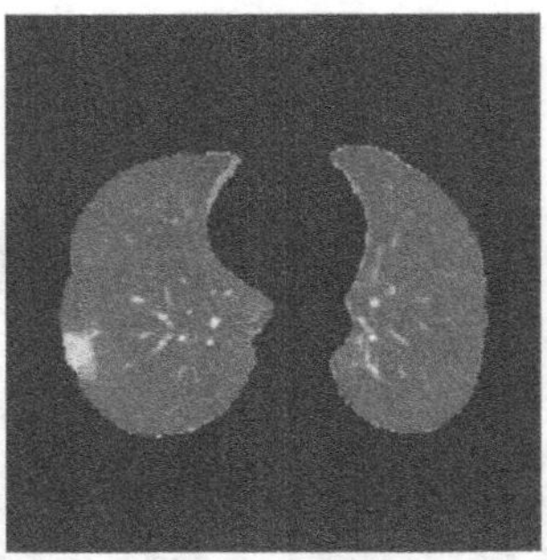

(c) Extracted area by the final contour (same as in Fig. 10 (g))

Fig. 12. The appropriate initial contour and the final contour for the CT slice #3 in Fig. 10 (c).

5. Concluding remarks

In this chapter, we have taken into account non-isolated nodules connected to the walls of the chest that cannot be detected by the conventional CAD systems for lung cancer. To detect such nodules, we have proposed a technique to transform the non-isolated nodules into the isolated ones by using an active contour model to extract the lung area from the original CT image. The promising results suggest that the detection accuracy of the CAD systems can be further improved by incorporating the proposed technique.

6. Acknowledgements

This work was partially supported by The Ministry of Education, Culture, Sports, Science and Technology under Grant-in-Aid for Scientific Research #19500413 and the Okawa Foundation.

7. References

T. Naruke, et al. (1988). Prognosis and survival in resected lung carcinoma based on the new international staging system, *J. Thorac Cardiovasc Surg*, Vol. 96, pp. 440-447, 1988.

Takeshi Iinuma, Yukio Tateno, Toru Matsumoto, Shinji Yamamoto, and Mitsuomi Matsumoto. (1992). Preliminary Specification of X-ray CT for Lung Cancer Screening (LSCT) and its Evaluation on Risk-Cost-Effectiveness, *Nippon Acta Radiologica*, Vol. 52, pp. 182-190 (in Japanese).

Shinji Yamamoto, Ippei Tanaka, Masahiro Senda, Yukio Tateno, Takeshi Iinuma, Toru Matsumoto, Mitsuomi Matsumoto. (1993). Image Processing for Computer Aided Diagnosis in the Lung Cancer Screening System by CT(LSCT), *Trans. Institute of Electronics, Information and Communication Engineers*, Vol. 76-D-2, pp. 250-260 (in Japanese).

M. Prokop and M. Galanski. (2003). *Spiral and Multislice Computed Tomography of the Body*, Thieme Medical Publishers, Stuttgart.

International Early Lung Cancer Action Program (I-ELCAP). (2006). Survival of Patients with Stage I Lung Cancer Detected on CT Screening, *NEJM*, Vol. 355, No. 17, pp. 1763-1771.

T. Okumura, T. Miwa, J. Kako, S. Yamamoto, M. Matsumoto, Y. Tateno, T. Iinuma and T. Matsumoto. (1998). Variable-N-Quoit filter applied for automatic detection of lung cancer by X-ray CT, *Proc. of Computer-Assisted Radiology*, pp. 242-247 (in Japanese).

Y. Lee, T. Hara, H. Fujita, S. Itoh and T. Ishigaki. (1997). `Nodule detection on chest helical CT scans by using a genetic algorithm, *Proc. of IASTED International Conference on Intelligent Information Systems*, pp. 67-70.

Shinji Yamamoto, Masato Nakayama, Masahiro Senda, Mitsuomi Matsumoto, Yukio Tateno, Takeshi Iinuma, Tohru Matsumoto. (1994). A Modified MIP Processing Method for Reducing the Lung Cancer X-ray CT Display Images, *Medical Imaging Technology*, Vol. 12, No. 6 (in Japanese).

Tomoko Miwa, Jun-ichi Kako, Shinji Yamamoto, Mitsuomi Matsumoto, Yukio Tateno, Takeshi Iinuma, Toru Matsumoto. (1999). Automatic Detection of Lung Cancers in Chest CT Images by the Variable N-Quoit Filter, *Trans. Institute of Electronics, Information and Communication Engineers*, Vol. 82-D-II, pp.178-187 (in Japanese).

N. Homma, K. Takei, and T. Ishibashi. (2008). Combinatorial Effect of Various Features Extraction on Computer Aided Detection of Pulmonary Nodules in X-ray CT Images, *WSEAS Trans. Information Science and Applications*, Vol. 5, Issue 7, pp. 1127-1136.

Michael Kass, Andrew Witkin, and Demetri Terzopoulos. (1998). Snakes: Active Contour Models, *International Journal of Computer Vision*, pp. 321-331.

National Cancer Imaging Archive (NCIA), https://imaging.nci.nih.gov/ncia/faces/baseDef.tiles

2

Informatics and Computerized Tomography Aiding Detection and Diagnosis of Solitary Lung Cancer

Aristófanes Corrêa Silva[1], Anselmo Cardoso Paiva[2], Rodolfo Acatauassu Nunes[3] and Marcelo Gattass[4]

[1,2]*Federal University of Maranhão, Applied Computing Group NCA/UFMA, Av. dos Portugueses, S/N, Campus do Bacanga, Bacanga, CEP 65085-580, São Luís - MA*
[3]*State University of Rio de Janeiro - UERJ, São Francisco de Xavier, 524, Maracanã, CEP 20550-900, Rio de Janeiro, RJ*
[4]*Pontiphical Catholic University of Rio de Janeiro - PUC-Rio, R. São Vicente, 225, Gávea, CEP 22453-900, Rio de Janeiro, RJ*
Brazil

1. Introduction

From all malignant tumors, except for non-melanoma skin cancer, lung cancer is the second most common type among men and the most frequent among women. The most worrying characteristic of this kind of cancer, however, is that it has caused more deaths that the sum of the deaths caused by prostate, breast and rectal cancer in developed countries. Patients with lung cancer have a five-year survival rate varying from 13% to 21% in developed countries and varying from 7% to 10% in emerging countries. Only in 2005, 1.3 million deaths were caused by lung cancer throughout the world. In this very same year, the National Institute of Cancer (INCA) registered on the official statistics that lung cancer caused the death of 14,715 people in Brazil. Estimations of this specialized Brazilian organism point that the number of new cases in 2010 will be 17,810 among men and 9,460 among women. Such incidence is still the result of the large consumption of tobacco in the past, and does not reflect the present scenario of reduction of the smoking habit by the people as a result of the preventive actions more recently implemented (INCA, 2009).

Such incidence is still the result of the large consumption of tobacco in the past, and does not reflect the present scenario of reduction of the smoking habit by the people as a result of the preventive actions more recently implemented through the world. One of the causes of the low survival rate from lung cancer is related to difficulty of its precocious diagnosis due to the absence of symptoms and to the poor diagnosis at more advanced stages of the disease (Jamnik et al., 2002). Due to these characteristics, several efforts have been made targeting precocious diagnosis of lung cancer.

The detection of lung cancer in an initial stage has been improved by a wider use of noninvasive image techniques, such as radiography and computerized chest tomography (CT). However, invasive techniques are still necessary to the diagnostic definition that occurs through the cytological and histopathological study of materials obtained via suction puncture or biopsy. In this scenario, where the application of non-invasive techniques gains special relevance, a large number of computational tools have been employed, such as Computer-aided Detection (CAD) and Computer-aided diagnosis (CADx), developed from image processing and computer vision techniques.

Using digital images generated in the process of acquisition of the CT, it is possible to identify the lung nodule and execute a series of measurements on it, in order to find some correlation among these measurements and its diagnose of malignancy or benignity (Silva et al., 2009). The need to obtain a precise diagnose of the lung nodule in order to provide longer survival to the patient, specially at the starting stage when the tumor still has small dimensions, has incited many researchers to look for new forms of detection and diagnosing with help of a computer (Matsuoka et al., 2005), (Khan et al., 1991), (Vittitoe et al., 1997) and (Wolf et al., 2005). The idea present in those tools is to provide an aid to the specialist doctor, whether to evince suspicious radiological artifacts or to offer a second opinion to the specialist in the diagnosing.

Works as those of (Jeong et al., 2005) and (Reeves & Kostis, 2000) have well demonstrated this task of detection and diagnosing of the lung nodule. There is a set of works in the area of pattern recognition that use texture and morphology as discriminative features of benign and malignant nodules in the diagnosing, such as in (Iwano et al., 2005) and (Seemann et al., 1999), that use the form of the nodule and in (Lo et al., 2003) that use morphology and texture together, aiming to classify the nodule as malignant or benign. Recent researches in the area of image processing with adoption of techniques of exploratory analysis of areas, largely used in geostatistics, have presented promising works, such as (Silva et al., 2005), (Silva et al., 2009) and (Silva et al., 2008), which extract certain texture measurements associated to the lung nodules and are able to discriminate them as malignant and benign with accuracy varying from 80% to 100%. However, this behavior is not perfectly noticed when using more than one CT image database containing a sufficiently large number of lung nodule cases. Given this, new measurements are being adapted to be used in lung nodule diagnosis, aiming to obtain the same behavior when using several CT image databases.

This work presents a methodology for recognition of directional patterns of spatial distribution, having the computer as a tool for diagnose aiding, especially in a precocious manner, when the classic initial characteristics of malignancy are not well defined

The chapter is divided in the following way: Section 2 gives the medical viewpoint of the characteristics of a lung nodule. In Section 3 we show the state of the art of works that do the detection and/or diagnosis of lung nodules. Section 4 exemplifies a tentative of our research team to automatically detect the lung nodule in a CT exam. In Section 5 we show the application of one geostatistical measure and geometric measurements to suggest a diagnosis for the lung nodule. In Section 6 we will give an ideia of how we expect CAD/CADx to be applied to CT images in the next years. Finally, in Section 7, we present some final considerations.

2. Medical viewpoint of the diagnosing of the solitary lung nodules by computerized tomography

Lung cancer, associated to the smoking habit in more than 90% of cases, is the leading cause of deaths and, in developed countries, it is responsible for a mortality rate bigger than that of breast, prostate and rectal-colon cancer together, which, despite the large incidence, are more controllable tumors from the therapeutic viewpoint. Perhaps the large amount of cancerous substances carried by the smoke of cigarettes propitiates multiple molecular ways, which represent a greater biological aggressiveness and more difficult therapeutic response. On the other hand, paradoxically, lung cancer is easier to prevent and decreases in parallel with the reduction of the use of tobacco, such as has been seen world-wide. Unfortunately, in less developed countries, the use of cigars has been increasing, bringing a disease of difficult control, whose five-year survival, after diagnosis, is about 10%, in those locations where health systems are weaker. The best chance to improve the survival in lung cancer is the precocious diagnosis, occasionally done by the detection of anomalies in the bronchial mucosa, the bronchoscopy and, more frequently, by finding the image of a lung nodule.

The solitary lung nodule is defined as an spherical image of up to 3 cm of diameter, not accompanied by lesions that could suggest metastasis or invasion of neighbor structures, traditionally obtained with a simple pulmonary radiography. Nevertheless, since the rise of the first Computerized Tomography prototypes, evolving to the helical technique with a detector and, more recently, multiple detectors (multi slice), it has been possible to diagnose lung nodules which were invisible to simple X-rays.

In general, the more frequent diagnosing, which correspond to more than 80% of the cases of lung nodules, but which can vary according to the characteristics of the population under study, are the tuberculous or fungal granulomas, primary or metastatic lung cancer, the harmatoma and the carcinoid tumor (Franquet et al., 2003). The main consequence of the diagnosing of small nodules is the increase of the possibility of catching lung cancer in a recent stage, what is known to increase the possibility of cure (Hanley & Rubins, 2003), (Lillington & Caskey, 2003). This fact has already its reflections in the present TNM staging system for lung cancer, modified in 2010, and which now covers the so called T1 (tumor with up to 3 cm in diameter) in two sub-categories: T1a (up to 2 cm) and T1b (ranging from 2 to 3 cm), created with the hope of stratify different survivals (Rami-Porta et al., 2009).

Together with all this benefic repercussion in the precocious detection of lung cancer, there appears, on the other hand, a greater diagnostic difficulty, since benign nodules constitute the majority of small nodules. Naturally, if there is not a correct judgment of the lung nodule image, there will be an unnecessary increase of the number of invasive diagnosing procedures, such as punctures with thin and cutting needles, transbronchial biopsy, video-assisted thoracic surgery (VATS) and thoracotomy, methods with several possibilities of complications, but in most cases with no mortality. Thus, all of the attributes of the image must be well evaluated, not only to detect the nodule, but also to help determining its nature. In this context, we may give emphasis to the screening of lung cancer, the measurement of texture and density of the nodule, the dynamical evaluation by the volumetry and contrast impregnation and the fusion of the images obtained by CT and positron emission (PET/CT). The computerized methods for aiding detection and diagnosis, central object of this chapter, are analyzed in the next section.

2.1 Tracking lung cancer through computerized tomography

Despite there is not a definitive proof that the screening by Computerized Tomography decreases the global mortality by lung cancer, various findings tend to serve as a indication that this goal can be achieved, maybe with the association to more than on advanced screening method, such as looking for antibodies in the peripheral blood (Patel et al., 2010).

Studies about screening lung cancer using low-dosage helical computerized tomography have advanced mainly in the USA, especially in New York City, which in a pioneer manner showed the first results in 1999, from an experiment started in 1993. Other studies have also been developed in Canada, Europe and Japan (I.Henschke & Yankelevitz, 2000). Despite some criticisms about the cost-effectiveness of the method and the lack of a control group, the works

have been multiplying and make clear the intention of coming to a standard of effectiveness in order to reduce the mortality by lung cancer (Bellomi et al., 2006).
Detection aiding software can, through well established algorithms, perform the automatic tracking of images with nodular profile, but still find difficulties in the segmentation of nodules close to vessels and the thoracic wall, which demand special techniques. A special advantage would be the diminishment og the errors caused by the radiologist's tiredness, since with modern devices the number of images to be analyzed increased significantly. However, a relatively large number of false positives have been observed and this also testifies that it will always be necessary the radiologist's interpretation. Selecting the group of risk for lung cancer, and in which can be different inclusion criteria, the percentage of lung nodules per patient has been very variable in the literature, achieving even 50%, due to the endemic pulmonary disorders. Nevertheless, most part of these nodules is constituted by benign nodules, about 90% of cases, and so the need for observation has been increasing. In parallel, new diagnosing programs (CADx systems) have been adopted, always intending to increase sensibility, specificity and accuracy in order to make the final judgment easier for the responsible medical (Way et al., 2010).

2.2 Texture of the lung nodule to the computerized tomography

With the rise of the tomographers with multiple detectors, the discovery of nodules has become more and more frequent. These nodules, besides small, have diverse textures. Screening programs have surprise entirely solid, non-solid (fosco glass texture) and mixed nodules, which may have different biological behaviors (Hasegawa et al., 2000). This way, for example, solid nodules are comprised into the whole spectrum between the carcinoma (small and non-small cells) while the non-solid ones are usually represented by adenocarcinomas of the bronchoalveolar subtype, with different biological behavior, normally more indolent. Recent works have showed that the frosted glass texture, though being unspecific, can be the starting form of lung cancer for computerized tomography. On the other hand nodules heavily calcified, with central calcification or popcorn-like calcifications are inherently benign. Nodules which alternate regions of fat density and rough calcifications suggest harmatoma, a benign nodule composed of cartilagenous, osseous and fat tissues, with normal histological aspect.
Nodules with predominance of density of soft parts, where cancer is more incident, need a deeper study, because the human sight is unable to observe the minimal differences on gray tones, which are actually the expression of a certain X-ray attenuation coefficient. Computer programs can do this separation by analyzing the texture of the lung nodules through the statistical study of the component voxels or eventual arrangements they form, each one with its value or intensity. Despite these programs are very promising, they remain under study in the literature being tested against a lung nodule database with known histopathological, cytological or microbiological diagnosis.

2.3 Dynamic evaluation of the lung nodule by the computerized tomography

The dynamic evaluation is characterized by a study in two distinct moments of the same nodule, with or without use of intravenous contrast. The commonest dynamic evaluation without use of contrast is the calculation of the so called doubling time, which implies two volumetric determinations after a certain time interval.
The volumetry of the lung nodule has been considered as an important attribute to study undetermined nodules, especially if there is a screening program. Due to the tri-dimensional

evaluation of the nodule, it establishes more precisely if there was a growing, involution or stabilization, conclusions which have traditionally be taken by the analysis of the diameters of a central tomographic cut, whose limitation is the incapacity to detect variations in other cuts and specially in the z axis. Given the sensibility of the CT, it is possible to make a second measurement in a short period, inclusively in the range below 30 days, and surprise the nodules with doubling time in the spectrum of growing of neoplastic disorders, indicating, so, its resection (Winer-Muram et al., 2002). Classically, doubling times inferior to 45 days have been associated to inflammatory processes and those ranging from 45 to 450 days have been associated to neoplasm (Nathan et al., 1962). Above 450 days the nodules has been considered benign. However, certain tumors of germinative genealogy can have doubling times below 45 days. For a neoplastic lesion, the smaller the doubling time the bigger the biological aggressiveness of the tumor.
The computerized tomography with contrast injection is based on the fact that the vascularization of the malignant nodule is much more prominent than that of the benign one, especially in its central portion, occurrence demonstrated in immunohistochemistry techniques with the use of antibodies anti-factor VIII. Made under standardization, the method featured by Swensen and partners, in 1996, showed, with a cutoff point of 20 Hounsfield Units, a sensibility of 98%, a specificity of 73% and an accuracy of 85% (Christensen et al., 2006). Presently, in a general manner, we consider that a raise of more than 15 to 25 Hounsfield Units (HU), after a contrast injection in standardized conditions to enable comparison, suggests malignancy, but some benign conditions, inflammatory, such as tuberculous granuloma and cryptogenic pneumonia, can also raise the radiologic intensity (Jeong et al., 2005). Lately, more value has been given to the impregnation curve (wash-in) and disimpregnation (wash-out) of contrast as a way to detail and help distinguishing the benign nodules from the malignant one. In practical terms, the absence of impregnation is the most useful dynamic feature, because it decreases significantly the possibility of malignancy, having elevated negative predictive value (Christensen et al., 2006). These conclusions are relativized in nodules smaller than 1 cm.

2.4 Association between computerized tomography and the positron emission tomography (PET)

It has been demonstrated that the PET/CT association (PET integrated to CT) is more adequate than the separate exams to diagnose the nature of the lung nodule. The same way as in other methods, with PET, one has been giving more value to the quantification obtained for the diagnosing, through the so called SUV max (Standardized Uptake Value) which measures the maximum intensity of consumption of the agent marked by the tumored cells in the region of interest. In the case of glucose it is used the 18-deoxi-fluoroglucose (FDG), admitting, usually, as cutoff point the value 2.5 (Martins et al., 2008). Nevertheless, despite the high sensibility, above 90%, the specificity in zones of high incidence of tuberculosis and histoplasmosis stay between 70% and 80%, revealing still a reasonable possibility of false positives, represented specially by the tuberculous granuloma. There has been some research aiming to change glucose, the commonest energetic substrate, by an amino acid to be incorporated to the DNA, as, for example, methionine (11 âĂŞ C- Methionine), obtaining a smaller incidence of false positives, without sensibility loss (Sasaki et al., 1999). What is special about the value of the PET is its contribution for the simultaneous staging in the case of the malignant nodule, since it has the capability of pointing metastasis in places where other image methods cannot find them. The incorporation of the study with PET has been recommended in the evaluation of the probability of malignancy by the Bayesian method (Meert, 2010).

3. CAD/CADx lung systems

The development of medical images acquisition techniques, in particular Computerized Tomography (CT), which may furnish more detailed information about the human body, has increased the capability and fidelity in the diagnosing of many diseases. On the other hand, the dimensions of these images are becoming bigger and bigger, increasing the need for computer vision techniques that can make interpretation easier. This Section aims to provide an overview of literature in automatic CT image analysis in the lung region.

The work of (Beigelman-Aubry et al., 2007) presented an evaluation of nodule detection and its response time when performed by radiologists with and without use of a computerized system. The work showed that the system improves the sensibility of the detection, what raised the trust interval in 2%. Among the experiments with 109 patients, there was a nodule which was not detected by one of the radiologists, but was detected by the system. Besides, the use of the system decreases considerably the time required by the specialists to analyze the exams.

This way, nodule detection systems have great importance in this process, despite they don't give the final diagnosis.

Nodule detection systems usually involve 4 steps: pre-processing, extraction of nodule candidates, reduction of false positives and classification. Pre-processing normally consists in restricting the search space, delimiting the lung, and reducing noises in the image. The region of the lung is segmented and nodule candidate objects are identified. Among these objects most of the non-nodules are discarded in the false positive reduction stage. The remaining objects are then classified into nodule and non-nodule. In some methods, the false positive reduction is performed after classification. Some works found in the literature involving these steps are presented next.

(III & Sensakovic, 2004) showed the importance of adequate segmentation of lungs in computer aided detection and/or diagnosing systems. His studies indicated that up to 17% of lung nodules can be lost during lung segmentation if the algorithm is not adjusted to the task of nodule detection.

A great challenge is the segmentation of lungs affected by high density pathologies connected to their bounds. Due to the lack of contrast between these pathologies and the tissues adjacent to the lung, density-based methods fail in this region. In this case, it is necessary some edition technique, but, even so, part of the lung is normally lost (Sluimer et al., 2006).

Due to the large amount of air in the lung, its interior has dark tonality in CT images, differing from the region around it. This way, contrast between lung and neighbor tissues is the basis for most lung segmentation methods. Most methods are based on rules (Hu et al., 2001), (Zheng et al., 2003), (Leader et al., 2003). The lung region can be found in two ways (Sluimer et al., 2006). The first one is by means of region growing starting at trachea. The second one, more usual, used thresholdings and constraints in size and location.

To find nodule candidates, the main techniques used are: multiple thresholding (Armato et al., 1999), (Ko & Betke, 2001), (Zhao & Yankelevitz, 1999), (Zhao et al., 2004), mathematical morphology (Ezoe et al., 2002), (Fetita et al., 2003), (Tanino et al., 2003), (Awai et al., 2004), clustering) (Kanazawa et al., 1998), (Gurcan et al., 2002) (Kubo et al., 2002), (Yamada et al., 2003), analysis of connected elements in thresholded images (Oda et al., 2002), (Saita et al., 2004), detection of circles in thresholded images (Wiemker et al., 2002) and use of emphasis filter with spherical structure elements (Chang et al., 2004), (Li & Doi, 2004), (Paik et al., 2004), (Paik, 2002).

In (Osman et al., 2007), for each slice, regions of interest (ROI) were found by using density values of the pixels and analyzing their eight directions. The joining of all slices formed 3D ROIs, which allows identifying the nodules when compared to a nodule model (template). Sensibility reached 100%, but the test data were restricted to six cases.

(Retico et al., 2008) proposed a system based on emphasis filters for spherical objects and a neural classification based on voxels of selected regions to reduce false positives. The system performance was evaluated in a set of data from 39 CT and reached 80-85% of sensibility and 10-13 FP/exam.

(Bae et al., 2005) developed a Computer Aided Diagnosis (CADx) for high-resolution CT images (HRCT - High-resolution computed tomography) using bi-dimensional and tri-dimensional analysis algorithms. This technique was tested in eight lung cancer cases and obtained 95% of sensibility and 0.91 FP/slice.

To improve the sensibility of the detection, (Li et al., 2008) used an emphasis filter in the identification stage and, to reduce false positives, used a rule-based classifier.

After the nodule candidate objects have been generated, characteristic features of these objects are calculated. Classifiers are then applied. These classifiers use the features to identify candidate objects either in the nodules set or in the non-nodule set.

Several techniques can be used as classifiers in the final stage of nodule detection: based on either rules or linear classifiers (Lee et al., 2001), (Mekada et al., 2003), (Chang et al., 2004), by combining models (template matching) (Brown et al., 2003), analysis of the nearest cluster (Ezoe et al., 2002), (Tanino et al., 2003), support vector machine (Lu et al., 2004), (Mousa & Khan, 2002), (Sousa et al., 2007), neural networks (Suzuki et al., 2008), (Lo et al., 2003), (Zhang et al., 2004) and Bayesian classifier (Farag et al., 2004), (McCulloch et al., 2004). The features mostly used for classification are those based on the density of voxels, description of shapes, spatial relation and size information.

(Sousa et al., 2007) proposed a set of three morphological features specially developed for characterization of lung nodules with which matching rates of 100% were achieved using support vector machine, despite this work used a small database.

In some works, the classifier presents good sensibility, but also a high number of false positives. This way, techniques have been sought, in order to reduce this number after the identification which, in some cases, work as filters before classification.

(Armato et al., 1999) presented a methodology for detection of lung nodules with just the pre-processing stages, detection of candidates and classification. Nodule candidates were found by through multiple thresholding and, next, using shape and density attributes and discriminant linear analysis, the classification detected 70% of the nodules indicated by specialists and 3 false positives per slice in average (approximately 80-90 false positives per exam). In later papers, Armato and co-authors has focused in rules to reduce the number of false positives: rule-based (III et al., 2001), (Arimura et al., 2004), discriminant analysis (Arimura et al., 2004), (III et al., 2002) and neural networks (Arimura et al., 2004), (Suzuki, 2003). The best result obtained by these techniques was of 80.3% in detection rate with 4.8 false positives per exam against 27.4 without false positives reduction (Suzuki, 2003).

(Saita et al., 2004) added to the nodules detection methodology proposed by (Oda et al., 2002) a false positives reduction stage.

(Lee et al., 2004) added the false positive reduction stage to the nodules detection method initially proposed by (Lee et al., 2001). To do this, they added five density attributes and

adjusted the thresholding parameters to the original model. The sensibility continued the same in 72.4% but the FP rate decreases from 30.8 to 5.5 per exam.
False positives reducing is important, because, even if sensibility keeps unaltered, the radiologist's final amount of work is reduced.

4. Lung nodule detection

This section presents, under the form of a sequence of stages, the procedures proposed to perform the detection of lung nodules in a CT in an incremental manner. Another important aspect of the methodology is the adoption of specific strategies for nodule detection in particular conditions, such as nodules linked to the chest wall, aggregated to the bronchi or blood trees, and the single ones.
The proposed methodology corresponds to the application of several successive stages of processing to CT images, eliminating portions of them which do not correspond to interesting areas, in this case, lung nodules. Figure 1 shows the methodology stages. Figure 2 presents a CT slice consecutively submitted to this process. More details about this method in (Sousa et al., 2010)

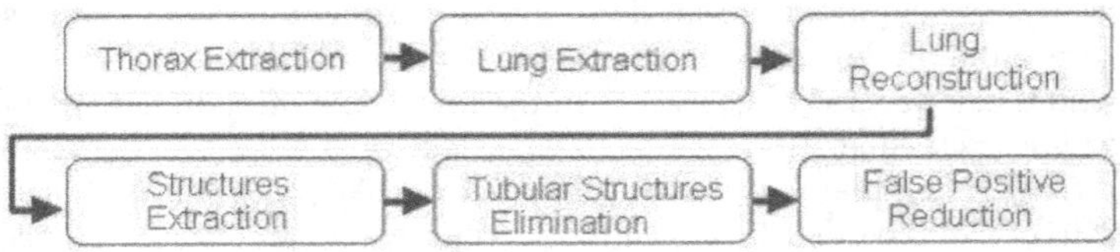

Fig. 1. Methodology Stages.

4.1 Thorax extraction

The process is started with thorax extraction. This stage comprises the removal of all artifacts external to the patient's body, among which are: bed sheets, the air that involves the patient and the surface on which he lies, as example of the items numbered in Figure 2(a).
These structures are identified by a region growing algorithm whose seeds are initially put on the four corners of each slice. The similarity criterion for the algorithm is based on gray tones of the voxels, since great part of the external region of the thorax (which we want to identify) is formed by low intensity voxels.

4.2 Lung extraction

The objective of lung extraction is to identify the thoracic wall and mediastinum voxels, making possible the work on the next stages with just the region which forms the pulmonary parenchyma. That is achieved again with use of the region growing algorithm, this time, however, identifying the high-intensity voxels with values greater than the threshold and with no need for tolerance. The final result, after the growing and elimination of the high intensity voxels can be seen in Figure 2(c).

4.3 Lung reconstruction

Occasionally the lung extraction stage erroneously eliminates some voxels which belong to the pulmonary parenchyma. These mistakes can lead to elimination, inclusively, of

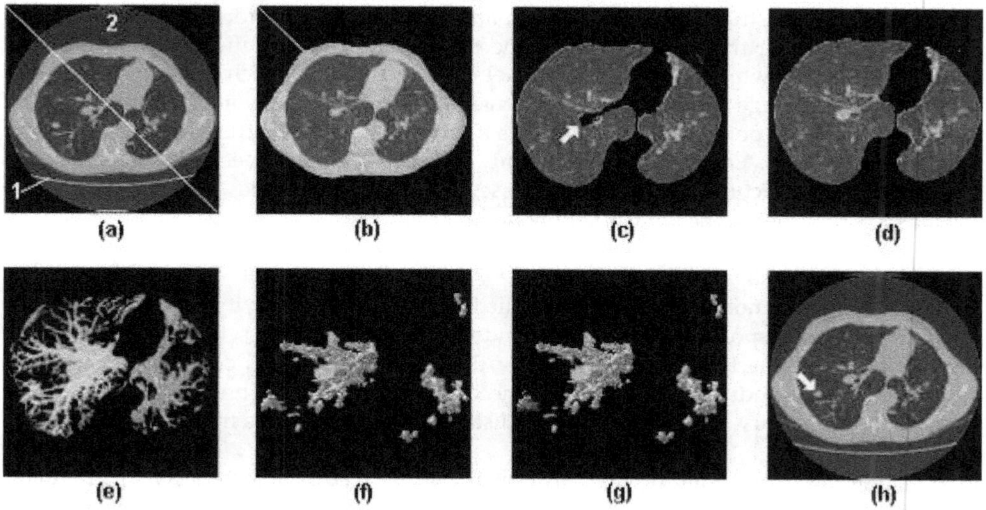

Fig. 2. Automatic lung nodule detection sequence. (a) Eliminates of all artifacts external to the patient's body, identified as 1 and 2 in the figure. (b) Removal of thorax, leaving just the parenchyma. (c) Shows an example of the internal lung region and the thoracic wall erroneously eliminated. (d) Parenchyma reconstructed with rolling-ball algorithm. (e) 3D visualization of the remaining structures after threshold application and identified with different colors. (f) 3D visualization of the structures after tubular elimination. (g) Shows the correct identification of a lung nodule among other normal lung structures which came from the previous stage. (h) Presents the same nodule identified in the original tomography image by an arrow.

possible nodules, inducing an error in detection. This way, the reconstruction stage has great importance for preservation of peripheral nodules.

Figure 2(c) shows an example of an internal lung region and the thoracic wall erroneously eliminated together, due to its high intensity voxels.

In order to recover the correct lungs outlines, this stage uses the rolling-ball algorithm (Gurcan et al., 2002), a mathematical morphology technique based on closing operations executed with a circular structuring element, whose radius, in this specific case, was of thirty pixels. Figure 2(d) shows the result after application this stage.

4.4 Parenchyma structures extraction

The previous stages had the main objective of detecting the pulmonary region, but only in this stage, in fact, the search for internal lung regions occurs. This stage is performed in two steps: the first one identifies and removes the less dense parenchyma tissue out from the image, keeping only its internal structures; the second one isolates each of the tri-dimensional structures found so that they can be individually processed.

The elimination of less dense tissues is performed by means of a thresholding process. The proper threshold is again obtained from the volume voxels histogram, being considered only the parenchyma-internal ones.

Nevertheless, these structures need to be separated individually, before the nodules can be identified. So, each tri-dimensionally connected structure is identified through a region growing algorithm which starts in each voxel of the structures which are not isolated yet. The result of this stage is that every tri-dimensionally connected region can be individually processed from this point. Figure 2(e) shows each tri-dimensional structure identified with distinguished colors. Each color was randomly chosen and has no special meaning. We can notice on it that structures such as blood vessels, bronchi and nodules are preserved, while the major part of the parenchyma is suppressed.

4.5 Tubular structures elimination

We observed that among the objects identified by the 3D connectivity property, there are structures that correspond to the bronchial and vascular trees. Besides, there are cases where each nodule is connected to one or more of these structures. This creates a problem for detection of these nodules, generating the need for identifying the bronchial and vascular trees of the pulmonary parenchyma so that distinguishing these trees from possible nodules can be possible.

Blood vessels are, as a rule, tubular. The depth of the medial axis varies very gradually, inclusively in ramifications. In other words, blood vessels have thickness almost constant in a certain location. Nodules have totally different characteristics. As they are compact structures, they present an abrupt increase in the depth of the medial axis. This is perceived more clearly in spicular nodules. The process consists in verifying to which of both patterns the structures match better. With this objective, observing the structures to be identified, we use an analysis based on their skeleton. This is possible since they resemble very much their medial axis, obtained by means of the 3D skeletonization algorithm proposed in (Sousa et al., 2007).

The bifurcations among the vessels possibly present an increase in the depth of the medial axis, but this increase, besides being small when compared with the diameter of the vessel, is gradual. On the other hand, in the case of aggregated nodules, the increase in the depth of the media axle is much more abrupt and intense. With the correct balance of cutoff thresholds it is possible to come to a stage that results in few false positives or false negatives, with a good sensibility. Anyway, errors generally occur in this stage, making necessary the posterior stage of reducing false negatives and false positives, which, in our case, was based on Support Vector Machine (SVM).

For each individual structure, the skeleton is calculated. After that, all of its segments are scanned sequentially. During the scan of each segment the maximum value of depth is selected and its neighborhood with the same pattern is also selected. The selection of the neighborhood must consider the average depth of the adjacent medial voxels and the variation from one to another, in sequence.

After the region is selected, it is previously evaluated. A very large rate between the length of the selected part of the branch and its thickness clearly indicates a tubular region. However, a great thickness in relation to the length indicates a compact structure, possibly a nodule. An example can be seen in Figure 3(a) where we can notice a nodule connected to several blood vessels. Figure 3(b), on the other hand, presents the same region after the elimination of these vessels.

4.6 False positives reduction

False positives reduction is the stage in which the detection is refined by eliminating the false lung nodules. For that, we used the SVM (Vapnik, 1998) previously trained to recognize the

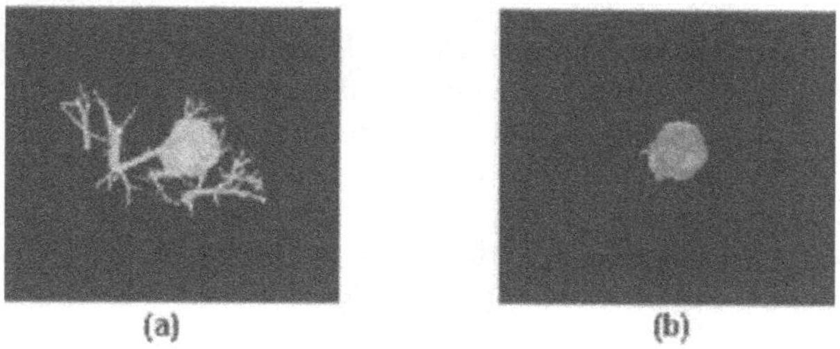

Fig. 3. Tubular Structures Elimination.

true nodules with basis on a series of descriptive features. This work used features commonly used in other works (Agam et al., 2005), (Lu et al., 2004) and (Peldschus et al., 2005) with the same objective, but with new features as well, especially developed for describing lung nodules and distinguishing them from other pulmonary structures.

The complete list of the studied features is: Geometry (spherical disproportion, spherical density, pondered radial distance, sphericity, elongation, Boyce-Clark radial shape index), Texture (contrast, energy, entropy, homogeneity, moment), histogram (average, standard deviation, skewness, kurtosis, energy, entropy), Gradient (average, standard deviation, skewness, kurtosis, energy, entropy) and Spatial (location of the candidate). More details for all those measurements can be found in (Sousa et al., 2007).

The set of features extracted from every candidate generates a vector which characterizes them. As each features, however, bears on one isolate aspect of the candidate, it occurs that many of them are in different units and frequently in disproportional scales.

To minimize the complexity of the model and speed up the process, we attempted to select a subset of features which are more significant for classification. We empirically tested several subsets of features and verified which one had the best performance. The starting model had 24 variables and after selecting the best subset, there were 8 variables left: geometry (spherical disproportion, spherical density), histogram (standard deviation, skewness, entropy), gradient (standard deviation, kurtosis), spatial (location of candidate).

The adoption of the vector, such as obtained after calculating these features would cause some of them to be overestimated by the SVM classifier due to the numerically greater value, while others, because they vary in smaller intervals, would be underestimated. This way, the features vector must be normalized so that all the features have the same representativeness.

After all candidates have been completely measured and described, each one by a normalized features vector, these vectors are passed to the SVM, which uses the previous knowledge, obtained by the analysis of other seemingly cases, to identify the real nature of each candidate, recognizing them as lung nodules or as normal lung structures. As SVM kernel, we used the radial basis function. The library LIBSVM (Chang et al., 2004) was used for training and validation of the SVM classifiers.

Figure 2(g) shows the correct identification of a lung nodule among other normal lung structures which came from the previous stage. Figure 2(h) presents the same nodule identified in the original tomography image by an arrow.

5. Lung nodule diagnosis

The proposed methodology aims to classify single lung nodules into two groups: benign and malignant. To perform this task, this methodology was based on the steps seen in Figure 4.

The first step is the acquisition of the image, which was obtained from a patient's chest CT exam. Step 2 is the segmentation of the tri-dimensional volume of the nodule using method describe in Section 4. Right after that, the representative features of the nodules are obtained by the use of the Simpson's Index, that is, the texture analysis stage combined with the geometric features extraction. This index has not been used in applications of analysis of medical images in order to diagnose. The last step is the classification of the nodules as either benign or malignant by a One-Class SVM. One-Class SVM was chosen because it was little used in such applications. For more information about this method see (Silva et al., 2009).

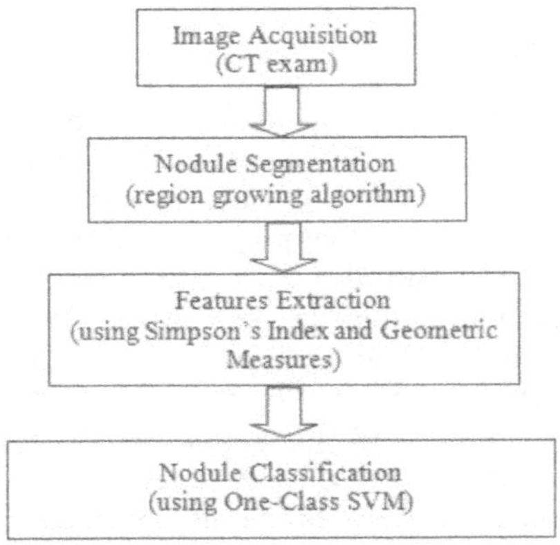

Fig. 4. Methodology Steps.

5.1 Simpson's index

Simpson's Index is a second order statistical spatial feature that has been used by Ecology specialists to determine the biodiversity of species in a region (Simpson, 1949). Its main functionality is to summarize the representation of this diversity in a single value capable of qualifying this region as either very heterogeneous or uniform.

Simpson's Index takes into consideration the richness of the species, that is, the number of species present in an area, and still, the regularity of such species, what is a measurement of the relative abundance of each species (Hill, 1973). With these considerations it is possible to analyze which community in a region is more diversified.

The Simpson's Index is the measurement of the probability of two individuals, randomly selected from a sample, to belong to the same species i among the existing species j in the sample, as in Equation 1 (Ricklefs, 1997).

$$D = \sum_{i=1}^{j} p_i^2 \tag{1}$$

where $p_i = \frac{n_i}{N}$. For each i,it is found the probability (p_i) for the occurrence of the species i; n_i represents the occurrence of individuals from the species i and N is the total of individuals in the sample. The index is normally used according to Equation 1 when the sample is obtained by sampling process, not being possible to exactly determine the number of individuals in this sample. For a finite sample, where the total amount of individuals is known, the Simpson's

Index can be obtained, still, through Equation 2 (Lyons et al., 2008).

$$D = \frac{\sum_{i=1}^{j} n_i(n_i - 1)}{N(N-1)} \tag{2}$$

The values obtained for the Simpson's Index are in the interval from 0 to 1, where the value 0 represents infinite diversity in the sample and 1 means that there's no diversity.

Our proposal is the extraction of Simpson's Index, as a measurement for texture, taking each voxel found in the volume a possible species under analysis. The distinguishing can be possible due to the morphological behavior of each kind of nodule: benign nodules present, in most cases, a round or well defined shape, while malignant nodules, due to their capability of spreading to other organs present a spicate or less defined shape. As the obtaining of the index will occur in areas of interest, the small occurrence of voxels in a certain area of interest can be related to the shape of this nodule. This way, the benign nodules have a tendency to show a more homogeneous behavior, that is, less diversified in a certain region of study.

5.2 Geometrical measures

The shape of a lung nodule may represent an important indicator of its malignancy or benignity, as we said before. With features geometrical measures is possible to extract and analyze further information identified or not identified by doctors. In this work, three 3D geometry features extracted from each nodule in our database. They are: Spherical Disproportion, Spherical Density and Sphericity. Spherical Disproportion is described in the Equation 3, Spherical Disproportion in Equation 4 and Sphericity in Equation 5. Other information about these measurements can be found in (Sousa et al., 2007).

$$S = \frac{A}{4\pi R^2} \tag{3}$$

$$\varphi = \frac{100.n}{V} \tag{4}$$

$$E = \frac{(6V)^{\frac{2}{3}} \pi^{\frac{1}{3}}}{A} \tag{5}$$

5.3 Validation the classification method

In order to evaluate the methodology with regard to its power of characterizing the proposed groups, we tried to obtain the sensibility (Se), specificity (Sp) and accuracy (Ac) measurements for all analysis performed in the study. Sensibility is given by $TP/(TP+FN)$, specificity is obtained by $TN/(TN+FP)$, and accuracy is given by $(TP+TN)/(TP+TN+FP+FN)$, where TP is true-positive, TN is true-negative, FP is false-positive and FN is false-negative. This way, the malignant lung nodules correctly computed are reported as true positives.

5.4 Experimental tests

We performed the extraction of the texture features by applying Simpson's Index where the area of interest was represented by circular rings as in Figure 5. Our objective with these forms of extraction is to evaluate the diversity in the edge regions determined by two concentric circles.

We have determined the size of the circles by finding the central point, mass center, of each nodule and then, calculated the distance of this central point to the most distant point of each

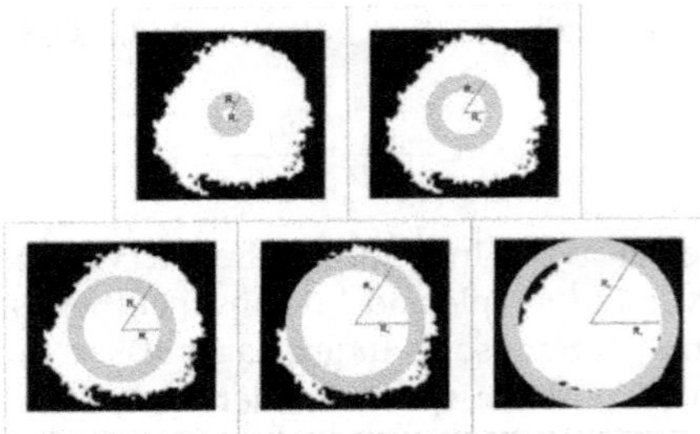

Fig. 5. Analysis applied to the nodule by means of circular rings containing 6 external radius.

nodule. This way, we get a R radius that represents a greater possible measurement for the construction of a circle or still, in the analysis by rings, the maximum allowed radius. From the radius R, we got the others values of radiuses as $1/6R$, $1/3R$, $1/2R$, $2/3R$ and $5/6R$. These are represented as R1, R2, R3, R4, R5 e R6 (value of R).

Next, Simpson's Index of Equation 2 was calculated in each region for a certain ring. We made use of this index because we have quantitative and exact knowledge of the total number of individuals in the sample, that is, the total of voxels in each nodule. In order to increase the discriminatory power of the methodology, we obtained geometry measurements of the nodules which were reported in Section 5.2. Then, we performed the classification considering the Simpson's Index extracted in each ring, for the analysis by rings aggregating to each analysis the geometry measurements.

A library for SVM, called LIBSVM (Chang & Lin, 2003), was used for training and testing the One-Class SVM classifier (Schölkopf et al., 2001). During the classification stage, four different proportions for the training and test subgroups were used: 50/50, 60/40, 70/30 and 80/20, where the first number represents the percentage of cases used in training(Tr) and the second number represents the percentage of cases used in test(Te). The cases used in each subgroup were randomly selected from the total number of database.

The results shown in Table 1 were obtained in each Tr/Te proportion for each region in analysis in rings and indicate that in ring A1 the best values of sensibility, specificity and accuracy were found: 100%, 80% and 90%, respectively in Tr/Te proportion of 80/20. The use of geometry aided to put this boundary region in evidence as discriminant between malignant and benign nodules.

	Tr/Te = 50/50			Tr/Te = 60/40			Tr/Te = 70/30			Tr/Te = 80/20		
	Se %	Sp %	Ac %	Se %	Sp %	Ac %	Se %	Sp %	Ac %	Se %	Sp %	Ac %
R1	0	100	50	50	70	60	100	3.33	51.67	**100**	**80**	**90**
R2	50	76.67	63.33	75	73.33	74.17	66.67	83.33	75	100	46.67	73.33
R3	25	90	57.5	25	90	57.5	100	63.33	81.67	100	63.33	81.67
R4	75	60	67.5	75	60	67	33.33	66.67	50	100	43.33	71.67
R5	50	63.33	56.67	75	63.33	69.17	66.67	40	53.33	50	83.33	66.67

Table 1. Results found for all group Tr/Te in each region in the analysis in rings.

The Table 2 display the results of the sensibility averages, specificity and accuracy obtained in each group Tr/Te for the analysis in rings. The best found result was of the group 80/20, which obtained values of 90% of sensibility, 63.33% of specificity and 76.67% of accuracy.

Tr/Te	Se (%)	Sp (%)	Ac (%)
50/50	40.00	78.00	59.00
60/40	60.00	71.33	65.67
70/30	73.33	51.33	62.33
80/20	**90.00**	**63.33**	**76.67**

Table 2. Results found to averages of the sensibility, specificity and accuracy obtained in group Tr/Te for the analysis in rings.

6. Future directions

Several researchers believe that Computer-aided Detection (CAD) and Computer-aided Diagnosis (CADx) systems will become an increasingly important tool for radiologists in the early detection of lung cancer using CT images. Besides this feeling, we may see that there are several challenges in the development and use of such systems.

One of the main challenges is the use of these systems for early detection of lung cancer reducing the number of false positive, that often lead to unnecessary invasive medical procedures and produce high levels of anxiety among patients who fear they have a tumor.

The challenges posed by CT-based lung CAD are exponential. With multidetector chest CT, which generates hundreds of images, lung CAD highlights multiple findings for each study. But we can notice that the newer developments in lung CAD technology for CT images have dramatically reduced the false positive rates.

The challenges posed by CT-based lung CAD are exponential. With multidetector chest CT, which generates hundreds of images, lung CAD highlights multiple findings for each study. But we can notice that the newer developments in lung CAD technology for CT images have dramatically reduced the false positive rates.

Eliminating the nuisance of false-positives makes the technology much more manageable in the clinical setting, especially with preferences for increased sensitivity.

Decreasing the false positive rate while maintaining a high degree of sensitivity in these systems is also a problem facing CAD/CADx systems. We may observe that in general the CAD/CADx systems report good sensitivity but at the expense of high false positive rates.

These systems are satisfactorially used as second readers. But, the sensibility must be improved if we intend, in the future, to use these systems as the first reader.

Although the introduction of low-dose helical computed tomography (CT) is considered to be one of the most promising clinical research developments, another direction in the development of CAD/CADx systems is the introduction of other imaging modalities for lung cancer detection, diagnosis, staging, and treatment monitoring.

Hence, great efforts have been made to develop new bronchoscopic imaging techniques (Yasufuku, 2010). Bronchoscopic imaging techniques capable of detecting preinvasive lesions and currently available in clinical practice include autofluorescence bronchoscopy (AFB), high magnification bronchovideoscope, and narrow band imaging (NBI). And also the combination of PET and CT.

Finally, we believe that CAD/CADx systems must be integrated into radiology training programs to help radiologists getting comfortable with such systems.

7. Final remarks

We have presented here a methodology to use CT images combined with computational methods (image processing, computational vision and pattern recognition) to aid the specialists in the detection and another for diagnosis of lung cancer.
The matching rates discussed demonstrate that there is technical viability for implantation of the methodologies. Concerning the needs for it, statistics related to lung cancer clearly indicate that methods for helping in precocious diagnosis of lung nodule may increase the patient's survival chances.
Due to the high sensitivity per exam, this tool has triage exam characteristics, that is, belongs to the first set of exams to be required, which identify the suspicious cases, but need to be confirmed later, by more strict exams, in this case, the medical analysis.
Since precocious diagnosis represents a considerable increase in the patient's survival chances, the proposal of methodologies that promotes this increase, as it is shown as a very useful tool for the specialist in the attempt to anticipate more and more the nodule identification.
Another point is that the public network of hospitals in some places suffers from the lack of specialists. The resources to increase the staff, however, are also limited. Redirecting qualified craft of the available specialists to less repetitive tasks may mean making better use of their skills. One step in that direction is to use the methodologies like these in the preliminary analysis of CT exams, being the specialist just in charge of validating the result.
Finally,we may verify that methodologies as described here in also is a financially attractive solution because it works on simple microcomputers, many of which are already available in the hospitals. Large investments in infrastructure would not be necessary for its implantation.
Actually, there is a debate on the magnitude of the impact of such systems currently in clinical use. But, on the other hand we may also see that we cannot afford to ignore their potential benefits.
We may observe that more emphasis must be given to the CAD/CADx observed studies, in order to allow them to reach their full potential. Also, we need the development of novel methods for reducing the number of false positive detections, and integrate these systems into medical education.
These systems are intended to assist radiologists, but not replace them. The radiologist should be the final judge in determining the final assessment. But all the effort to develop technologies that assist then in making more accurate interpretations should be encouraged, as this will generate several benefits to women's health.

8. References

Agam, G., III, S. G. A. & Wu, C. (2005). Vessel tree reconstruction in thoracic ct scans with application to nodule detection., *IEEE Trans. Med. Imaging* 24(4): 486–499.

Arimura, H., Katsuragawa, S., Suzuki, K., Li, F., Shiraishi, J., Sone, S. & Doi, K. (2004). Computerized scheme for automated detection of lung nodules in low-dose CT images for lung cancer screening, *Academic Radiology* 11: 617–629.

Armato, S. G., Giger, M. L., Moran, C. J., Blackburn, J. T., Doi, K. & MacMahon, H. (1999). Computerized detection of pulmonary nodules on CT scans, *Radiographics* 19(5): 1303–1311.

Awai, K., Murao, K., Ozawa, A., Komi, M., Hayakawa, H., Hori, S. & Nishimura, Y. (2004). Pulmonary nodules at chest ct: Effect of computer-aided diagnosis on radiologists detection performance, *Radiology* 230: 347–352.

Bae, K. T., Kim, J.-S., Na, Y.-H., Kim, K. G., & Kim, J.-H. (2005). Pulmonary nodules at chest ct: Effect of computer-aided diagnosis on radiologists detection performance, *Radiology* 236: 286–293.

Beigelman-Aubry, C., Raffy, P., Yang, W., Castellino, R. A. & Grenier, P. A. (2007). Computer-aided detection of solid lung nodules on follow-up mdct screening: evaluation of detection, tracking, and reading time., *AJR. American journal of roentgenology* 189(4): 948–955.
URL: *http://dx.doi.org/10.2214/AJR.07.2302*

Bellomi, M., Rampinelli, C., Funicelli, L. & Veronesi, G. (2006). Screening for lung cancer, *Cancer Imaging* 6: S9ŰS12.

Brown, M. S., Goldin, J. G., Suh, R. D., McNitt-Gray, M. F., Sayre, J. W. & Aberle, D. R. (2003). Lung micronodules: Automated method for detection at thin-section CT-initial experience 1, *Radiology* 226: 256–262.

Chang, C.-C. & Lin, C.-J. (2003). LIBSVM – a library for support vector machines. Available at http://www.csie.ntu.edu.tw/ cjlin/libsvm/.

Chang, S., Emoto, H., Metaxas, D. & A., L. (2004). Pulmonary micronodule detection from 3-d chest ct, *Lecture Notes in Computer Science - Medical Image Computing and Computer-Assisted Intervention* 3217: 821–828.

Christensen, J. A., Nathan, M. A., Mullan, B. P., Hartman, T. E., Swensen, S. J. & Lowe, V. J. (2006). Characterization of the solitary pulmonary nodule: 18-fdg pet versus nodule enhancement CT., *Am J Roentgenology* 187(5): 1361–1367.

Ezoe, T., Takizawa, H., Yamamoto, S., Shimizu, A., Matsumoto, T., Tateno, Y., Iimura, T. & Matsumoto, M. (2002). Automatic detection method of lung cancers including ground-glass opacities from chest x-ray ct images, Vol. 4684, SPIE, pp. 1672–1680.
URL: *http://link.aip.org/link/?PSI/4684/1672/1*

Farag, A., El Baz, A., Gimel'farb, G. & Falk, R. (2004). Detection and recognition of lung nodules in spiral ct images usingdeformable templates and bayesian post-classification, *ICIP04*, pp. V: 2921–2924.

Fetita, C. I., Prêteux, F., Beigelman-Aubry, C. & Grenier, P. (2003). 3d automated lung nodule segmentation in hrct, *Medical Image Computing and Computer-Assisted Intervention - MICCAI 2003* 2878(2878): 626–634.

Franquet, T., Muller, N., Gimenez, A., Martinez, S., Madrid, M. & Domingo, P. (2003). Infectious pulmonary nodules in immunocompromised patients: usefulness of computed tomography in predicting their etiology., *J Comput Assist Tomogr* 27: 461–8.

Gurcan, M. N., Sahiner, B., Petrick, N., Chan, H. P., Kazerooni, E. A., Cascade, P. N. & Hadjiiski, L. M. (2002). Lung nodule detection on thoracic computed tomography images: Preliminary evaluation of a computer-aided diagnosis system, *Medical Physics* pp. 2552–2558.

Hanley, K. S. & Rubins, J. B. (2003). Classifying solitary pulmonary nodules. new imaging methods to distinguish malignant, benign lesions, *Postgraduate medicine* 114(2): 29–35.

Hasegawa, M., Sone, S., Takashima, S., Li, F., Yang, Z.-G., Maruyama, Y. & Watanabe, T. (2000). Growth rate of small lung cancers detected on mass CT screening, *The British Journal of Radiology* 73: 1252–1259.

Hill, M. O. (1973). Diversity and evenness: a unifying notation and its consequences., *Ecology* 54: 427–432.

Hu, S., Hoffman, E. A. & Reinhardt, J. M. (2001). Automatic lung segmentation for accurate quantitation of volumetric x-ray ct images, *IEEE Transactions on Medical Imaging* 20: 490–498.

I.Henschke, C. & Yankelevitz, D. F. (2000). Ct screening for lung cancer, *Radiologic Clinics of North America* 38(3): 487–495.

III, S. G. A., Giger, M. L. & MacMahon, H. (2001). "Automated detection of lung nodules in CT scans: Preliminary results", *Medical Physics* 28: 1552–1561.

III, S. G. A., Li, F., Giger, M. L., MacMahon, H., Sone, S. & Doi, K. (2002). Lung cancer: Performance of automated lung nodule detection applied to cancers missed in a CT screening program, *Radiology* 225: 685–692.

III, S. G. A. & Sensakovic, W. F. (2004). Automated lung segmentation for thoracic ct: Impact on computer-aided diagnosis, *Academic radiology* 11: 1011–1021.

INCA, N. I. (2009). Estimativa 2008: Incidência de câncer no Brasil. Instituto Nacional do Cancer. In Portuguese. URL: www.inca.gov.br.

Iwano, S., Nakamura, T., Kamioka, Y. & Ishigaki, T. (2005). Computer-aided diagnosis: A shape classification of pulmonary nodules imaged by high-resolution ct, *Computerized Medical Imaging and Graphics* 29(7): 565–570.

Jamnik, S., Santoro, I. L. & Uehara, C. (2002). Comparative study of prognostic factors among longer and shorter survival patients with bronchogenic carcinoma, *Pneumologia [online]* 28(5): 245 – 249.

Jeong, Y. J., Lee, K. S., Jeong, S. Y., Chung, M. J., Shim, S. S., Hojoong, K., Kwon, O. J. & S, K. (2005). Solitary pulmonary nodule: characterization with combine wash-in and washout features of dynamic multidector row CT., *Radiology* 2(237): 675–683.

Kanazawa, K., Kawata, Y., Niki, N., Satoh, H., Ohmatsu, H., Kakinuma, R., Kaneko, M., Moriyma, N. & Eguchi, K. (1998). Computer-aided diagnosis for pulmonary nodules based on helical CT images, *Computered Medical Imaging and Graphics* 22: 157–167.

Khan, A., Herman, P. G., Vorwerk, P., Stevens, P., Rojas, K. A. & Graver, M. (1991). Solitary pulmonary nodules: comparison of classification with standard, thin-section, and reference phantom ct, *Radiology* 179(2): 477–481.
URL: *http://radiology.rsna.org/content/179/2/477.abstract*

Ko, J. P. & Betke, M. (2001). Chest CT : Automated nodule detection and assessment of change over time - preliminary experience, *Radiologic Clinics of North America* 218: 267–273.

Kubo, M., Kubota, K., Yamada, N., Kawata, Y., Niki, N., Eguchi, K., Ohmatsu, H., Kakinuma, R., Kaneko, M., Kusumoto, M., Mori, K., Nishiyama, H. & Moriyama, N. (2002). Cad system for lung cancer based on low-dose single-slice ct image, *in* M. Sonka & J. M. Fitzpatrick (eds), *Society of Photo-Optical Instrumentation Engineers (SPIE) Conference Series*, Vol. 4684 of *Presented at the Society of Photo-Optical Instrumentation Engineers (SPIE) Conference*, pp. 1262–1269.

Leader, J. K., Zheng, B., Rogers, R. M., Sciurba, F. C., Perez, A., Chapman, B. E., Patel, S., Fuhrman, C. R. & Gur, D. (2003). Automated lung segmentation in x-ray computed tomography: development and evaluation of a heuristic threshold-based scheme, *Academic Radiology* 10(11): 1224–1236.

Lee, Y., Hara, T., Fujita, H., Itoh, S. & Ishigaki, T. (2001). Automated detection of pulmonary nodules in helical ct images based on an improved template-matching technique.

Lee, Y., Tsai, D.-Y., Hara, T., Fujita, H., Itoh, S. & Ishigaki, T. (2004). Improvement in automated detection of pulmonary nodules on helical x-ray ct images, *in* J. M. Fitzpatrick & M. Sonka (eds), *Society of Photo-Optical Instrumentation Engineers (SPIE) Conference*

Series, Vol. 5370 of *Presented at the Society of Photo-Optical Instrumentation Engineers (SPIE) Conference*, pp. 824–832.

Li, Q. & Doi, K. (2004). "New selective nodule enhancement filter and its application for significant improvement of nodule detection on computed tomography", *in* J. M. Fitzpatrick & M. Sonka (eds), *Society of Photo-Optical Instrumentation Engineers (SPIE) Conference Series*, Vol. 5370 of *Presented at the Society of Photo-Optical Instrumentation Engineers (SPIE) Conference*, pp. 1–9.

Li, Q., Li, F. & Doi, K. (2008). Computerized detection of lung nodules in thin-section ct images by use of selective enhancement filters and an automated rule-based classifier, *Academic radiology* 15(2): 165–175.

Lillington, G. A. & Caskey, C. I. (2003). Evaluation and management of solitary and multiple pulmonary nodules, *Clinics in chest medicine* 114: 111–9.

Lo, S.-C. B., Hsu, L.-Y., Freedman, M. T., Lure, Y. M. F. & Zhao, H. (2003). Classification of lung nodules in diagnostic ct: an approach based on 3d vascular features, nodule density distribution, and shape features, Vol. 5032, SPIE, pp. 183–189.
URL: *http://link.aip.org/link/?PSI/5032/183/1*

Lu, X., Wei, G.-Q., Qian, J. Z. & Jain, A. K. (2004). Learning-based pulmonary nodule detection from multislice ct data, *CARS*, p. 1356.

Lyons, D. J., P.M.Dunworth & Tilbury, D. W. (2008). Simpson's diversity index, Available at http://www.countrysideinfo.co.uk/simpsons.htm.

Martins, R. D. C., Almeida, S. A. A. D., Siciliano, A. A. A. D. O., Landesmann, M. C. P. P., Silva, F. A.-c. B.D., Franco, C. A. d. B. & Fonseca, L. M. B. d. (2008). Valor do fdg [18f]-pet/tc como preditor de ca em nodulo pulmonar solitario, *Jornal Brasileiro de Pneumologia* 34: 473 – 480. In Portuguese.
URL: *http://www.scielo.br/*

Matsuoka, S., Kurihara, Y., Yagihashi, K., Niimi, H. & Nakajima, Y. (2005). Peripheral solitary pulmonary nodule: Ct findings in patients with pulmonary emphysema1, *Radiology* 235(1): 266–273.
URL: *http://radiology.rsna.org/content/235/1/266.abstract*

McCulloch, C. C., Kaucic, R. A., Mendonça, P. R., Walter, D. J. & Avila, R. S. (2004). Model-based detection of lung nodules in computed tomography exams1: Thoracic computer-aided diagnosis, *Academic radiology* 11(3): 258–266.

Meert, A.-P. (2010). Pulmonary nodule: a bayesian approach, *Revue medicale de Bruxelles* pp. 117–21.

Mekada, Y., Kusanagi, T., Hayase, Y., Mori, K., ichi Hasegawa, J., ichiro Toriwaki, J., Mori, M. & Natori, H. (2003). Detection of small nodules from 3d chest x-ray ct images based on shape features, *CARS*, pp. 971–976.

Mousa, W. & Khan, M. (2002). Lung nodule classification utilizing support vector machines, *ICIP02*, pp. III: 153–156.

Nathan, M. H., Collins, V. P. & Adam, R. A. (1962). Differentiation of benign and malignant pulmonary nodules by growth rate, *Radiology* 79: 221–32.

Oda, T., Kubo, M., Kawata, Y., Niki, N., Eguchi, K., Ohmatsu, H., Kakinuma, R., Kaneko, M., Kusumoto, M., Moriyama, N., Mori, K. & Nishiyama, H. (2002). "Detection algorithm of lung cancer candidate nodules on multislice CT images", *in* M. Sonka & J. M. Fitzpatrick (eds), *Society of Photo-Optical Instrumentation Engineers (SPIE) Conference Series*, Vol. 4684 of *Presented at the Society of Photo-Optical Instrumentation Engineers (SPIE) Conference*, pp. 1354–1361.

Osman, O., Ozekes, S. & Ucan, O. N. (2007). Lung nodule diagnosis using 3d template matching, *Comput. Biol. Med.* 37(8): 1167–1172.

Paik, D., Beaulieu, C., Rubin, G., Acar, B., Jeffrey, R., Yee, J., Dey, J. & Napel, S. (2004). Surface normal overlap: A computer-aided detection algorithm withapplication to colonic polyps and lung nodules in helical ct, *MedImg* 23(6): 661–675.

Paik, D. S. (2002). *Computer Aided Interpretation of Medical Images*, PhD thesis, Stanford University.

Patel, K., EC, F., AW, K., BS, L., S, B., JS, C., D, D., L, T., KA, W., C, F., C, C., SH, C., LP, F., P, B., MJ, L. & JA, B. (2010). Enhancement of a multi-analyte serum biomarker panel to identify lymph node metastases in non-small cell lung cancer with circulating autoantibody biomarkers, *International journal of cancer. Journal international du cancer* .

Peldschus, K., Herzog, P., Wood, S. A., Cheema, J. I., Costello, P. & Schoepf, U. J. (2005). Computer-aided diagnosis as a second reader: Spectrum of findings in ct studies of the chest interpreted as normal, *Chest* 128: 1517–1523.

Rami-Porta, R., ley, J. J., JJ, C. & Goldstraw, P. (2009). The revised tnm staging system for lung cancer., *Ann Thor. Cardiovasc. Surg.* 15: 4–9.

Reeves, A. P. & Kostis, W. J. (2000). Computer-aided diagnosis of small pulmonary nodules, *Seminars in Ultrasound, CT, and MRI* 21(2): 116 – 128. The Solitary Pulmonary Nodule.

Retico, A., Delogu, P., Fantacci, M. E., Gori, I. & Preite Martinez, A. (2008). Lung nodule detection in low-dose and thin-slice computed tomography, *Comput. Biol. Med.* 38(4): 525–534.

Ricklefs, R. E. (1997). *Estrutura da comunidade*, 3 edn, Guanabara Koogan, Rio de Janeiro, chapter 22, pp. 344–346.

Saita, S., Oda, T., Kubo, M., Kawata, Y., Niki, N., Sasagawa, M., Ohmatsu, H., Kakinuma, R., Kaneko, M., Kusumoto, M., Eguchi, K., Nishiyama, H., Mori, K. & Moriyama, N. (2004). "Nodule detection algorithm based on multislice CT images for lung cancer screening", *in* J. M. Fitzpatrick & M. Sonka (eds), *Society of Photo-Optical Instrumentation Engineers (SPIE) Conference Series*, Vol. 5370 of *Presented at the Society of Photo-Optical Instrumentation Engineers (SPIE) Conference*, pp. 1083–1090.

Sasaki, M., Kuwabara, Y., Ichiya, Y., Akashi, Y., Yoshida, T., Nakagawa, M., Murayama, S. & Masuda, K. (1999). Differential diagnosis of thymic tumors using a combination of 11c-methionine pet and fdg pet., *J Nucl Med* 40(10): 1595–601.

Schölkopf, B., Platt, J., Shawe-Taylor, J., Smola, A. & Williamson, R. (2001). Estimating the Support of a High-Dimensional Distribution, *Neural Computation* 13(7): 1443–1471.

Seemann, M. D., Staebler, A., Beinert, T., Dienemann, H., Obst, B., Matzko, M., Pistitsch, C. & Reiser, M. F. (1999). Usefulness of morphological characteristics for the differentiation of benign from malignant solitary pulmonary lesions using hrct, *European Radiology* 9(3): 409–417.
URL: *http://www.springerlink.com/content/bwmmf72udk9nfa4x/*

Silva, A. C., da Silva, E. C., de Paiva, A. C. & Nunes., R. A. (2005). Diagnosis of lung nodule using Moran's Index and Geary's Coefficient in computerized tomography images. Submitted to Pattern Analysis and Applications.

Silva, C. A., Silva, A. C., Netto, S. M. B., de Paiva, A. C., Junior, G. B. & Nunes, R. A. (2009). Lung nodules classification in ct images using simpson's index, geometrical measures and one-class svm, *MLDM*, pp. 810–822.

Silva, E. C., Silva, A. C., de Paiva, A. C., Nunes, R. A. & Gattass, M. (2008). Diagnosis of solitary lung nodules using the local form of ripley's k function applied to three-dimensional ct data, *Computer Methods Programs in Biomedicine.* 90(3): 230–239.

Simpson, E. H. (1949). Mensurement of diversity., *Nature* 163: 688.

Sluimer, I., Schilham, A., Prokop, M. & van Ginneken, B. (2006). Computer analysis of computed tomography scans of the lung: a survey, *Medical Imaging, IEEE Transactions on* 25(4): 385–405.
URL: *http://dx.doi.org/10.1109/TMI.2005.862753*

Sousa, J. R. F. S., Silva, A. C. & Paiva, A. C. (2007). Lung structure classification using 3d geometric measurements and svm., *Progress in Pattern Recognition, Image Analysis and Applications*, Vol. 4756, Springer Berlin / Heidelberg, pp. 783–792. Book Series: Lecture Notes in Computer Science.

Sousa, J. R. F. (2007). *Metodologia automática para detecção de nódulos pulmonares*, Master's thesis, Universidade Federal do Maranhão. In Portuguese.

Sousa, J. R. F., Silva, A. C., de Paiva, A. C. & Nunes, R. A. (2010). Methodology for automatic detection of lung nodules in computerized tomography images, *Computer Methods and Programs in Biomedicine* 98(1): 1 – 14.
URL: *http://www.sciencedirect.com/science/article/B6T5J-4X30C13-1/2/a002a6f4726e17552c7290b1d27ed137*

Suzuki, K. (2003). Massive training artificial neural network (mtann) for reduction of false positives in computerized detection of lung nodules in low-dose computed tomography, *Medical Physics* 30: 1602–+.

Suzuki, K., Shi, Z. & Zhang, J. (2008). Supervised enhancement of lung nodules by use of a massive-trainingartificial neural network (mtann) in computer-aided diagnosis (cad), *ICPR08*, pp. 1–4.

Tanino, M., Takizawa, H., Yamamoto, S., Matsumoto, T., Tateno, Y. & Iinuma, T. (2003). A detection method of ground glass opacities in chest x-ray ct images using automatic clustering techniques, *in* M. Sonka & J. M. Fitzpatrick (eds), *Society of Photo-Optical Instrumentation Engineers (SPIE) Conference Series*, Vol. 5032 of *Presented at the Society of Photo-Optical Instrumentation Engineers (SPIE) Conference*, pp. 1728–1737.

Vapnik, V. N. (1998). *Statistical Learning Theory*, Wiley-Interscience.
URL: *http://www.amazon.ca/exec/obidos/redirect?tag=citeulike04-20&path=ASIN/0471030031*

Vittitoe, N. F., Baker, J. A. & Floyd, C. E. (1997). Fractal texture analysis in computer-aided diagnosis of solitary pulmonary nodules, *Academic Radiology* 4(2): 96–101.

Way, T., Chan, H.-P., Hadjiiski, L., Sahiner, B., Chughtai, A., Song, T. K., Poopat, C., Stojanovska, J., Frank, L., Attili, A., Bogot, N., Cascade, P. N. & Kazerooni, E. A. (2010). Computer-aided diagnosis of lung nodules on ct scans: Roc study of its effect on radiologists' performance, *Academic radiology* 17(3): 323–332.

Wiemker, R., Rogalla, P., Zwartkruis, A. & Blaffert, T. (2002). Computer-aided lung nodule detection on high-resolution ct data, *in* M. Sonka & J. M. Fitzpatrick (eds), *Society of Photo-Optical Instrumentation Engineers (SPIE) Conference Series*, Vol. 4684 of *Presented at the Society of Photo-Optical Instrumentation Engineers (SPIE) Conference*, pp. 677–688.

Winer-Muram, H. T., Jennings, S. G., Tarver, R. D., Aisen, A. M., Tann, M., Conces, D. J. & Meyer, C. A. (2002). Volumetric growth rate of stage i lung cancer prior to treatment: serial ct scanning, *Radiology* pp. 798–805.

Wolf, M., Krishnan, A., Salganicoff, M., Bi, J., Dundar, M., Fung, G., Stoeckel, J., Periaswamy, S., Shen, H., Herzog, P. & Naidich, D. P. (2005). Cad performance analysis for pulmonary nodule detection on thin-slice mdct scans, *International Congress Series* 1281: 1104–1108. CARS 2005: Computer Assisted Radiology and Surgery.

Yamada, N., Kubo, M., Kawata, Y., Niki, N., Eguchi, K., Omatsu, H., Kakinuma, R., Kaneko, M., Kusumoto, M., Nishiyama, H. & Moriyama, N. (2003). Roi extraction of chest ct images using adaptive opening filter, *in* M. Sonka & J. M. Fitzpatrick (eds), *Society of Photo-Optical Instrumentation Engineers (SPIE) Conference Series*, Vol. 5032 of *Presented at the Society of Photo-Optical Instrumentation Engineers (SPIE) Conference*, pp. 869–876.

Yasufuku, K. (2010). Early diagnosis of lung cancer, *Clinics in Chest Medicine* 31(1): 39–47.

Zhang, X., McLennan, G., Hoffman, E. A. & Sonka, M. (2004). Computerized detection of pulmonary nodules using cellular neural networks in ct images, *Medical Imaging 2004: Image Processing*, San Diego, CA, USA.

Zhao, B., Ginsberg, M. S., Lefkowitz, R. A., Jiang, L., Cooper, C. & Schwartz, L. H. (2004). Application of the ldm algorithm to identify small lung nodules on low-dose msct scans, Vol. 5370, SPIE, pp. 818–823.
URL: *http://link.aip.org/link/?PSI/5370/818/1*

Zhao, B. & Yankelevitz, D. (1999). Two-dimensional multi-criterion segmentation of pulmonary nodules on helical CT images, *Medical Physics* 26(6): 889–895.

Zheng, B., III, J. K. L., Maitz, G. S., Chapman, B. E., Fuhrman, C. R., Rogers, R. M., Sciurba, F. C., Perez, A., Thompson, P., Good, W. F. & Gur, D. (2003). A simple method for automated lung segmentation in x-ray ct images, Vol. 5032, SPIE, pp. 1455–1463.
URL: *http://link.aip.org/link/?PSI/5032/1455/1*

3

Computer-aided Analysis and Interpretation of HRCT Images of the Lung

Zrimec Tatjana[1] and Sata Busayarat[2]
[1]*Centre for Health Informatics*
[2]*School of computer science and engineering Wales, NSW 2052*
University of New South Wales
Australia

1. Introduction

High Resolution CT (HRCT) techniques developed in the last decade have become invaluable tools for the detection of subtle diffuse lung disease patterns and for their characterisation into multiple possible diseases. HRCT imaging protocols produce 3D volume data and enable accurate visualisation of imaged anatomy and much better visualisation of the disease patterns than conventional X-rays. However, the amount of information produced by today's HRCT scanners is beyond the ability of a radiologist to process in normal clinical practice. Single detector scanners generate up to 40 images per study and multi-slice detectors generate 300-600 high-resolution axial images. Furthermore, the number of images is rapidly growing. It is difficult and time consuming to analyse images accurately and efficiently by hand. Systems for computerised image analysis are needed to help with the large number of images and to draw radiologist's attention to fewer, diagnostically useful images.
The goal of computerised medical image analysis and interpretation is to detect abnormal appearance of the imaged anatomy and to assist radiologists in identifying and integrating all the useful information available in an image (Brown & McNitt-Gray, 2000). There is a growing number of computer-aided diagnosis (CAD) systems aimed at automating the analysis of lung CT images and supporting diagnosis (Uppaluri, et al., 1999; Uchiyama et al., 2003; Sluimer, 2005; Zrimec et al., 2007; Tolouee et al., 2008). Uppaluri *et al.* (1999) presented a CAD system for detecting six lung tissue patterns using textural features. A multiple feature method was used to determine the optimal subset among 22 textural features calculated for each 31x31 pixel square region of interest in an image. A Bayesian classifier was trained to use the optimal subset of features to recognize six different tissue patterns. They reported that the automated system performed as well as experienced human observers who were told the diagnosis in advance. Uchiyama et al. (2003) also divided the lung into square regions and employed neural networks to perform classification of HRCT images into six textural classes. The neural network, trained with examples of different tissue patterns, was able to automatically detect images containing abnormalities and to provide good classification. In the work reported by Sluimer (2005), a multi-scale filter bank was used to represent the local image texture and structure. They used various classifiers to

train the system. They reported that the CAD ROC curve showed very similar performance compared to that of two radiologists.

Various combinations of wavelet transforms, in combination with support vector machines (SVM's), were also used to discriminate among several texture patterns from patients affected by interstitial lung diseases. Two sets of over-complete wavelet filters, discrete wavelet frames (DWF) and rotated wavelet frames (RWF) were used to extract the features, which best characterise the lung tissue patterns (Tolouee et al., 2008). The system was able to successfully classify four different lung patterns with the best multi-class accuracy achieved when combining DWF and RWF. Depeursinge (2010), described a texture classification system based on discrete wavelet frames (DWF) and quincunx wavelet frames (QWF) together with grey level histogram (GLH). After testing the performance of five different classifiers from the Weka machine learning environment (Witten & Frank, 2005), it was shown that the SVM classifier was the best in companions to Naive Bayes, k-NN, J48 and Multi Layer Perceptron (MLP), for correctly classifying instances into six classes of lung tissue patterns (Depeursinge, 2010).

Almost all existing CAD systems divide the image into small, usually square regions, applying classical image processing techniques to calculate the image features. They do not take advantage of existing anatomical knowledge. Accurate interpretation of medical images requires a detailed understanding of normal lung anatomy and of pathological changes that occur in the presence of disease (Webb *et al.*, 2000). In our approach to computer-aided detection, we first segment and extract anatomical features and landmarks from the images and then use them to help detecting abnormalities caused by disease processes. This approach enabled us to develop, for the first time, a digital model of the lung anatomy that incorporates regional information crucial for correct diagnosis. This is particularly important for lung diseases because the same disease patterns located in a different region of the lung or distributed in a different way can be linked to different pathologies (Webb *et al.*, 2000). Lung regions are extensively used in clinical reporting for indicating the location of detected disease patterns.

This chapter presents a methodology for building a computer system for interpreting HRCT images of the lung. The system is aimed at:

- automating the analysis and understating of lung CT scans,
- detecting lung disease patterns associated with diffuse lung diseases,
- providing radiologist with Computer-Aided Diagnosis as a second opinion.

To achieve these goals, the system is required to perform image analysis and interpretation, which includes:

a. *Segmentation* of the organs of interest;
b. Detection, classification and labelling of possible disease patterns;
c. Combination of disease patterns into a list of *differential diagnosis.*

Segmentation in image processing is defined as the separation of an image into regions that are meaningful for a specific task (Sonka, 2000). It is one of the first steps leading to image analysis and interpretation. In medical imaging, the segmented regions usually refer to organs, such as the heart, liver or lungs, or disease patterns, such as brain tumours or fibrosis in the lungs. Different image segmentation algorithms are used deepening on the type of object or feature of interest. Image segmentation usually involves image normalisation or pre-processing and low-level image processing to segment regions of interest from the image. Each region can be one to several pixels in size. It often involves higher-level candidate selection or ranking, where domain knowledge about the segmented object is used. In medical imaging, such knowledge can be about the anatomy or the specific disease patterns. The low-level image processing, often used in segmentation, includes thresholding, region growing, connected-component labelling, and mathematical morphology. Good descriptions of segmentation methods can be found in image processing text books (Gonzalez & Woods, 1993, Shapiro & Stockman, 2001) or books that are specific to medical image segmentation, such as (Sonka, 2000, Suetens, 2008). In this chapter we present our knowledge-based approach to segmentation lung anatomy and other anatomical landmarks. We also present the way in which the landmarks are used for generating regional information needed for image interpretation.

Detection, classification and labelling of possible disease patterns are the major tasks of the system and often are performed iteratively to achieve satisfactory results. There is a large class of disorders known as Diffuse Parenchymal Lung Disease (DPLD) that primarily affect the lung parenchyma and can be best diagnosed using HRCT. They are characterised by specific abnormal findings mostly texture-like in appearance (Webb, Muller & Naidich, 2000). Consequently, most of the systems for computerised analysis of HRCT images of the lung are texture based and are trained to detect and classify abnormal tissue patterns into several textural categories. The system for computer-aided interpretation of HRCT images, presented here, differs from existing systems by using knowledge about the disease patterns, their appearance and distribution, in addition to texture information. The rules for classifying detected patterns are automatically generated using machine learning. Two examples of pathology detection are presented to demonstrate the different detection techniques required for different disease patterns.

Differential diagnosis (DDx), the process of weighing the probability of one disease versus that of other diseases, is a particularly challenging task even for experienced radiologist since the combination of several abnormal findings can be associated with a specific diagnosis (Webb *et al.*, 2000). It requires good detection of disease patterns and substantial experience in radiology. Consequently, there is a relatively small number of publications on this topic. We present our preliminary results on differential diagnosis.

2. High-resolution CT and the human lung

Detailed understanding of lung anatomy is a prerequisite for successful image interpretation. We will look at the lung anatomy and it appearance on HRCT images. We will also learn what is used for image interpretation by radiologists.

2.1 Lung anatomy

There are two lungs, one on each side of the thoracic cavity, which are protected by the rib cage. Between the two lungs lies a space called the mediastinum, which is occupied by the heart, the trachea (the main airway), the oesophagus (tube to the stomach) and large blood vessels. In healthy people, each lung is elastic and conical in shape (Figure 1a). The hilum is the area on the medial surface of each lung, where the main bronchus, pulmonary artery, pulmonary vein and nerves enter and leave the lung. Each lung has a major or oblique fissure that divides the lung into upper and lower lobes. The right lung has also a minor or horizontal fissure that further divides the upper lobe. The lung consists of bronchi (or pulmonary airways), pulmonary blood vessels and connective tissue that support the structure of the lung; together these are called parenchyma. The pulmonary-arterial and the bronchial trees run alongside each other and branch simultaneously in a tree-like structure. The branches are of similar size in a healthy lung.

2.2 High-resolution CT images of the lung

Computer tomography (CT) is currently the best imaging modality for diagnosing lung diseases. High resolution CT scanners generate a three dimensional view of the imaged organs with sub-millimetre resolution in axial sections. It provides detailed information regarding the lung parenchyma and can delineate structures down to the level of the secondary pulmonary lobule, the smallest structure in the lung. It is particularly useful for image-based diagnosis, since alteration of the lung anatomy, caused by a disease, can be clearly seen in a thin-slice CT image (Webb et al., 2000). Figure 1 shows examples of a lung (a), an HRCT series of axial images (b) and an axial image with normal anatomy (c).

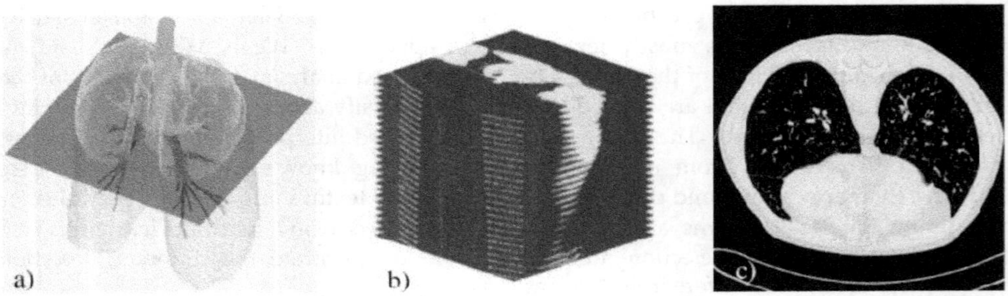

Fig. 1. Examples of a human lung (a), a series of HRCT images (b) and an axial image with normal anatomy (c).

In patients with diffuse lung disease, contiguous scanning is usually not necessary, since diffuse lung abnormalities can be adequately sampled with the acquisition of interspaced sections (Muller, 1991). In a routine HRCT protocol, 1 mm thick images are acquired with 10 to 20 mm inter-slice spacing.

To develop and evaluate our system, HRCT scans from three radiology practices in Sydney, Australia were used. The images were taken using a SIEMENS CT scanner with a tube voltage of 140kVp, current between 180 and 280 mAs, and exposure time of 750 ms. Data were reconstructed as 512x512 matrices with a slice thickness of 1.0 mm and 15 mm inter-slice spacing. The data are stored as DICOM 16-bit greyscale images with the pixel intensity proportional to tissue density represented in Hounsfield Unit[1] (HU).

2.3 Image marking and semantic labelling

We use machine learning to train a computer to recognise disease patterns in an HRCT image and to correctly classify them into different diseases. Supervised learning requires examples of lungs with labelled disease patterns and areas with normal appearance. Although the disease patterns are clearly visible to a trained human eye, it is not obvious how to provide an appropriate description that can be used by a computer. To enable easy

[1] Hounsfield unit (HU) is a unit used in medical imaging (CT or MRI scanning) to describe the amount of x-ray attenuation of each "voxel" (volume element) in the three-dimensional image.

communication with the radiologists while acquiring knowledge about different disease appearance in the HRCT images, we used a web-based interactive tool for image labelling.
The LMIK image labeller, developed for the Learning Medical Image Knowledge project (Rudrapatna *et al.*, 2004), was designed for easy access, marking and semantic labelling of images. It automatically downloads images from a hospital picture archiving and communication system (PACS) and stores them in a local LMIK database. The web-based interface enables access to the image database, provides interactive image display and a variety of semantic labelling facilities. Radiologists are able to remotely access cases from the local database, select and delineate representative examples of different lung diseases patterns (see Figure 2).

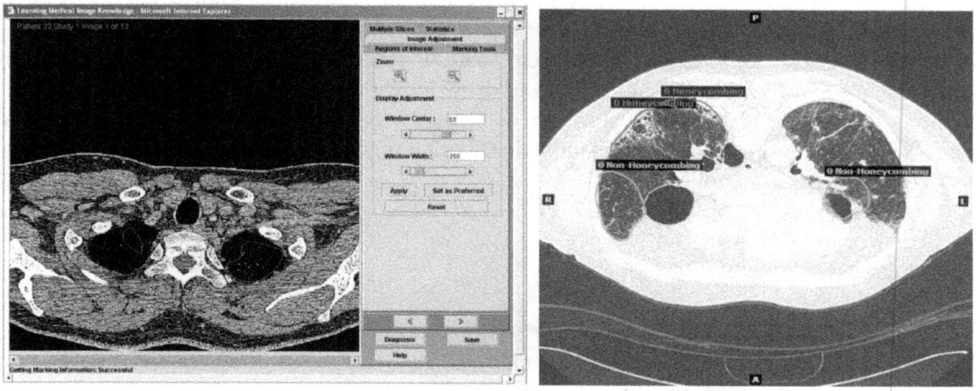

Fig. 2. LMIK Image labeler for Web-based semantic marking and labeling.

Every marked example consists of a delineated region of interest (ROI) containing a pattern, a label indicating the name of the pattern and the pattern severity, ranging from normal, moderate to severe.
The LMIK image labeller was used to provide ROIs with disease patterns as well as ROIs with normal lung tissue by at list two radiologist for the same cases. Radiologists were also able to compare their marking and labelling with each other and to agree on consistent marking for some difficult cusses.

2.4 Observing radiologists interpreting HRCT images

We had three experienced radiologist in our project group. They provided us with the latest textbooks and the books they are using when reporting on images (Webb *et al.*, 2000) as well as multimedia educational tools for interpretation of HRCT images of the lung,. We also had a few sessions observing the radiology reading and reporting HRCT cases in radiology practice.
The information used in the interpretation process can be summarised as:

a. knowledge of the imaged anatomy being investigated
b. landmarks
c. regional descriptions

Knowledge of the imaged anatomy being investigated - Radiologists use knowledge of anatomy when inspecting HRCT images. For example, knowledge about the shape of the lung in a cross sectional HRCT image helps to understand which part of the lung is captured in the image or knowledge of a broncho-arterial pair appearance helps to detect the presence or absence of a bronchial disease.

Landmarks - Radiologists make extensive use of anatomical landmarks, which are objects or features that help determine the location of the imaged part of the body. Selected landmarks are usually consistent, despite variations in the patient's position during scanning, or changes due to disease progression (Betke *at al*, 2003).

Regional descriptions - Knowledge of the regional distribution of lung diseases also assists in detecting pathology. In textbooks on interpreting HRCT images of the lung, it is noted: "When attempting to reach diagnosis using HRCT, the practitioner should not only be focused on the morphology of the structures appearing in the HRCT, but on their distribution, location and appearance" (Webb *et al.*, 2000). Many lung diseases show specific regional distributions or preferences. The same features located in a different region of the lung or distributed in a different way can be linked to different pathologies (Webb *et al.* 2000). Preferential predominant involvement of one or more lung regions is commonly seen in HRCT, even in patients with chest radiographs showing a "diffuse" abnormality (Muller, 1999). For the purpose of interpreting HRCT the regional distribution can be categorised in several ways:

- central lung vs. peripheral lung
- upper lung vs. lower lung
- anterior lung vs. posterior lung
- unilateral vs. bilateral.

2.5 Knowledge based analysis of HRCT images of the lung

To take advantage of the wealth of medical knowledge in lung image analysis, a computerised lung model or atlas, depicting the lung anatomy and lung appearance on the HRCT images is required. In the absence of such a model, we built a digital model from a nearly normal case of HRCT images taken with contiguous scanning, i.e., without inter-slice spacing, to represent the structure and anatomy of the lung and to record regional information. Literature on the visual interpretation of HRCT images of the lungs (Webb *et al.*, 2000) was used to acquire knowledge and create rules about disease appearance and behaviour. Machine learning was employed to automatically generate rules for detecting anatomical features and disease patterns during image analysis.

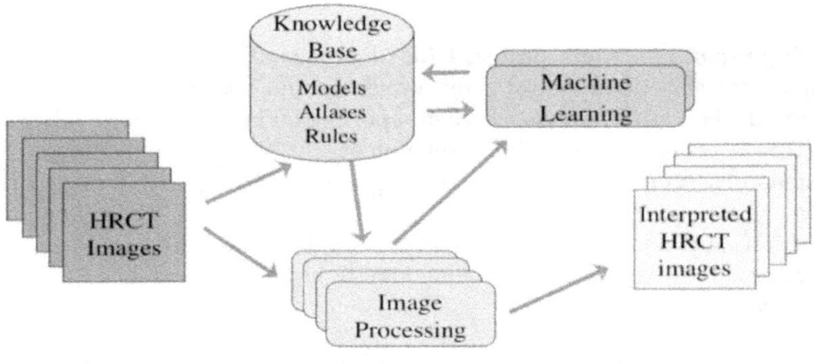

Fig. 3. System overview. Images are processed and interpreted using image processing algorithms, adapted for medical images, and knowledge that is mostly automatically generated and stored in the knowledge base.

An overview of the main modules involved in the computer aided detection and interpretation system is shown in Figure 3. An example of the use of the knowledge base is in providing spatial constraints indicating where an algorithm should be applied and semantic constraints to segment the correct objects. The knowledge includes a lung model, several HRCT lung atlases and a set of heuristic rules. The image processing module contains a variety of image processing algorithms that are able to work in cooperation with the knowledge from the knowledge base. The image processing module together with the machine-learning module are used to generate new knowledge that is stored in the knowledge base.

3. Segmentation of lung anatomy

Segmentation in medical imaging is particularly challenging largely because the appearance of organs and diseases differ from person to person. Other factors, such as acquisition artefacts, poor image quality or different scanning protocols, also make the task nontrivial. For automated segmentation to be successful, image processing needs to incorporate domain-specific knowledge as used by radiologist.

The set of anatomical features segmented by our system are grouped into:

- *Lung segmentation* - this includes features that help determine the lung structure, for example, lung boundaries, fissures;
- *Segmentation of broncho-vascular structures* - features that are part of the normal lung anatomy, for example, airways and vessels;
- *Landmarks segmentation* - this includes features within the lung and the lung surroundings, for example, the trachea and the ribcage.

3.1 Lung segmentation

Segmenting the lung fields is the primary task in any CT pulmonary image analysis. Automated and semi-automated segmentation of CT and HRCT has been an active area of research over the past decade. Armato and Sensakovi (2004) emphasised the importance of lung segmentation as a pre-processing step of a CAD system. Similarly, the bronchial tree is one of the most important and most prominent structures inside the lung. Kuhnigk *et al.* (2005) recognised the importance of the bronchial tree segmentation as a way to divide the lung lobes into smaller regions and use them to evaluate the distribution of diseases.

A number of authors have reported high accuracy for segmenting lung fields. Most of those approaches are based on grey-level thresholding, seeded region or volume growing or a combination of both. Examples that fall into this category are (Brown, et al., 1997; Hu, Hoffman, & Reinhardt, 2001; Garnavi, *et al.*, 2005; Sluimer, 2005; Lee, et al., 2004). Various techniques were used to overcome shortcomings of the basic thresholding and region growing algorithms. Another approach uses active contouring such as energy-minimising snakes to find the lung contour, for example (Papalousis, 2003; Li & Reinhardt, 2001). Active contours have a better ability to deal with irregular shapes than thresholding and region growing (Kass *et al.*, 1987). This is because they use their own shape as an input, instead of the pixel intensity alone.

In lung segmentation 3D lung surfaces and 2D lung boundaries are determined to separate the pixels belonging to the lung parenchyma from the background. Some issues need addressing when segmenting the lungs on 2D cross-sectional images. First, the two lungs are close to each other in the posterior part of the body and a simple thresholding or morphology method often connects the two lungs. Merged lung need to be separated to determine the left and the right lung. The second issue is that segmentation sometimes includes the main bronchi as part of the lung since the bronchi also have low intensity and enter the lung in the hilum region. Main bronchi are generally not considered part of the lung and they also create irregularities in the hilum surface. The last issue occurs in the anterior part of the lung. Gas in the stomach also appears as a low density region on the image so the segmentation often includes it as part of the lung as well.

A method for automatic lung boundary segmentation, described here, addresses all the above-mentioned issues. It uses a combination of the thresholding and morphology operators followed by active contours to achieve both robustness and smooth contour. Lung segmentation consists of the following steps:

- *Pre-processing* – reduces noise and removes the large bronchi and CT background.
- *Segmentation* – extracts the lung from the image using a combination of thresholding, morphology and other image processing techniques.
- *Post-processing* – ensures the two lungs are separate, removes remaining false-positives and smoothes the contour using active contour snakes.

3.1.1 Pre-processing

The number of noisy pixels in an HRCT image may vary depending on the CT machine and the parameters used. A 3×3 median filter is used to reduce the noisy pixels by averaging them with the 3×3 neighbouring pixels. Even though the sharpness decreases as a result of the median filter, its effect is insignificant for large objects like the lungs. The large bronchi are segmented and removed from the image to prevent inclusion in the lung boundary.

3.1.2 Segmentation

Thresholding generally works well for lung segmentation because of the great intensity difference between the lung and the surrounding tissues in the thorax. Initially, a fixed threshold of −500 HU (middle point between air and water density) was used, but it was found inappropriate for some special cases. In some lung diseases, the density range of lung parenchyma is wide so a fixed threshold may not be optimal in all cases. Consequently, a histogram analysis is used to select a threshold. After removing the CT background, the

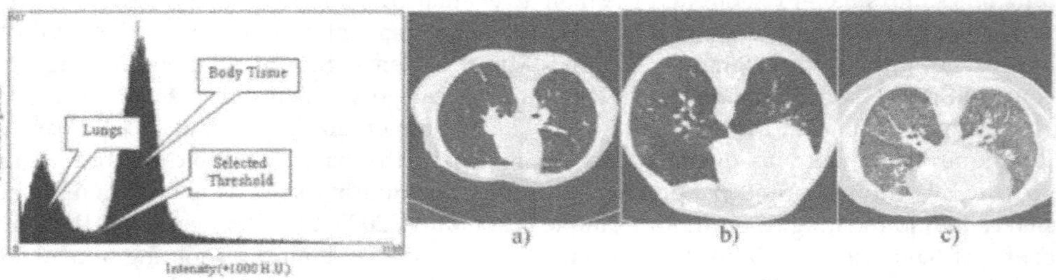

Fig. 4. Intensity histogram of an HRCT image of the lung. The first peak corresponds to low intensity pixels in the lung and the second peak corresponds to high-intensity pixels in the body. The threshold used for lung segmentation is the midpoint between the two peaks. Lungs with different densities: normal density lungs (a), low-density lungs (b) and high-density lungs (c).

intensity distribution of an HRCT image is bimodal, as shown in the histogram in Figure 4. The first peak in the histogram corresponds to pixels inside the lungs and the second peak corresponds to the pixels in the body tissue. The threshold selected for lung segmentation is the midpoint between the two peaks, ensuring that most of the pixels in the two groups are correctly separated.

In some high-density disease cases, the lung may be broken into multiple regions after thresholding. A sequence of morphological operators is applied to smooth the lung contour and to merge multiple regions into one large region.

3.1.3 Post-processing

A special strategy is used to address the issue of two connected lungs (see Figure 5). After the thresholding and morphology, the following heuristic rule is applied to test whether the two lungs are merged:

If

there is only one segmented object **and**
its size is over 1220 mm^2 **and**
its centre-of-mass lies within 40 mm width from the image centre line

then the lungs are merged

The lung pleura are used to help separate the lungs. The lung pleura are thin layers of membrane covering the lungs. While the pleura have the same density as other tissues, their intensity on HRCT is lower because of the HRCT volume-averaging effect. As a result, the pleura line separating the two lungs is often not detected by the globally optimal threshold. A threshold of −750 HU is used to segment the pleural line lying between the spinal cord and the sternum, as shown in Figure 5(c). The detected pleural line and the final result is shown in Figure 5(d).

Active Contour Models, or snakes, are used as the final post-processing step to smooth the lung contour. Snakes are dynamic, energy minimising curves, first introduced by Kass *et al.* (1987). A snake is a special form of deformable model, which is moved under the influence of internal forces and the curve itself, and external forces calculated from the image data. Generally, the internal force discourages bending the curve and the external force potentially pulls the curve toward the image contour. The deformation of snakes is

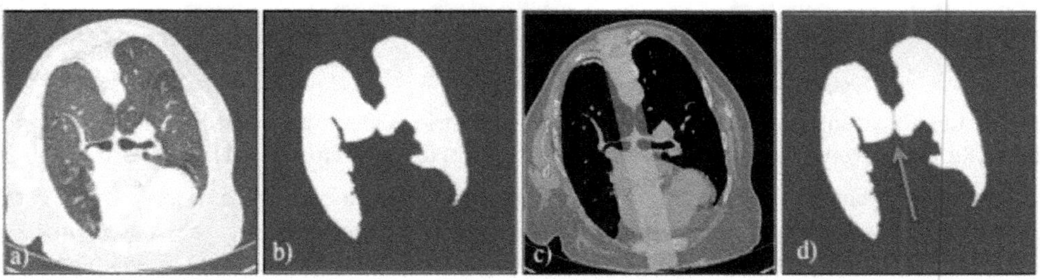

Fig. 5. An image of two lungs that are close to each other: appearance on HRCT (a), and the merged region resulted from the thresholding and morphology during the segmentation (b). The potential lung touching area, the 60-pixel-witdh bar between the spinal cord and the sternum (c), and the two lungs separated, indicated by the arrow, using the detected plural line (d).

controlled by an energy function that incorporates the internal and external forces and defines their weights. More specifically, the energy function is defined as:

$$E = \int_c \alpha(s)E_{cont} + \beta(s)E_{curv} + \gamma(s)E_{image} ds \qquad (1)$$

where the contour, *c*, is parameterised by its arc length, *s*. The first two terms define the internal energy and the last term defines the external energy. The coefficients $\alpha(s)$, $\beta(s)$, and $\gamma(s)$ are user-defined constants used to balance the smoothness and fitness of the contour. Normal Push force proposed by Papasoulis (2003) helps push the snakes into a concavity, which is common in lung contours near hilum. The snakes are initialised to be two circles centred at the centroids of the two lungs. The circles' radii are determined by the size of the lungs. The circles are clipped so that they do not lie outside the image. The entire deformation requires up to 200 iterations but the algorithm may stop early if no change occurred during the last iteration. Figure 6 shows intermediate steps and the final result of the lung segmentation.

3.2 Fissure segmentation

Fissures divide the lung into lobes that are relatively independent functional units. Lung pathology may be confined to one lobe, which in some cases can be surgically removed. There are several reports on segmenting pulmonary fissures. A method described by Kubo, et al. (2001) used a linear detector to segment fissures from thin CT scans and used surface curvature calculation and morphology filters to improve the results around pulmonary lesion. A fuzzy set approach with a fixed threshold was used by Zhang and Reinhardt, (1999) to segment the fissures. Wang *et al.* (2006) proposed a method for fissure segmentation using a 2D-shape-based curve-growing model with a semi-automatic initialisation.

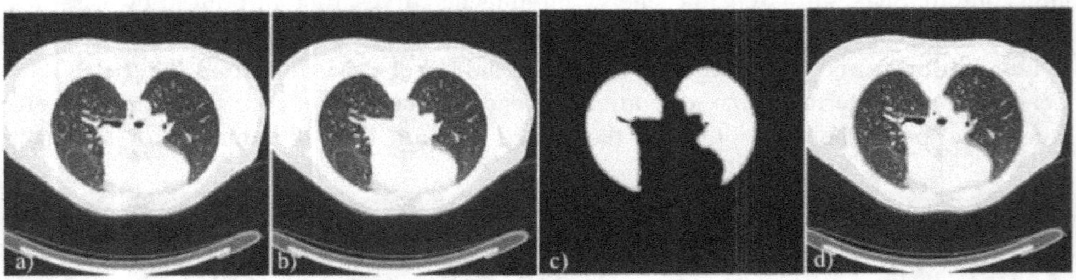

Fig. 6. Results of lung boundary pre-processing at various steps: an input lung HRCT image (a), after large bronchi removal (b), after non-body pixel removal (c) and final result (d).

A knowledge-based method for fissure detection, developed in our previous work, performs well in cases where fissures are fully visible (Zrimec & Busayarat, 2004; Zrimec *et al.*,2004). However, in almost 30% of the images, the fissures are only partially visible or are not visible at all (Eenakshi *et al.*, 2004). Using information from the lung model, it was possible to successfully determine fissures in the cases where fissures were partially visible or missing. The model guided fissure detection by predicting its expected location. The detected fissures were used to determine the lung lobes in 2D images (see Figure 7(a) and (b)) and in 3D models of patient data (see Figure 7(c)).

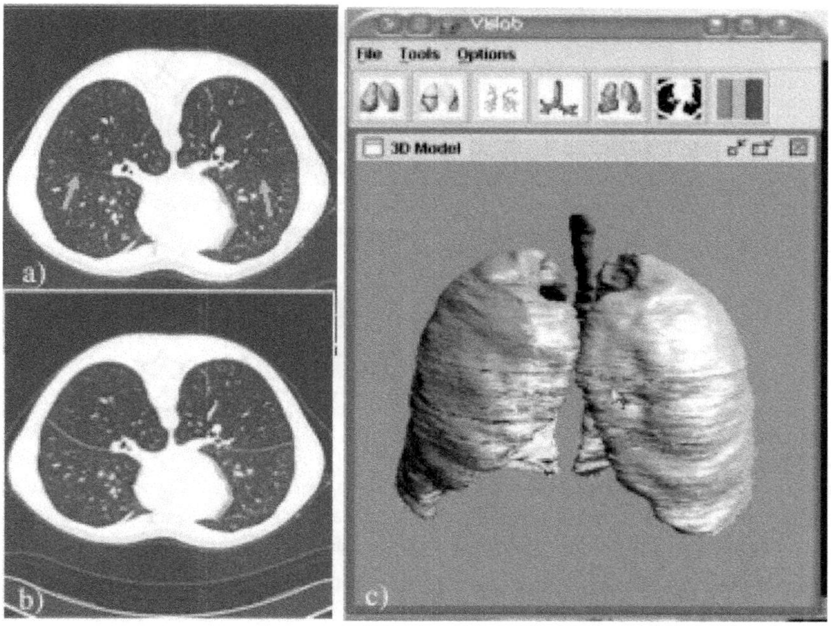

Fig. 7. Majors fissures visible on both lungs, (arrows) (a), segmented fissures (b) and a 3D model with four lung lobes (c).

3.3 Segmentation of broncho-vascular structures

Pulmonary airways, or bronchi, are amongst the most important structures in the lungs. They distribute inhaled air to the alveoli where oxygen and carbon dioxide exchange between air and blood takes place. The bronchial tree is complemented by a system of arterial blood vessels and pulmonary veins that transport the blood. From a clinical point of view, the identification of bronchi CT images provides valuable clinical information in patients with suspected airways diseases including bronchiectasis and constrictive obliterative bronchiolitis (Webb *et al.*, 2000). One of the main signs of a respiratory disease is the dilation of the bronchi. From an image processing point of view, bronchi can be used as landmarks for image registration, because their branching pattern is relatively static for the first four generations (Tschirren *et al.*, 2002).

Several publications discuss segmentation of bronchi in HRCT. Because the bronchi exhibit a tree-like structure, 3D approaches such as volume growing or tree-skeleton detection have been employed (Chiplunkar, et al., 1997; Aykac, et al., 2003). Their method was based on a 2D segmentation using an eight-connected seeded region growing with an adaptive threshold and a 3D connectivity analysis. The work was extended to be capable of determining the bronchial tree skeleton, detecting the branching points and matching them (both intra and inter-subject). A group from France also reported research on bronchial tree segmentation (Preteux, Fetita, & Grenier, 1997; Fetita & Preteux, 1999; Fetita & Preteux, 2000; Fetita & Preteux, 2001). Their method also consisted of 2D segmentation and 3D analysis of the 2D results. Their 2D segmentation was based on the connection cost algorithm, which filled all the local intensity minima (i.e. bronchi lumens). The 3D analysis involved stacking

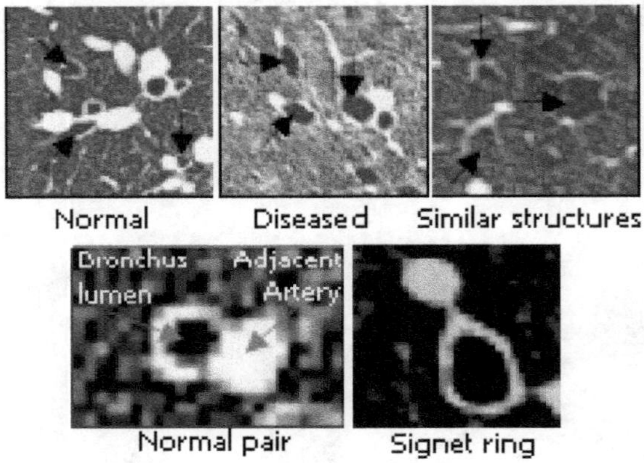

Fig. 8. Broncho-vascular pairs. Top left: an example of normal boncho-vascular structure, top middle: an example of diseased boncho-vascular structure with enlarged bronchi, top right: structures within the lungs with similar appearance; left bottom: enlarged pair; right bottom: an example of bronchial dilatation – "signet ring".

the 2D segmented results and filling up the gap where a bronchus is missing. They also constructed a 3D descriptive structure of the bronchial tree from the 3D stack.

In axial cross-sectional images, vertically oriented bronchi appear as high-attenuation circular or elliptical rings. Radiologists usually use this type of bronchus for diagnosing airway diseases, such as bronchiectasis. Figure 8 shows examples of a normal broncho-vascular pair and an abnormal pair with dilated bronchus. Automatic identification of bronchi, running nearly perpendicular to the scan plane, consists of potential candidate generation and candidate classification based on knowledge in the lung model. After thresholding, edge and radius analysis is performed to find all potential bronchi candidates, all dark rounded objects with bright walls. P-tile thresholding was used to handle inter-subject lung tissue density variability. Each object in the candidate bronchi list is represented by nine attributes. Knowledge of bronchial appearance in HRCT images is used to derive a heuristic function for ranking the candidates. The knowledge includes their average intensity, size, shape and position. Knowledge from the lung model, which includes a fully segmented bronchial tree, provides the expected number of bronchi for each lung in each cross-sectional image. The heuristic function, which is a weighted sum of all attributes, is used to remove all objects that are not bronchi. The final segmentation of the bronchi is done by region growing and rule-based classification to distinguish bronchi from other structures with similar appearance (Busayarat et al., 2005a).

Each bronchus has an accompanying artery. The arteries appear as high-attenuation solid circles or ellipses. An automatic method for detecting arteries based on (Chabat, et al., 2001) had problems with the ambiguous appearances of the adjacent arteries, which presents difficulties even for an experienced radiologist. It also had problems in providing accurate measurements of the size of small arteries due to the pixel rounding effect. A new technique was developed that uses knowledge-directed template matching to approximately locate the adjacent artery (Busayarat et al., 2005b). Knowledge of broncho-arterial anatomy helps locate the adjacent artery when there is more than one possible candidate nearby. Even though there is a high contrast between artery and lung parenchyma, an artery often contacts with other similar-density structures, such as bronchial wall and other vessels. This causes the growing region to leak into those structures. A specially developed region-growing algorithm, with leak correction, was used to accurately segment the arteries and to calculate their sizes. In contrast to other template matching techniques, where predefined templates are used, here the templates are generated on the fly using the detected bronchi in an image.

3.3.1 Trachea segmentation and carina detection

The trachea appears in an axial slice as a circular black object located in the middle of the body contour. To segment the trachea in an HRCT image, a fixed value of -400HU threshold is applied. After morphological filtering and connected component labelling, the trachea is segmented using knowledge about its expected location and size. Since the oesophagus can sometimes be misclassified as the trachea, the rules for trachea segmentation also include knowledge about the appearance of the oesophagus. The trachea is traced until the point at which it starts to bifurcate into two main bronchi. This bifurcation is known as carina (Figure 9). In a sparse scan (with 15 mm gap between consecutive slices), the exact location of the carina may not be visible. In that case, the slice before the trachea bifurcation is used as the carina position. We use carina as a landmark.

3.4 Detecting lung landmarks

Anatomical landmarks that are used to help determine the location of the imaged part of the lung include landmarks that are located on the ribcage and landmarks that are part of the lungs. The sternum, vertebrae and spinal canal are located on the ribcage. The trachea bifurcation - carina, hilum and the lung root are part of the lungs. These landmarks are often consistent and stable even in a presence of a disease. For example, the sternum and the vertebrae are good anatomical landmarks because they are bones and their position is relatively fixed within the chest. The sternum and the vertebrae have been used before for a different task, namely for inter-patient image registration (Archip, *et al.*, 2002; Betke, *et al.*, 2003). Radiologists use the carina, the bifurcation point of the trachea and the hilum, as a landmark. The hilum, as a landmark, defines the base of the lung, which is comparable between patients. Figure 9 shows examples of the landmarks.

Archip *et al.* (2002) used a knowledge-based approach to identifying the spinal cord. The knowledge base consists of an anatomical structures map and a task-oriented architecture, which is represented by a frame-like system. Deglint *et al.* (2007) uses a different approach to segment the spinal cord, based on 3D-seeded region-growing to detect the bones. The initial seed voxels are automatically obtained by an image processing procedure. The Hough transform is then applied on each image to find the best fitting circle inside the backbone, which represents the spinal cord. Betka *et al.* (2003) used an attenuation-based template matching approach to detect the sternum and spine. The sternum and spine were used to compute the optimal rigid-body transformation that aligns two CT scans of the same patient.

3.4.1 Sternum segmentation

The sternum and the spine are good landmarks in the chest HRCT images because they are bones outside the lungs. Their density (~1000 HU) is significantly higher than the surrounding soft tissue (30 to 40 HU) so they are relatively easy to segment. The spinal cord is inside the spine and because of its smaller size, provides an accurate landmark. Figure 9(a) shows HRCT appearances of the sternum, spine and spinal canal.

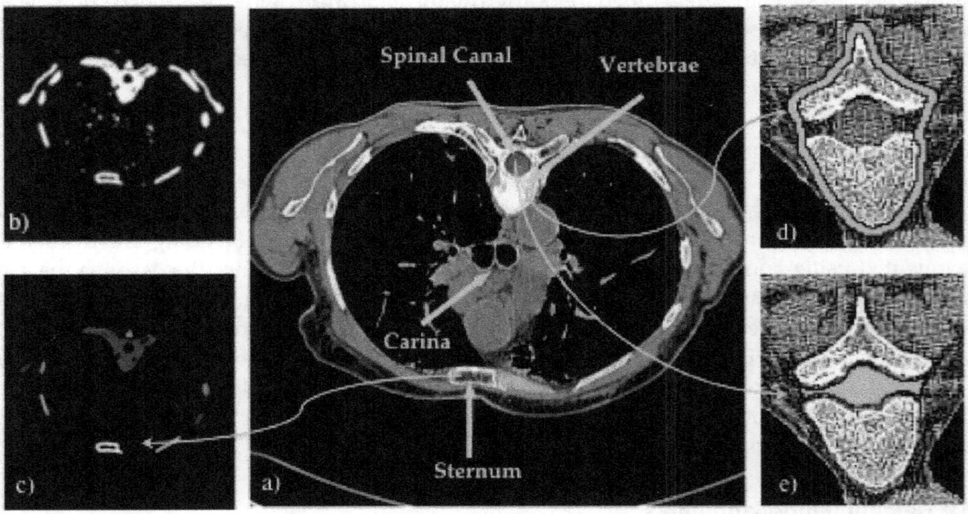

Fig. 9. HRCT appearances of carina, sternum, vertebrae and spinal canal (a); Segmented bones, sternum candidates (b), Segmented sternum (c); Segmented vertebrae using snakes (d) and segmented spinal canal (e). The image (a) is displayed using soft-tissue window setting (mean=40, width=500).

Our method uses intensity-based thresholding and morphological operators to segment the bones. A simplified version of the knowledge base presented in (Archip, et al., 2002) is also used to distinguish the sternum and the spine from other bone structures. The knowledge, encoded as parameters in the image processing script consists of knowledge about the sizes of the sternum and spine and their approximated positions, relative to the body. Once the spine is detected, a template-matching method is used to search for the spinal cord inside it. Sternum segmentation starts by removing the pixels outside the body in the image. Next, thresholding is used to segment bony pixels in the image. The bone density ranges from 400 HU, which is significantly higher than the surrounding soft tissues. The threshold value chosen for segmenting bone pixels is 300 HU, which is low enough to compensate the partial volume effect, and high enough to not include the tissues. Binary dilation and connected-component labelling are then applied to separate each bony region and remove noise. Every connected region that is smaller than 50 pixels is considered noise and removed from the image. The remaining connected regions are candidates for the sternum selection during the post-processing step. An example of an image with all candidates is shown in Figure 9(b).

In the post-processing step, knowledge of the location of the sternum is used for candidate selection. Specifically, the expected location of the sternum is near the middle and anterior part of the body. This is represented as a distance between the candidate sternum and the body. The Manhattan or city-block distance, between the candidate midpoint and the middle and most anterior point of the body-bounding box, is used to rank the candidates using Equation 2:

$$sternum\_distance(C,B) = \left|mid_x(C) - mid_x(B)\right| + \left|mid_y(C) - \max_{p \in B} p_y\right| \qquad (2)$$

$$mid_{axis}(obj) = \frac{\min_{p \in Obj} p_{axis} + \max_{p \in Obj} p_{axis}}{2}$$

where B and C are sets of pixels belonging to a candidate and the body region, respectively. The candidate with the lowest distance is selected is the sternum (Figure 9(c)).

3.4.2 Spine and spinal cord segmentation

The spine detection algorithm is almost identical to the sternum segmentation algorithm because they are both bones and their locations can be assumed. The obvious difference is the location constraint because the spine appears in the posterior whereas the sternum is in the anterior part of the body. Therefore, the distance function is changed to Equation 3.

$$spine\_distance(C,B) = \left|mid_x(C) - mid_x(B)\right| + \left|mid_y(C) - \min_{p \in B} p_y\right| \qquad (3)$$

One problem with spine detection is that it sometimes connects with the rib. We overcome this problem by removing all pixels that are further from the component's middle axis than the empirically determined distance of 37.5 millimetres. We set the upper limit of a spine diameter to be 75 millimetres using the guideline from Madden (2001). The spine outline is defined using active contour snakes. The snake is required because the spinal cord is not always completely surrounded by bones. The snake wraps around the spine and makes it a close-shape object (see Figure 9(d)). The snake is configured to rely more on the internal elastic and bending forces, than the external imaging force.

For segmentation, we defined the spinal cord's appearance in HRCT as the biggest circular and low-density object inside the spine (Figure 9(e)).

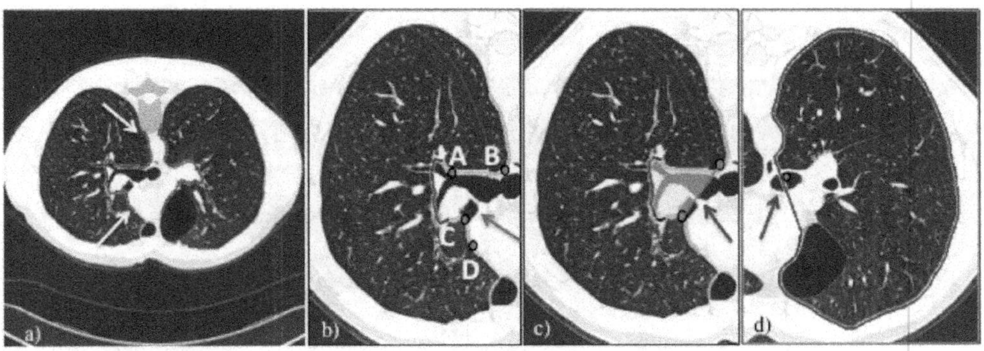

Fig. 10. The mediastinal part of the lung with potential hilum regions (white arrows) (a); candidates for hilum end points (b), detected hilum (arrow) (c); lung root (arrow) (d).

3.5 Hilum detection

The hilum is a wedge-shaped depression of the mediastinal surface of each lung, where the bronchi, blood vessels, nerves, and lymphatics enter or leave the viscus (Webb *et al.*, 2000).

On axial HRCT images, the hilum appears in the mediastinum as a high-density hole surrounded by low-density lung parenchyma. It can be used as an anatomical landmark in many applications, such as lung region separation and image registration.
The method for hilum detection is based on curvature analysis of the lung boundaries and proceeds as follows. To restrict the curvature analysis, a potential hilum region is determined (see Figure 10(a) marked with arrows). The hilum region is only the mediastinal part of the lung boundaries. A curvature analysis is performed in that region to detect the most concave curved section of the lung boundaries (see Figure 10(b) blue arrow). Four points, two on each side, with maximum slopes that are close to the section with maximum curvature, are chosen as candidates for hilum end points (see Figure 10(b), A, B, C, D). Two of those points are selected to be the hilum end points by using heuristic rules. The rules use, among other information, the relative position of the points with respect to the medial axes.

3.6 Lung root detection

Generally, the root of the lung is understood to be the entire hilum surface, where many structures enter or leave the lung (Betke *et al.*, 2003). However, we need a more specific definition of the lung root to use it as a landmark for other image analyses. After discussions with radiologists, the point where the main bronchus passes through the hilum surface is chosen to represent the lung root. Figure 10(d) illustrates the lung root point, which is the midpoint of the first intersection between the bronchi and the hilum surface.

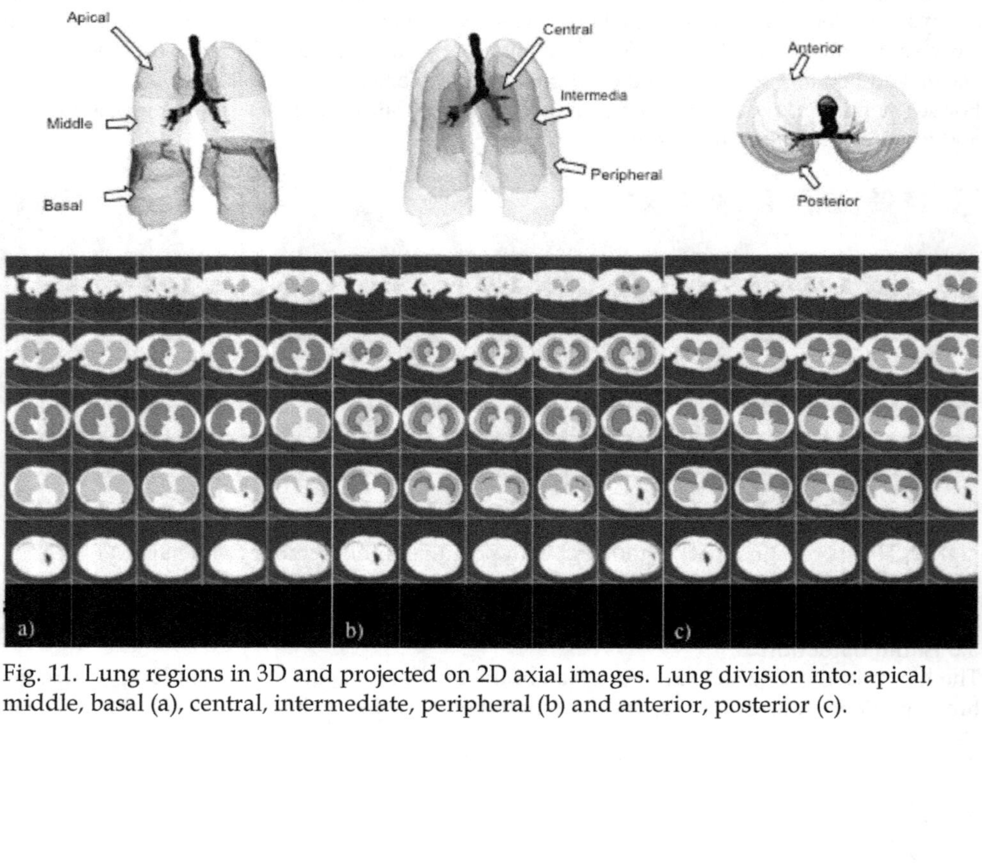

Fig. 11. Lung regions in 3D and projected on 2D axial images. Lung division into: apical, middle, basal (a), central, intermediate, peripheral (b) and anterior, posterior (c).

3.7 Dividing lung into pulmonary regions

A novel approach for dividing the lung and parenchyma into multiple clinically meaningful regions is as follows. The entire lung parenchyma is divided into three axes: apical-middle-basal, anterior-posterior and peripheral-intermediate-central, which creates eight overlapping regions. For the purpose of HRCT image integration, the lung regions are mapped to each 2D axial image.

Each lung is vertically divided into *apical, middle* and *basal* regions. The images above the hilum belong to the *apex* of the lung, the images in the region of hilum belong to the *middle* region of the lung and the images bellow the hilum belong to the *base* of the lung. Figure 11(a) shows an example of the apical-basal division. The apical, middle, and basal regions in 2D are displayed in green, red, and blue colour, respectively.

The coronal plane, which runs through the centre of the carina, is used to divide the lung into two parts: *anterior* and *posterior.* However, not all HRCT scans are taken in a perfectly prone-supine orientation (i.e. the subject does not lie perfectly flat). Two additional landmarks, namely the *spinal cord* and *sternum,* are used for the alignment. The coronal plane needs to be perpendicular to the medial plane that runs through the centre of the spinal cord and the sternum. An example of the resulting anterior-posterior division is shown in Figure 11(c). The anterior and posterior regions are displayed in green and red colour, respectively.

To divide the lung into *central, medial* and *peripheral* regions, the following 3D algorithm, developed together with a radiologist from our group, was used. A three-dimensional position of the lung root and voxels belonging to the lung surface are used. For each lung, a line is drawn between the lung root and each lung surface voxel. Since the lung root is outside the lung, the line will pass the lung surface twice, in and out. The line section between the first and the second crossing points are then divided into three parts equally. The first part, closer to the lung root, is the *central* region, the second part is *intermediate* region and the last third is *peripheral* region. The central, intermediate and peripheral divisions are projected onto 2D axial images (Figure 11(b)). After segmenting the anatomy, landmarks and lung regions, the images are prepared for detecting abnormal findings.

4. Computer-aided detection and interpretation of disease patterns

There is a substantial number of different disease patterns that can be visually identified in HRCT images of the lungs. In this chapter, we report on the detection of two kinds. One shows structural deformation of the bronchi by bronchial dilatation and bronchial wall thickening and the other shows fibrous changes of the lung parenchyma, represented by honeycombing. Bronchial dilatation and bronchial wall thickening patterns are associated with Bronchiectasis and honeycombing is associated with Interstitial Diffuse Lung Diseases (IDLD) or Diffuse Parenchymal Lung Disease (DPLD). The two examples described here were chosen to demonstrate the different detection techniques required by different disease patterns.

Rules for classifying the detected patterns were built automatically using supervised machine learning. In supervised learning, a set of pre-classified training examples is used to generate classification rules. We used J48, the Weka (Witten *et al.*, 2005) implementation of the C4.5 decision tree induction algorithm. The input to J48 was a set of classified examples of disease patterns represented by a set of image attributes. The result of learning is a classification tree in which the most informative attributes are used to determine the correct class.

4.1 Bronchial dilatation as a direct sign for Bronchiectasis

Bronchiectasis is defined as localised, irreversible bronchial dilatation, often with thickening of the bronchial wall (Webb, et al., 2000). Dilation of a bronchus is detected by comparing its size with the size of the accompanying artery. Bronchiectasis is considered present when the internal diameter of a bronchus is greater than that of the adjacent pulmonary artery. The typical appearance of this pattern is known as the "signet ring sign" (see Figure 8). Webb *et al.* (2000) reported that subjective visual criteria are most often used in the interpretation of HRCT images and a few different scoring systems are used to assess bronchaectasis extend and severity. We have used an HRCT bronchiectasis scoring system (Webb *et al.*, 2000) that provides ranges for bronchial dilatation and the bronchial wall thickening.

A set of parameters, calculated to compare the bronchus and its accompanying artery, includes lumen area, shortest diameter and the ratios of the lumen areas and the shortest diameters of a broncho-vascular pair.

Machine learning was used to automatically determine the severity thresholds and to determine which parameters to use in assessing the severity for different sizes of bronchi (Zrimec *et a*l., 2003; Busayarat & Zrimec, 2005). Figure 12 shows radiologist's marked examples of bronchial dilatation and results of the detected and classified by a computer.

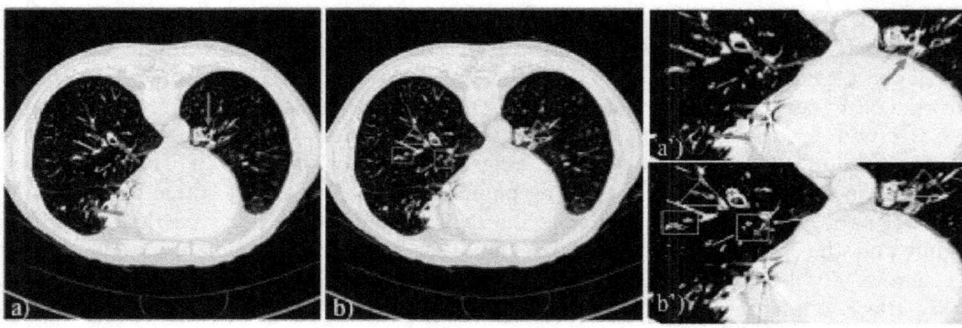

Fig. 12. Results of bronchial dilatation detection and severity assessment. Radiologist's marked broncho-arterial pairs (a), red arrows dilated (a'); computer detection results with severity assessment (b), green rectangle: normal, yellow triangle: mild dilatation (b').

4.2 Honeycombing as a sign for interstitial lung diseases

Honeycombing indicates a disease process characterised by a cluster of air-filled cysts divided by thick walls. The cysts range from a few millimetres to several centimetres and occur predominantly in the periphery of the lung (Webb, et al., 2000). Honeycombing is common in patients with idiopathic pulmonary fibrosis (IPF) and other interstitial diseases. In an HRCT image, honeycombing can be seen as a cluster of roughly circular dark patches surrounded by white walls (see Figure 13). Because of its characteristic appearance, honeycombing is a challenging pattern to detect by a computer. For example, broncho-vascular structures have similar appearance (see Figure 13).

Honeycombing is present in many disorders that primarily affect the lung parenchyma. They are characterised by specific abnormal findings, mostly texture-like in appearance. Consequently, most of the automated detection algorithms, being developed to analyse CT scans are texture based. The classical approach is to use a set of image features to describe the image content and to use some classification scheme to distinguish between different patterns. Initially, we adopted a similar approach. After experimenting with different attribute subsets for describing the content of the image and with different learning schemes for improving the system's performance, the results reveal that classical pattern detection approaches do not perform satisfactorily. The problem is that texture descriptors, alone, do not capture information that is pertinent to medical images, i.e. the disease appearance and distribution. Therefore, we incorporated knowledge of the lung regions and anatomy as well as specialist's knowledge of disease appearance, which help improve the detection.

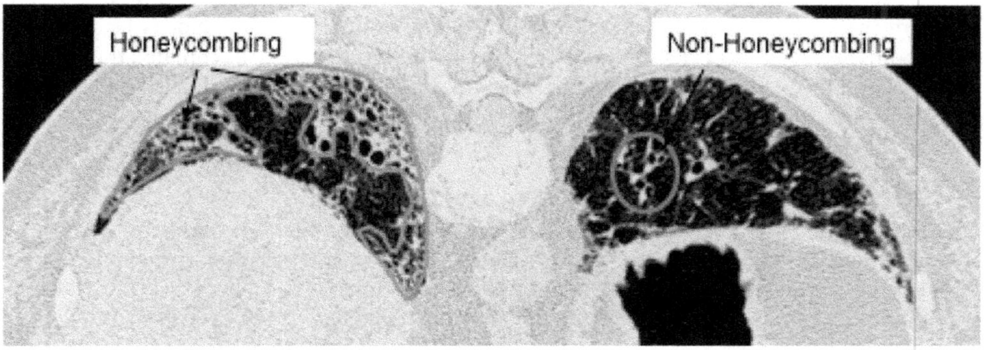

Fig. 13. Left lung - outlined region with honeycombing. Right lung - outlined example of broncho-vascular structures, which has similar appearance as honeycombing.

Rules for discriminating between honeycombing and non-honeycombing patterns were created automatically by supervised machine learning. The training examples were obtained from the images with labelled regions provided by radiologists. The regions with representative examples of honeycombing and other lung diseases patterns, marked by the radiologists as described in section 2.3, were processed to extract statistical features from the images that best represent the underlying texture. The marked regions were subdivided into blocks of size 7x7 and 15x15 pixels. Adjacent blocks overlapped such that the centres of adjacent blocks were three pixels apart. A set of attributes was calculated for each central pixel and it's neighbours in the block. Two block sizes were used to capture the characteristics of small and larger honeycombing cysts.

First and second order texture attributes and grey-level difference were calculated for each block (Haralick, 1979; Wong & Zrimec, 2007). The first order texture attributes measure the grey-level distribution within the block. Those attributes include: the mean HU, variance, skewness, kurtosis, energy and entropy. The second order features describe the spatial distribution of the grey-levels within these blocks. A co-occurrence matrix is calculated that specifies the frequency of a particular grey-level occurring near another grey-level. The co-occurrences of the grey-levels for four different directions were measured: 0°, 45°, 90°, 135°. Each pixel, with its surrounding area, is represented by 63 attributes per window, resulting in a feature vector with 126 attributes (63 for blocks of 7x7 pixels and 63 for blocks of 15x15pixels).

Correlation-based Feature Selection (CFS) (Hall, 2000) was used to reduce the dimensionality of the feature vector. CFS selects subsets of attributes that are highly correlated with the class and that have low inter-correlation.

A subset of features that best discriminates honeycombed and non-honeycombed regions was selected and used for learning. J48 decision tree learning produced rules for recognising honeycombing regions. Figure 14(a) shows an example of applying the classification rules.

We used expert knowledge about the appearance of honeycombing to improve the classification results. An example of such knowledge is that "Honeycombing results in cysts ...which have a peripheral predominance" (Webb, at al., 2000. pp 91). We implemented a post-processing step using knowledge about the lung regions (section 3.7). Masks with peripheral, intermediated and central regions were used to guide the classification algorithm. The classification algorithm classifies potential blocks as honeycombing only if they are in the periphery of the lung or in close proximity to other blocks classified as honeycombing. Results of the detection are shown in Figure 14, which contains the original image (Fig 14(a)), image with overlaid lung regions (Fig 14(b)), to determine the lung periphery, and regions with detected honeycombing (Fig 14(c)).

5. Results

Results of the methods developed to detect abnormalities in airways indicating Bronchiectasis and honeycombing are presented. The performance was compared against the manual reference set using the following three measures:

$$accuracy = \frac{TP+TN}{P+N} \quad sensitivity = \frac{TP}{TP+FN} \quad specificity = \frac{TN}{TN+FP} \quad precision = \frac{TP}{TP+FP}$$

where TP is the true positive rate, i.e., the number of pixels correctly classified. TN is true negative rate. FP is the false positive rate and FN is false negative rate. P and N indicate the total number of positives and the number of negatives. *Accuracy* is the degree of closeness of measurements of a quantity to its actual (true) value. *Sensitivity* determines the proportion of actual disease pattern that has been detected. *Specificity* measures the amount of non-disease pattern that has been classified as non-disease pattern. *Precision* - reproducibility or repeatability is the degree to which repeated measurements under unchanged conditions show the same results.

5.1 Evaluation of the success of detection of bronchial dilation and bronchial wall thickening singes

The success of the disease patterns detection depends on quality of feature segmentation. This evaluation consisted of the following experiments:

- the success of the automatic segmentation of bronchi,
- the success of correctly identified broncho-arterial pairs,
- the success of detection of the extent of baronial dilatation,
- the success of detection of bronchial wall thickening.

The result of the automatic detection of bronchi was compared with the 711 manually identified bronchi from 67 images of 18 subjects. It achieved 73% sensitivity and 83% accuracy on the unseen data. Most of the false negatives occur with small bronchi, which radiologists also have difficulty in identifying.

The experiment for evaluating artery detection and bronchial-dilatation assessment was performed on 324 HRCT images from 64 subjects. Ground truth or the reference set consisted of 442 broncho-arterial pairs manually marked and verified by experienced

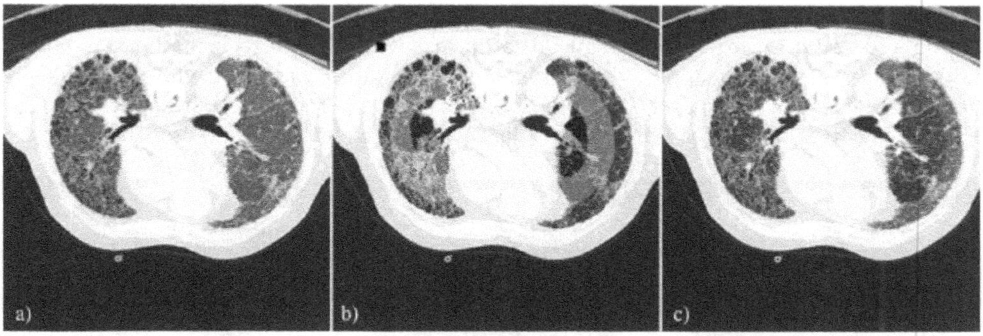

Fig. 14. Results of honeycombing detection (a) (red – honeycombing and green – non-honeycombing), image with regional information (b), final results after post processing (c).

radiologist PW. The artery detection was considered as correct if the centre was detected with error < 2 pixels. Artery detection achieved 90% accuracy (400/442). Figures 12(b) and 12(b') show the results of the broncho-arterial pairs detection.

To evaluate the performance of the severity of the bronchi dilation, 194 broncho-arterial pairs were manually classified as normal (94), mild (64) or severe (36). The experiment for baronial dilatation assessment only used samples that have correctly detected arteries. On 10-fold cross-validation, the system achieved 82% accuracy.

Bronchial wall thickening was evaluated on 12 broncho-arterial pairs marked by radiologists. The system demonstrated 83% correct detection. Examples of bronchial wall thickening and severity assessment are shown in Figure 15.

5.2 Evaluation of honeycombing detection

The performance of rules generated by machine learning is tested by cross-validation and by applying them to previously unseen cases. This evaluation consisted of the following experiments:

- Creation of the classifier and evaluation of its performance with 10 fold cross validation;
- Evaluation the success of classifying unseen cases.

The detection of honeycombing was tested on 42 HRCT images from 10 patients. The training data set consisted of 30 images with 110 marked and labelled regions by radiologists. Those regions were used to generate 2964 blocks with honeycombing and 2569 blocks with non-honeycombing training examples. Using tenfold cross validation, the method achieved 98% accuracy.

A set of 12 unseen images was used for evaluation. In the evaluation set, there were 28 regions with honeycombing and 20 regions without honeycombing. This resulted into 1240 blocks with honeycombing and 876 blocks with non-honeycombing regions. The evaluation on the unseen data achieved 94.6% accuracy. The evaluation was performed on the radiologist's marked regions.

6. Discussion

To validate the robustness of the algorithm in real clinical practice, the dataset is selected to have variations that reflect the real data. There are variations in four difference aspects: number of slices, slice gap, slice thickness and spatial pixel size. The slice gap, or distance between two adjacent slices, in our data set is a constant of 15 milimeters. Another aspect we considered was the variety of patients. The dataset was selected to include scans with a wide range of abnormalities. In particular, it includes subjects with high-density abnormalities, such as ground glass opacity, and with low-density abnormalities, such as emphysema. It also includes a few cases of airways abnormalities, such as bronchiectasis.

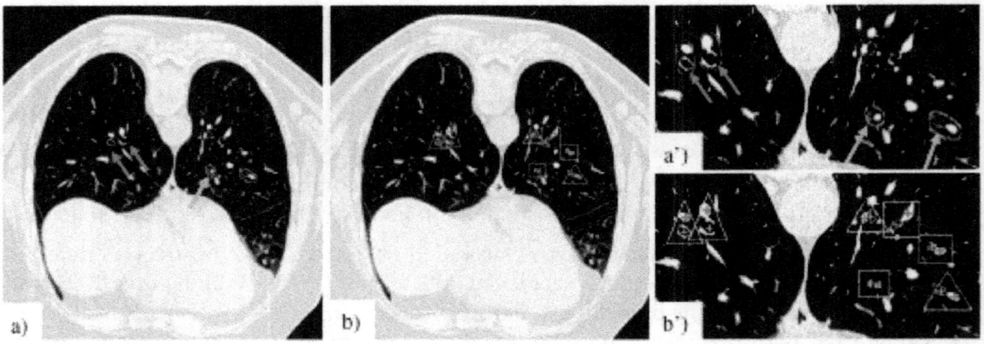

Fig. 15. Results of bronchial wall thickening detection and severity assessment. Radiologist's marked broncho-arterial pairs (a), green arrows - normal and red arrows dilated (a'); computer detection results with severity assessment (b), green rectangle: normal, yellow triangle: mild dilatation (b').

To evaluate the performance of the segmentation algorithms a set of scans from 84 subjects was used. Each scan contained a series of cross-sectional images in the axial plane. There were a total number of 1685 images. The evaluation was performed on a manually segmented data set, verified by a radiologist. The evaluation showed that the segmentation algorithms were quite successful with the sensitivity shown in Table 1. From the results presented in Table 1, we can see that the chosen landmarks are very stable across patients.

Our segmentation algorithms have mostly been developed for processing two-dimensional axial images rather than 3D because the radiology practices that supplied the data routinely use images with 15 mm gaps for analysing diffuse interstitial lung diseases. There is a trend, in the recent years, to move from two-dimensional to three-dimensional processing (Sluimer, 2005). A three-dimensional data set is necessary for bronchial and arterial three segmentation and we have already experimented on a limited data set of 20 subjects to segment both structures.

A major problem in the evaluation was the creation of a reference dataset, which required manual tracing of outlines. To assist in the creation of the reference dataset, we developed interactive tools for annotating regions, lines and points in the images that represent anatomical structures (Rudrapatna, et al., 2004) . The reference standard or the ground truth, used for evaluating the anatomy segmentation was manually created by an observer who is familiar with lung anatomy. The reference standard was verified and corrected by three expert radiologists to ensure accuracy of the data. These tools enforce consistency of manual segmentation amongst radiologists. The same tools can be used in clinical practice for manually correcting cases where the automatic segmentation was not successful.

The tasks of detecting, classifying and labelling possible disease patterns were demonstrated on two kinds of diseases patterns, one related to structural deformation of the bronchial tree and one showing fibrotic changes of the lung parenchyma. The results show that the system is able to recognise potential lung abnormalities and indicate their size and location. Computer analysis and evaluation of bronchial morphology, especially bronchial thickness, is important, because bronchi are responsive to treatment. This system can help assess treatment outcomes as well as assist in studies of the effects of new drugs.

Differential diagnosis in the case of interstitial lung disease is difficult even for experienced chest radiologists. Radiologists inspect the appearance of lung regions in all images and based on the pattern of pathology and its distribution, along with the patient's history, an evaluation of the case is reported. Although the current system does not have access to the patient's history we have preliminary results from automated methods for calculating the percentage of affected lung and for assessing the distribution of the decease patterns. The system provides a list of possible diagnoses with their probability, based on the patterns detected in the images. Radiologists then combine the suggested differential diagnosis with the patient history for the case report.

7. Conclusions and future work

We have presented a system for computer-aided detection of disease patterns. In the proposed framework, normal anatomy and anatomical landmarks are segmented and used to detect disease patterns. Recognising normal anatomy helps in detecting many diseases that have similar appearance. For example, the appearance of honeycombing is similar to normal bronchi and vessels. Because we know the expected location of the bronchi and vessels, they can be eliminated, leaving the honeycombing. Most of the methods developed are knowledge-guided. Knowledge of anatomy comes from a model of the lung. Specific knowledge, related to HRCT images, was acquired via machine learning from examples. Knowledge about disease appearance and its distribution in the lungs was encoded in heuristic rules. Having learned the lung anatomy and having developed a model of the lung, we are now concentrating on building systems for recognising patterns created by other lung diseases.

Landmark	Trachea	Carina	Sternum	Spinal Cord	Hilum
%Sensitivity	100%	99%	99%	96%	93%

Table 1. Results of the automatic segmentation of anatomical landmarks.

Although there is an increasing number of publications on computer added CT analysis of DILD, it is difficult to compare the results form different groups. One of the problems is the absence of a common, carefully annotated and representative database for benchmarking algorithms (Sluimer, 2005) similar to the Lung Image Database Consortium for nodule detection (Armato *et al.*, 2004). We are already making efforts in developing similar data sets for interstitial lung diseases detection.

8. Acknowledgment

We thank Claude Sammut for his comments and Medical Imaging Australia for providing images. We also thank radiologists Peter Wilson, Michael Jones Daniel Moses and Pravati Panigrahi for providing clinical resources, image annotation and inspection of the results.

9. References

Archip, N., Erard, P. J., Egmont-Petersen, M., Haefliger, J. M., & Germond, J. F. (2002). A knowledge-based approach to automatic detection of the spinal cord in CT images. IEEE Transactions on Medical Imaging, pp. 1504-1515.

Armato, S. G., & Sensakovic, F. W. (2004). Automated lung segmentation for thoracic CT. Academic Radiology , 11 (9), 1011-1021.

Armato SG, McLennan G, McNitt-Gray MF, et al. (2004). The Lung Image Database Consortium: developing a resource for the medical imaging re- search community. Radiology 2004; 232:739–748.

Aykac, D., Hoffman, E. A., McLennan, G., & Reinhardt, J. M. (2003). Segmentation and analysis of the human airway tree from three-dimensional X-Ray CT images. IEEE Transactions on Medical Imaging, 2(8), 940-950.

Betke, M., Hong, H., Thomas, D., Prince, C., & Ko, J. (2003). Landmark detection in the chest and registration of lung surfaces with an application to nodule registration. Medical Image Analysis , 7, 265–281.

British Thoracic Society, (1999). BTS guidelines on the diagnosis, assessment and treatment of diffuse parenchymal lung disease in adults, Thorax, vol. 54, no. Supplement 1, pp. S24–S30.

Brown, M. S., McNitt-Gray, (2000). Medical Image Interpretation, Handbook of Medical Imaging, Volume 2. Medical Image Processing and Analysis, ISBN 9780819477606, SPIE Press, 399-440.

Brown, M. S., McNitt-Gray, M. F., Mankovich, N. J., Goldin, J. G., Hiller, J., Wilson, L. S., et al. (1997). Method for segmenting chest CT image data using an anatomical model: Preliminary results. IEEE Transaction on Medical Imaging , 16 (6), 828-839.

Busayarat, S., & Zrimec, T. (2005a). Knowledge-directed automatic bronchi detection method for sparse HRCT scans of the lungs. Image and Vision Computing New Zealand, (pp. 369-374).

Busayarat, S., & Zrimec, T. (2005b). Automatic detection of pulmonary arteries and assessment of bronchial dilatation in HRCT images of the lungs. Computational Intelligence: Methods & Applications, Istanbul, pp. 5-10.

Chiplunkar, R., Reinhardt, J. M., & Hoffman, E. A. (1997). Segmentation and quantitation of the primary human airway tree. Society of Photographic Instrumentation Engineers- Medical Imaging, SPIE 3033, pp. 403-414.

Chabat, F., Hu, X., Hansell, D. M., & Yang, G.-Z. (2001). ERS transform for the automated detection of bronchial abnormalities on CT of the lungs. IEEE Transactions on Medical Imaging , 20 (9), 942-952.

Depeursinge, A., (2010). Affine–invariant texture analysis and retrieval of 3D medical images with clinical context integration, Phd Thesis, Unicersity Geneva.

Depeursinge, A., de Ville, D. V., Unser, M. , & M¨uller, H.(2008). Lung tissue analysis using isotropic polyharmonic B-Spline wavelets. In MICCAI '08: Proceedings of the First International Workshop on Pulmonary Image Analysis, New York, September, Springer, pp.125–133.

Depeursinge, A., Iavindrasana, J. , Hidki, A., Cohen, G., Geissbuhler, A., Platon, A., Poletti, P.-A. & M¨uller, H. (2008). A classification framework for lung tissue categorization. In K. P. Andriole and K. M. Siddiqui, editors, Medical Imaging 2008: PACS and Imaging Informatics, SPIE 6919, pp. 69190C- 69190C12.

Deglint, H. J., Rangayyan, R. M., Ayres, F. J., Boag, G. S., & Zuffo, M. K. (2007). Three-dimensional segmentation of the tumor in computed tomographic images of neuroblastoma. Digital Imaging , 20 (1), 72-87.

Eenakshi, S., Manjunath, K.Y., Balasubramanyam, V. (2004). Morphological variations of the lung fissures and lobes, Indian J. Chest Dis. Allied Sci., Vol. 46(3): 179-182.

Fetita, C., & Preteux, F. (1999). Three-dimensional reconstruction of human bronchial tree in HRCT. Proceedings of the International Society for Optical Engineering, *3646*, pp. 281-29.

Fetita, C., & Preteux, F. (2000). Bronchial tree modeling and 3D reconstruction. Society of Photographic Instrumentation Engineers, pp. 16-29.

Fetita, C., & Preteux, F. (2001). CT data-driven 3D airway model synthesis. World Multi Conference on Systemics, Cybernetics and Informatics, pp. 111-116.

Garnavi, R., Baraani-Dastjerdi, A., Moghaddam, H. A., Giti, M., & Rad, A. A. (2005). A new segmentation method for lung HRCT images. Digital Image Computing on Techniques and Applications, (p. 52).

Gonzalez, R. C., & Woods, R. E. (1993). Digital image processing. Addison Wesley.

Hall, M. A. (2000). Correlation-based feature selection for discrete and numeric class machine learning. In: ICML '00: Proceedings of the Seventeenth International Conference on Machine Learning, San Francisco, CA, USA, Morgan Kaufmann Publishers Inc. pp. 359–366.

Haralick, R. M., (1979). Statistical and Structural Approaches to Texture, Proceedings of the IEEE 67, pp. 786– 804.

Hu, S., Hoffman, E. A., & Reinhardt, J. M. (2001). Automatic lung segmentation for accurate quantitation of volumetric X-ray CT images. IEEE Transcation on Medical Imaging, 20 (6), 490-498.

Jain, R., Kasturi R. & Schunk, B. (1995). Machine vision, McGraw Hill.

Kass, M., Whitkin, A., & Terzopoulos, D. (1987). Snakes: active contour models. Proceedings of 1st International Conference on Computer Vision, London, pp. 259-269.

Kubo, M., Kawata, Y., Niki, N., Eguchi, K., Ohmatsu, H., Kakinuma, R., et al. (2001). Automatic extraction of pulmonary fissures from multidetector-row CT images. Internation Conference on Image Processing IEEE, pp. 1091-1094.

Kuhnigk, J. M., Dicken, V., Zidowitz, S., Bornemann, L., Kuemmerlen, B., Krass, S., et al. (2005). New tools for computer assistance in thoracic CT. part 1. functional analysis of lungs, lung lobes, and bronchopulmonary segments. Radio Graphics , 25, 525-536.

Lathi, B. P. (1998). Singal processing and linear systems. Berkeley-Cambridge.

Li, B. (2004). The construction of a normative human lung atlas by inter-subject registration and warping of CT images. PhD Thesis, University of Iowa.

Li, B., & Reinhardt, J. M. (2001). Automatic generation of object shape models and their application to tomographic image segmentation. Society of Photographic Instrumentation Engineers, 4322, pp. 311-322.

Madden, M. E. (2001). Introduction to sectional anatomy. Lippincott Williams & Wilkins.

Moore, K., & Dalley, A. (1999). Clinically oriented anatomy. Lippincott Williams and Wilkins.

Muller, N. (1991), Clinical value of High-Resolution CT in chronic diffuse lung disease, American Journal of Roentgenology, vol. 157, pp. 1163-1170.

Papalousis, J. (2003). LMIK - Anatomy and lung measurements using active contour snakes. Undergraduate Thesis, University of New South Wales.

Preteux, F., Fetita, C., & Grenier, P. (1997). Modeling, segmentation, and caliber estimation of bronchi in high-resolution computerized tomography. Society of Photographic Instrumentation Engineers, 3026, pp. 58-69.

Rudinsky, S., & Smirniotopoulos, J. G. (2006), Retrieved September 23 from Radiology glossary: http://rad.usuhs.mil/glossary.html

Rudrapatna, M., Sowmya, A., Zrimec, T., Wilson, P., Kossoff, G., Wong, J., Busayarat, S. , Misra, A., Lucas, P. (2004). LMIK – Learning Medical Image Knowledge: An Internet-based medical image knowledge acquisition framework", Electronic Imaging Science and Technology, IS&T/SPIE's 16th Annual Symposium, Jan 2004, San Jose, CA.

Shapiro, L., & Stockman, G. (2001). Computer vision. Prentice Hall.

Sluimer, I. C. (2005). Automated image analysis of the pathological lung in CT. PhD Thesis, Utrecht University.

Sonka, M. (2000). Handbook of medical imaging, volume 2. medical image processing and analysis. SPIE.

Suetens, P. (2008). Fundamentals of medical imaging. Second Edition, Cambridge University Press.

Tschirren, J., Palagyi, K., Reinhardt, J. M., Hoffman, E. A., & Sonka, M. (2002). Segmentation, skeletoniztion, and branchpoint matching -- a fully automated quantitative evaluation of human intrathoracic airway trees. Medical Image Computing and Computer-Assisted Intervention. Springer, 2489, pp. 12-19.

Tolouee, A., Abrishami-Moghaddam, H., Garnavi, R., Forouzanfar, M., & Giti, M. (2008). Texture analysis in lung HRCT images. 2008 Digital Image Computing: Techniques and Applications, dicta, pp.305-311.

Uchiyama, Y., Katsuragawa, S., Abe, H., Shiraishi, J., Li, F., Li, Q., Zhang, C.-T., Suzuki, K., and Doi, K. (2003). Quantitative computerized analysis of diffuse lung disease in high-resolution computed tomography", Medical Physics, Vol. 30(9): 2440–2454.

Uppaluri, R., Hoffman, E. A., Sonka, M., Hartley, P. G., Hunninghake, G.W., & McLennan, G. (1999). Computer recognition of regional lung disease patterns", American Journal of Respiratory and Critical Care Medicine, 160 (2): pp. 648–654.

Wang, J., Betke, M., & Ko, J. P. (2006). Segmentation of pulmonary fissures on diagnostic CT. Medical Image Analysis , 10, 530.

Webb, R. W., Muller, N., & Naidich, D. P. (2000). High-resolution CT of the lung, third edition. Lippincott Williams & Wilkins.

Witten, I.H., & Frank, E., (2005). Data mining: practical machine learning tools and techniques, Morgan Kaufmann Series in Data Management Sys, Morgan Kaufmann, second ed., June.

Wong, J., & Zrimec, T. (2007). Efficient detection of diffuse lung disease. Medical Imaging 2007: Computer-Aided Diagnosis Maryellen L. Giger; Nico Karssemeijer, Editors, SPIE Vol: 6514, pp. 651425-651431

Zhang, L., & Reinhardt, J. M. (1999). Detection of lung lobar fissures using fuzzy logic. Society of Photographic Instrumentation Engineers-Medical Imaging , 3660, 188-198.

Zhang, L., Hoffman, E. A., & Reinhardt, J. M. (2003). Atlas-driven lung lobe segmentation in volumetric x-ray CT images. SPIE. 5031, p. 308.

Zrimec, T., & Busayarat, S. (2004). 3D modelling and visualization of the human lung. Proceedings of the 2nd International Symposium on 3D Data Processing: Visualization and Transmission, pp. 110-115.

Zrimec, T., & Wong, J. (2007). Methods for automatic honeycombing detection In Hrct images of the lung. Mediterranean Conference on Medical and Biological Engineering (pp. 830-833). Springer, pp. 830-833.

Zrimec, T., Busayarat, S., & Wilson, P. (2004). A 3D model of the human lung. Proceedings of the International Society and Conference Series on Medical Image Computing and Computer-Assisted Intervention Springer, pp. 1074–1075.

Zrimec, T., Busayarat, S., & Wilson, P. (2003). A knowledge based approach for automatic detection and measurement of bronchial dilatation and Wall Thickening on HRCT Images of the Lungs. World Congress on Medical Physics and Biomedical Engineering. Springer, Sydney.

4

Prediction Models for Malignant Pulmonary Nodules Based-on Texture Features of CT Image[1]

Guo Xiuhua, Sun Tao[1], Wang huan and Liang Zhigang[2]
[1]*School of Public Health and Family Medicine, Capital Medical University, Beijing, 100069*
[2]*Department of Radiology, Xuan Wu Hospital, Capital Medical University, Beijing 100050*
China

1. Introduction

Lung cancer is one of the most harmful forms of cancer, which is the leading cause of cancer death in many regions of the world (Ahmedin JI et al.,2005). The overall 5-year survival rate of lung cancer patients is only 14%, and remained at this level for the past two decades. However, when lung cancer is found at the early stage I or II, 5-year survival rates can be as high as 60-70% (Beadsmoore CJ et al.,2003). Early diagnosis of lung cancer was only 15%(Li YR et al., 2007). Although histology diagnosis is the most accurate detection method in the medical environment, it is an aggressive invasive procedure that involves risks, discomfort and trauma, which restrict it to be used in the clinical practice. Digital CT (Computed Tomography), overcoming the shortages of histology diagnosis, has gradually become the best imaging diagnosis method of lung cancer. CT enables us to visualize lung anatomy in great detail and has been used to accurately diagnose lung diseases since the 1980s (Ye X et al.,2006).Detecting and diagnosing solitary pulmonary nodules (SPNs, referring to the lesion of lung field ≤ 3 cm in diameter), the most common manifestation of lung cancer, are critical since early identification of malignant nodules is crucial to the chance for successful treatment. But pulmonary nodules of lung cancer in CT images share similarity with benign cases to some extent, such as tuberculosis, inflammatory pseudotumor, hamartoma, and aspergillosis(Jee WC et al.,2008), which makes it difficult to distinguish, especially for the doctors who are not rich in clinical experience. With technique of computer rising, the computer-aided diagnosis (CAD) has become an auxiliary diagnosis tool (Jiang J et al.,2007), especially in diseases that can not be diagnosed efficiently. To improve the accuracy and efficiency of CT screening programs for the detection of early-stage lung cancer, a number of

---

[1] Program of Funds: The program of Natural Science Fund of China (Serial Number: 30972550); the program of Natural Science Fund of Beijing (Serial Number: 7092010); the program of Academic Human Resources Development in Institutions of Higher Learning Under the Jurisdiction of Beijing Municipality (Serial Number: PHR201007112)

research projects, such as texture analysis(Liu YN et al.,2008) and image segmentation(Sun XJ et al.,2006), have been done to assist radiologists in diagnosing lung cancer.

2. Protocols of CT scan

In this study, the chest CT examinations were performed by using 64 detector-row helical CT (Cardiac-64, Siemens Medical systems, Germany) with the following parameters: 0.5s tube rotation and 1.5 pitch. A caudal-cranial direction scan was performed during an aspiratory breathhold and no contrast was used. Images were obtained from the level of the lung bases (posterior recesses) to the lung apex with the help of a scout view. Exposure settings were 150 mAs and 120 kVp. The fields-of-view were large enough to cover the complete lung cross-section. Each chest CT examination was reconstructed using two different settings immediately after imaging with the following three combinations of section thickness/increment and kernel: (A) 1.0mm/1.0 mm and a soft kernel (Siemens B30 filter), (B) 1.0 mm/1.0 mm and a sharp kernel (Siemens B60). The Siemens B30 kernel is the standard soft-tissue reconstruction kernel, and B60 is the bone reconstruction kernel, widely used in high resolution chest CT at normal. Images were displayed with a lung (level, −600 HU and width, 1500 HU) and mediastinal (level, 30 HU and width, 400 HU) window settings. Slice thickness and reconstruction intervals for routine scanning were 1-5mm.Data were reconstructed with a matrix of 512×512. Diameter range is 1.0-3.0 cm.

3. Methods of texture extraction

Nowadays, the methods of texture extraction can be classified into four parts: statistical method, model method, spectrum method and structural method. The basic procedure of texture analysis is to extract texture of images using different methods and then run a set of mathematical texture operators to produce a corresponding set of texture feature values in order to describe character of images.

Co-occurrence is one category of Statistical methods, which is a measure of the relative frequency or joint probability of two image properties occurring under predefined constraints, across the domain of an image. Gray level co-occurrence matrix (GLCM) is the most widely used texture analysis method in biological imaging (Ondimu SN et al.,2008). GLCM holds potential for analyzing segmented images of biogenic sedimentary structures because it can be used to analyze multi-scale differences in image texture (Honeycutt CE, et al.,2008)· ROIs (small pulmonary nodules) were segmented using gray level threshold algorithm(Chou YC et al.,2007). Fig. 1 shows an example CT scan and a segmented slice of small pulmonary nodule. Using this segmentation algorithm, the small pulmonary nodules images were generated.

Curvelet transform, a kind of spectrum method, stems from Wavelets theory, but it overcomes the weakness of traditional multiscale representations using wavelets, and is suitable to capture more directional features in an image.

The main formulas offering to Curvelet transform are as followed:

$$\phi_{j,l,k}(X) = \phi_j(R_{\theta_1}(X - X_k^{(j,l)})) \tag{1}$$

where R_θ is the rotation by θ radians and R_θ^{-1} its inverse

Variable	Description	Formula
Energy	1 if Energy>0.20 0 otherwise	$f_1 = \sum_i^M \sum_j^N P^2(i,j)$
Inertia	1 if Inertia≤0.45 0 otherwise	$f_2 = \sum_{i=0}^{K-1} \sum_{j=0}^{K-1} (i-j)^2 c_{ij}$
Inverse Difference Moment	1 if Inverse Difference Moment >0.87 0 otherwise	$f_3 = \sum_i^M \sum_j^N \frac{P(i,j)}{\lvert i-j \rvert^k}, i \neq j$
Entropy	1 if Entropy≤0.89 0 otherwise	$f_4 = -\sum_{i=0}^{l-1} \sum_{j=0}^{l-1} p(i,j) \log_2 p(i,j)$
Correlation	1 if Correlation>0.98 0 otherwise	$f_5 = \frac{\sum_{i=0}^{l-1} \sum_{j=0}^{l-1} ijp(i-j) - \mu_1 \mu_2}{\sigma_1{}^2 \sigma_2{}^3}$
Cluster Tendency	1 if Cluster Tendency≤11.65 0 otherwise	$f_6 = \sum_i^M \sum_j^N (i+j-2\mu)^k P(i,j)$
Contrast	1 if Contrast≤0.45 0 otherwise	$f_7 = \sum_i^M \sum_j^N (i-j)^2 P(i,j)$
Homogeneity	1 if Homogeneity>0.88 0 otherwise	$f_8 = \sum_i^M \sum_j^N (\frac{P(i,j)}{1+\lvert i-j \rvert})$
Variance	1 if Variance≤42.36 0 otherwise	$f_9 = \frac{1}{2} \sum_i^M \sum_j^N ((i-\mu)^2 P(i,j) + (j-\mu)^2 P(i,j))$
Maximum probability	1 if Maximum probability≤0.36 0 otherwise	$f_{10} = \underset{i,j}{\overset{M,N}{Max}} P(i,j)$
Sun-mean	1 if Sun-mean≤11.66 0 otherwise	$f_{11} = \frac{1}{2} \sum_i^M \sum_j^N (iP(i,j) + jP(i,j))$
Difference-mean	1 if Difference-mean≤0.33 0 otherwise	$f_{12} = \frac{1}{2} \sum_i^M \sum_j^N (iP(i,j) - jP(i,j))$
Sum-Entropy	1 if Sum Entropy≤2.43 0 otherwise	$f_{13} = -\sum_{k=0}^{2K-2} c_{x+y}(k) \log\{c_{x+y}(k)\}$
Difference-Entropy	1 if Difference Entropy≤0.45 0 otherwise	$f_{14} = -\sum_{k=0}^{K-1} c_{x-y}(k) \log\{c_{x-y}(k)\}$

Table 1. Descriptions and formulas of fourteen Image-level texture features as variables used in the analysis

$$R_\theta = \begin{pmatrix} \cos\theta & \sin\theta \\ -\sin\theta & \cos\theta \end{pmatrix},\ R_\theta^{-1} = R_\theta^T = R_{-\theta}$$

A curvelet coefficient is the inner product between an element
$f \in L^2(R^2)$ and a Curvelet $\phi_{j,l,k}$

$$c(j,l,k)" := \int_{R^2} f(X)\overline{\phi_{j,l,k}(X)}dx \tag{2}$$

where R denotes the real line. Curvelet transform obeys an anisotropy scaling relation, length ≈ $2^{-j/2}$, width = 2^{-j}, so, width≈length^2. This equation called a curve scaling law.
Based on Curvelet transform, we extracted fourteen texture features of pulmonary nodules of CT images, including Entropy, Mean ,Correlation, Energy, Homogeneity, StdDev, MP, IDM, ClustTend, Inertia, SumMean, DiffMean, SumEntr, and DiffEntr. The meanings of some texture features are as follows.
Energy is defined to measure the number of repeated pairs, which is expected to be high if the occurrence of repeated pixel pairs is high. In statistical mechanics, entropy is defined as a factor or quantity that is a function of the physical state of a mechanical system and is equal to the logarithm of the probability of the occurrence of the particular molecular arrangement in that state. Inverse Difference Moment tells us about the smoothness of the image, like homogeneity. The IDM is expected to be high if the gray levels of the pixel pairs are similar. Inertia reflects the roughness of texture, which is expected to be low if the more elements are near to diagonal line of matrix when texture is rougher. Correlation is expected to measure the relevance of the gray of pixel. Sun–mean (mean) and Difference-mean provide the mean of the gray levels of the image. The sum–mean is expected to be large if the sum of the gray levels of the image is high. Standard deviation tells us how to spread out the distribution of gray levels . The variance is expected to be large if the gray levels of the image are spread out greatly. Results in the pixel pair is most predominant in the image. The Maximum probability (MP) is expected to be high if the occurrence of the most predominant pixel pair is high. The mean of the gray reflects the central tendency of the gray. Cluster tendency measures the grouping of pixels that have similar gray level values. Homogeneity measures the local homogeneity of a pixel pair. The homogeneity is expected to be large if the gray levels of each pixel are similar.
Curvelet transform is a new image representation approach that codes image edges more efficiently than wavelet transform. Curvelet will be better than wavelet in following cases (Candes EJ et al.,2006) :

1. Optimally sparse representation of objects with edges.
2. Optimal image reconstruction in severely ill-posed problems.
3. Optimal sparse representation of wave propagators.

Some studies have been done using Curvelet transform in image processing. Dettori and Semler(Lucia D et al.,2007)presented a comparative study between Wavelet, Ridgelet and Curvelet transform on some computed tomography (CT) scans. The comparative study indicated that Curvelet yields better results than Wavelet or Ridgelet.

4. Prediction models

Using texture feature values, we can establish model to predict the characteristics of pulmonary nodules. The methods of establishing prediction model are variable, such as logistic regression, discriminant analysis, artificial neural networks, and support machine vector. Because the same patient has many CT images, that is, there is correlation among CT images of one patient. Common mathematical methods, such as logistic regression, discriminant analysis, are not appropriate to predict the characteristics of pulmonary nodules.

Multilevel modeling techniques are appropriate when there is correlation among clusters of subjects. It is the presence of within-cluster correlation that justifies the use of a multilevel (hierarchical) model, and correlation multilevel modeling without within-cluster does not provide benefit (Kim DG et al.,2007). Now we take establishing prediction model of CT images for example. The authors identified there is correlation among CT images of one patient, so multilevel models were fitted to a two-level hierarchy and used to identify factors affecting texture features of benign and malignant CT images for individual casualties. By establishing a multi-level model of texture features of pulmonary nodules, the characteristics of pulmonary nodules in the CT images could be better described , which profit early identification of small pulmonary nodules.

We make small pulmonary nodules CT images as level 1 and SPN patients as level 2. With two-level structure data, three different equations can be formulated: individual-level model(image—level model, level 1 model), organization-level model(patient-level model, level 2 model), and combined model. Assuming normally distributed errors, for subject ij we have level 1 model, level 2 model and combined model (Wolfinger R et al.,1993), as

$$Y_{ij} \sim N(\hat{Y}_{ij}, \sigma^2{}_{ij});\; r_{ij} \sim N(0,\sigma^2);\; \hat{Y}_{ij} = \hat{\beta}_{0j} + \hat{\beta}_{1j}X_{ij};$$

$$Y_{ij} = \beta_{0j} + \beta_{1j}X_{ij} + r_{ij} \quad \text{(level 1 model)} \tag{3}$$

$$\beta_{oj} = \gamma_{00} + \gamma_{01}W_j + \mu_{0j} \quad \text{(level 2 model)} \tag{4}$$

$$\text{and } \beta_{1j} = \gamma_{10} \quad \text{(level 2 model)} \tag{5}$$

Substituting Eqs.(4)and(5) into Eq.(3) yields the combined model:

$$Y_{ij} = \gamma_{00} + \gamma_{01}W_j + \gamma_{10}X_{ij} + \mu_{oj} + r_{ij} \quad \text{(combined model)} \tag{6}$$

If the observed outcomes Y_{ij} are binary, a binomial logistic model is appropriate. A multilevel binomial logistic model for outcome probabilities of benign and malignant pulmonary nodules on CT image data used in this study is formulated as follows:

$$\log\left(\frac{p_{ij}}{1-p_{ij}}\right) = \gamma_{00} + \sum_{q=1}^{Q}\gamma_{0q}W_{qj} + \sum_{p=1}^{P}\gamma_{p0}X_{pij} + u_{0j} \tag{7}$$

Where P is the probability that malignant pulmonary nodules on CT image will occur (Y_{ij} =1), γ_{00} the intercept, W_{qj} a vector of patient-level characteristics, X_{pij} a vector of image-level characteristics, and the regression coefficients associated with the patient-level characteristics and the image-level characteristics, respectively, and u_{0j} is the random effect at level 2,where $u_{0j} \sim N(0,\sigma_u{}^2)$.

SVM is a popular classifier based on structural risk minimization principle (Vapnik VN.,1998), which could minimize the generalization error of the classifier. Recently, SVM has gained much attention as a useful tool for image recognition. Youngjoo Lee(Youngjoo L et al.,2009) investigated the performance of Bayesian classifier, ANN (artificial neural net) and SVM (support vector machine) for differentiating obstructive lung diseases using texture analysis. Results showed that SVM showed the best performance for classification. The same result had been got by Michael E. Mavroforakis(Michael EM et al.,2006) .

Compared with other classifiers, such as Artificial Neural Networks, SVM aims to find the hyperplane that maximizes the distance from the hyperplane to the nearest examples in each class. An attractive feature of SVM is that it can map linearly inseparable data into higher dimensional space so that SVM can make them to be linearly separable. There are two types of SVM, linear and non-linear. The training data of linear SVM may be analyzed as either linearly separable or linearly non-separable. Given a set of training vectors (l in total) belonging to separate classes (x_1,y_1), (x_2,y_2), (x_3,y_3), … ,(x_1,y_1) , where $x_j \in R^n$ denotes the ith input vector and $y_j \in \{+1,-1\}$ is the corresponding desired output. The maximal margin classifier aims to find a hyperplane w: wx+b=0 to separate the training data. In the possible hyperplanes, only one maximizes the margin (distance between the hyperplane) and the nearest data point of each class. The support vectors denote the points lying on the margin border (Huang YL,2005). The solution to the classification is given by the decision function

$$f(x) = sign\left(\sum_{j=1}^{N_{sv}} \alpha_j y_j (s_j, x) + b\right) \tag{8}$$

where α_j is the positive Lagrange multiplier, s_j is the support vectors (N_{sv} in total), and $k(s_j,x)$is the function for convolution of the kernel of the decision function. Such kernels must hold Mercer´s condition(V V,1982) which tells us whether or not a perspective kernel is a dot product in some space. The polynomial, radial, anova kernels are now often seen choices in SVM-based CAD applications.

5. Examples

In the rest of the paper, we will provide two practical examples to explain the use of prediction model for small pulmonary nodules, which based on texture extraction to predict the characteristics of pulmonary nodules.

5.1.Example1: Multilevel binomial logistic prediction model for malignant pulmonary nodules based on texture features of CT image.

The digitized CT image set used in this study contains 2171 ROIs (Region of Interests) extracted from 185 patients with small solitary pulmonary nodules, with 61 benign nodules and 124 malignant tumors. There were 107 men and 78 women (range of age, 19-80 years; mean ages, 58 years). The final diagnosis of 124 small peripheral lung cancers (diameter range, 1.0-3.0 cm; mean diameter, 2.0cm) was determined by either operation or biopsy. All the images were provided by the radiology department of Beijing Friendship Hospital affiliated to Capital University of Medical Science.

The structure of data from 185 patients is postulated as hierarchical data, which consists of two different levels: level-1 consisting of image-level characteristics and level-2 consisting of patient-level characteristics. Image-level characteristics contain detailed information associated with individual images such as Energy, Contrast, and Inverse Difference Moment and the patient-level characteristics include sex and age. Fourteen image-level and two patient-level variables are used as independent variables in the analysis, and the benign and malignant pulmonary nodules as the dependent variables, 1 malignant, and 0 benign. Sex and age are patient-level variables (1 man, 0 woman ; 1 age >50.00 0 others). The descriptions of the fourteen image-level variables used in the study are provided in Table 1. Besides, Table 1 gives formulas of fourteen GLCM textural features in the study (Dettori L et al.,2007; Yogesan1 K et al.,1996; Guo XH et al.,2008).

In this example, we used gray level co-occurrence matrix to get fourteen textural features and establishd multilevel binomial logistic prediction model (Wang H et al.,2010). combining patient and image characteristics of textural features Results showd that Five texture features, including Inertia, Entropy, Correlation, Difference-mean, Sum-Entropy, and age of patients own aggregating character on patient-level, were statistically different (P<0.05) between benign and malignant small solitary pulmonary nodules.

For multilevel binomial logistic models, the variance at the lowest level is completely determined by the population proportion (Kim DG et al.,2007). SAS software (version 9.1, SAS Institute (Shanghai) Co., Ltd.) was used to perform the estimation of multilevel binomial logistic models.

For obtaining estimates of between- and within-organization (or cluster) variance, null models were estimated (Table 2). The intra-class correlation coefficient (ICC) is 0.1795 for CT images, indicating that 17.95% of the total variation in images exists between patients, and therefore may be explained using patients-level predictors. As a result, the patients-level predictors are useful for estimating statistical models for texture features of CT images. In other words, multilevel models for texture features of CT images are necessary. It should be noted that roughly 18% of the total variation in texture features of CT images is attributable to the variability between patients, which suggesting that texture features of CT images are significantly influenced by patient's characteristics.

	external segmentation
Fixed effect	
Intercept	0.6766 (0.0100)
Random effect	
Images-level	0.03928(0.0066)
Patients-level	0.1795 (0.0000)
ICC	0.1795
-2 Log Likelihood	2861.9

Note. For parameter estimates, standard errors appear in parentheses.

Table 2. The estimation results of null models

Based on the results of null model estimation, one binomial logistic regression model and multilevel binomial logistic regression model can be used to estimate the texture features of CT images.

Table 3 presents the estimation results of CT images model, in which image and patient features are included as predictors. For logistic regression models, the odds ratio is used to interpret the actual effects of estimated coefficients. Odds ratios are also provided in Table 3. The results show that malignant pulmonary nodules in CT image are more likely to occur while Inertia is lower than 0.4435 (odds=1.494–1), Difference-mean is lower than 0.3315 (odds=1.332–1) or Inverse Difference Moment is higher than 0.8662 (odds=1.156–1) compared to benign pulmonary nodules. The results also show that malignant pulmonary nodules in CT image are less likely to occur while Entropy is lower than 0.8939 (odds =0.757–1), Sum- Entropy is lower than 2.4314 (odds =0.877–1) or Correlation is higher than 0.9754 (odds = 0.779–1) compared to benign pulmonary nodules. Malignant pulmonary nodules in CT image belongs to young patients (≤50) are less likely (odds= 0.503–1) than old patients (>50). These findings are consistent with warrants for old patients of the effects of small solitary pulmonary nodules. That means old patients are 49.7% ((1-0.503) ×100) more likely to get earlier period lung cancer than young patients. The sensitivity of multilevel binomial logistic prediction model was 90.6% for another 50 patients with small solitary pulmonary nodules, which had a good effect on prediction of small pulmonary nodules. The result of prediction would be improved with the enhancement of doctors' clinical experience.

5.2 Example 2: Support vector machine prediction model for small pulmonary nodules based on Curvelet transform to extract texture features of CT image

In this example, we explore the use of Curvelet transform to extract texture features of pulmonary nodules in CT image and support vector machine to establish prediction model of small solitary pulmonary nodules in order to promote the ratio of detection and diagnosis of early-stage lung cancer. Results show that the classification consistency, sensitivity and specificity for the model are 81.5%, 93.8% and 38.0% respectively.

2461 CT images used in this study are extracted from 129 patients with small solitary pulmonary nodules, including 537 CT images (25 benign cases) related to benign nodule and 1924 CT images (104 malignant cases) to malignant tumors. The final diagnosis of malignant cases was determined by either operation or biopsy. The diagnosis of benign cases was confirmed by operation, CT diagnosis or follow-up. The original format is DICOM, and diameters of the chest nodules were from 0.3 cm to 3 cm. 129 cases were provided by four hospitals, and details are as follows: Beijing Xuanwu Hospital of Capital Medical University (26 malignant cases, 11 benign cases), Beijing Friendship Hospital affiliated to Capital Medical University (35 malignant cases,6 benign cases), Chaoyang Hospital affiliated to Capital Medical University (20 malignant cases,7 benign cases) and Fuxing Hospital affiliated to Capital Medical University (23 malignant cases,1 benign cases). Based on Curvelet transform, we extracted fourteen texture features of pulmonary nodules of CT images. Every image could be decomposed into 18 sub-images. The 18 sub-images could be classified into three parts: inner layer, middle layer and outer layer. So 252 texture features were extracted from every image. Among those texture features, 158 texture features showed statistically significant differences between benign and malignant cases

	Estimate	Odds ratio	95% Confidence Limits
Fixed effects			
Intercept (γ_{00})	-0.0638 (0.1204)	0.9382	(-0.2997 0.1721)
Image-level			
Energy (γ_{10})	0.0776 (0.0683)	1.0807	(-0.0562 0.2114)
Inertia (γ_{20})	0.4014*** (0.1316)	1.4940	(0.1434 0.6594)
Inverse Difference Moment (γ_{30})	0.1450* (0.0813)	1.1560	(-0.0143 0.3043)
Entropy (γ_{40})	-0.2779*** (0.0603)	0.7574	(-0.3960 -0.1597)
Correlation (γ_{50})	-0.2493 *** (0.0956)	0.7793	(-0.4366 -0.0620)
Cluster Tendency (γ_{60})	0.0174 (0.0631)	1.0176	(-0.1062 0.1410)
Contrast (γ_{70})	-0.0461 (0.0743)	0.9549	(-0.1919 0.0996)
Homogeneity (γ_{80})	0.0904 (0.1425)	1.0946	(-0.1889 0.3696)
Variance (γ_{90})	0.0971 (0.0676)	1.1020	(-0.0353 0.2296)
Maximum probability (γ_{100})	0.1098 (0.0686)	1.1161	(-0.0247 0.2443)
Sun-mean (γ_{110})	0.0174 (0.0631)	1.0176	(-0.1062 0.1410)
Difference-mean (γ_{120})	0.2863** (0.1386)	1.3315	(0.0146 0.5580)
Sum-Entropy (γ_{130})	-0.1311** (0.0648)	0.8771	(-0.2581 -0.0041)
Difference-Entropy (γ_{140})	-0.1755 (0.1595)	0.8390	(-0.4881 0.1370)
Patient-level			
sex(γ_{01})	0.0781 (0.0581)	1.0812	(-0.0359 0.1920)
age(γ_{02})	-0.6871*** (0.0611)	0.5030	(-0.8069 -0.5674)
Random effects			
τ_{00} (μ_{0j})	0.4583*** (0.0280)		

Note. For parameter estimates, standard errors are within parentheses. *P< 0.10; **P< 0.05; ***P< 0.01

Table 3. Estimation results for CT images

through two independent samples tests of nonparametric test or two independent samples t-test

The 2461 images were divided into two parts: one part was as a training sample (80%) and the other part was as a test sample (20%). The training sample was used to establish the database and the test sample was used to evaluate the validity of prediction model of SVM (Table 4).

Samples	Benign	Malignant	Total
Training sample	429	1539	1968
Test sample	108	385	493
Total	537	1924	2461

Table 4. Benign and Malignant Cases Distribution

Based on Curvelet transform, 252 texture features we extracted were as parameters to establish prediction model for small pulmonary nodules (Table 5).

SVM	Pathological Diagnosis		Total
	Benign	Malignant	
Benign	41	24	65
Malignant	67	361	428
Total	108	385	493

Table 5. Prediction Results of Pulmonary Nodules Based On SVM

The validity of prediction model of SVM is evaluated by the following three indexes: sensitivity (93.8%), specificity (38.0%) and consistency (81.5%). The high sensitivity (93.8%) can reduce the false negative rate of early-stage lung cancer effectively.

There are other methods used in published papers to select texture features. Wavelet transform was used to extract the texture features of chest radiography, and the Energy was as the only parameter to establish the prediction model (Huang PW. et al.,2004). Lucia Dettori(Lucia D et al.,2007) selected Mean, StaDev, Energy and Entropy to establish the prediction model. Principal component analysis, a very useful tool to deal with colinearity, has various applications in texture extraction and tumor recognition(Zhang J et al.,2008). Mohamed Meselhy Eltoukhy(Mohamed ME et al.,2010) used Curvelet transform to decompose mammogram images into 4 levels, then selected the largest 100 texture features as parameters.

In order to select texture features which are more accurate to reflect characteristics of pulmonary nodules, we have made many attempts. Results were showed in table 6.

In order to promote sensitivity and specificity, we had made some attempts to select proper texture features. Compared with other methods, 252 texture features were used as parameters to establish prediction model is more satisfying.

Based on published reports, characteristics of pulmonary nodules can been detected by texture features. However, 2D images are irregular when decomposed, and the Curvelet transform is more suitable than the wavelet transform to extract texture features. The methods to establish prediction model are variable, such as multiple linear regression, logistic regression, discriminant analysis, artificial neural networks, but the result of support vector machine is better (Zheng Z et al.,2007).In this research, we establish support vector machine prediction model for small pulmonary nodules using Curvelet transform to extract texture features of CT image, which has not been reported to our knowledge.

	Sensitivity(%)	Specificity(%)	Consistency(%)
Using Energy As The Only Parameter	93.2	29.6	79.3
Using Texture Features of Inner Layer As Parameters	96.4	31.5	82.2
Using Texture Features of Middle Layer As Parameters	94.8	25.0	79.5
Using Texture Features of Outer Layer As Parameters	100.0	0.0	78.1
Using Mean, StaDev, Energy and Entropy As Parameters	94.8	29.6	80.5
Using Principal Component Analysis	100.0	0.0	78.1
Using 158 Texture Features As Parameters	94.5	34.3	81.3
The Largest 100 Texture Features As Parameters	93.8	28.7	79.5

Table 6. Prediction Results of Pulmonary Nodules Using Other Methods

6. Summary

In recent years, the incidence of lung cancer has been the top of cancers in the most countries. Because of the difficulty to diagnosis, more attention has been paid to lung cancer.

Now the most accurate diagnosis method of lung cancer is histology diagnosis, but this method is traumatic, which restricts it to be used in clinical practice. In the decades, digital CT has been the main diagnosis tool of lung cancer for its convenience and safety, and widely used in clinical practice. However, it is difficult to distinguish between benign and malignant cases in the CT images of pulmonary nodules, especially for the doctors who were lack of experience. From two examples, we can make the conclusion that the prediction model is so sensitive that it can diagnose early-stage lung cancer effectively, reduces the difficulty of distinguishing characteristics of pulmonary nodules and improves accuracy rate of diagnosing early-stage lung cancer.

7. References

Ahmedin JI, DVM, PhD, Taylor M, Elizabeth W, PhD, Alicia S, MPH, Ram CT, PhD, Asma G, MPH, Eric JF, PhD, MJT, MD, MS. (2005). Cancer statistics 2005, A Cancer Journal for Clinicians Vol.55(No.1):10-30.

Beadsmoore CJ, Screaton NJ. (2003). Classification, staging and prognosis of lung cancer, European Journal of Radiology Vol.45(No.1):8-17.

Chou YC, Teng MM, Guo WY, Hsieh JC, Wu YT. (2007). Classification of hemodynamics from dynamic susceptibility contrast magnetic resonance (DSC-MR) brain images using noiseless independent factor analysis, Medical Image Analysis Vol.11(No.3): 242–253.

Dettori L, Semler L. (2007). A comparison of wavelet, ridgelet, and curvelet-based texture classification algorithms in computed tomography, Computers in Biology and Medicine Vol.37(No.4): 486—498.

Guo XH, Zhang Y, Wang H, Li KC, Yao XY, Liang ZG.(2008). Exploring the Risk Factors of Lung Pulmonary Nodules with Cancer Using Sandwich Logistic Regression Analysis, Journal of Mathematical Medicine Vol.22(No.1): 66-68.

Honeycutt CE, Plotnick R. (2008) Image analysis techniques and gray level co-occurrence matrices (GLCM) for calculating bioturbation indices and characterizing biogenic sedimentary structures, Computers & Geosciences.

Huang PW., Dai SK. (2004). Design of a two-stage content-based image retrieval system using texture similarity, Information Processing & Management Vol.40 (No.1): 81–96.

Jee WC, Chin AY, Dae-Soon S, Naeyun C, Jinseon L, Hong KK, Yong SC, Kyung SL, Jhingook K.(2008). Prediction of lymph node metastasis using the combined criteria of helical CT and mRNA expression profiling for non-small cell lung cancer, Lung Cancer.

Jiang J, Yao B, Wason AM. (2007). A genetic algorithm design for micro calcification detection and classification in digital mammograms, Computerized Medical Imaging and Graphics Vol.31(No.1):49–61.

Kim DG, Lee Y, Simon W, Keechoo C. (2007). Modeling crash outcome probabilities at rural intersections: Application of hierarchical binomial logistic models. Accident Analysis and Prevention Vol.39(No.1):125-134

Li YR, Yang XF. (2007) The Progress on Clinical Early Diagnostic Methods of Lung Cancer, Journal of Clinical Pulmonary Medicine Vol.12(No.2):130-132.

Liu YN, Wang H, Guo XH, Liang ZG, He Q. (2008). Application of artificial neural networks in prediction model of early-stage lung cancer, Chinese journal of Medical Statistics Vol.1(No.1): 30–33.

Lucia D, Lindsay S. (2007). A comparison of wavelet, ridgelet, and curvelet-based texture classification algorithms in computed tomography, Computers in Biology and Medicine. 486-498.

Michael EM, Harris VG, Nikos D, Dionisis C, Sergios T. (2006). Mammographic masses characterization based on localized texture and dataset fractal analysis using linear, neural and support vector machine classifiers, Artificial Intelligence in Medicine. 145-162.

Mohamed ME, Ibrahima F, Brahim BS. (2010). A comparison of wavelet and curvelet for breast cancer diagnosis in digital mammogram, Computers in Biology and Medicine. 384–391.

Ondimu SN, Murase H. (2008). Effect of probability-distance based Markovian texture extraction on discrimination in biological imaging, Computers and Electronics in Agriculture Vol.63(No.1): 2-12.

Sun XJ, Zhang HB, Duan HC. (2006). 3D computerized segmentation of lung volume with computed tomography, Academic Radiology Vol.13(No.6):670–677.

Vapnik VN. (1998). Statistical learning theory. New York: Wiley.

V V. (1982). Estimation of Dependencies based on Empirical Data, Springer Verlag, New York.

Wang H, Guo XH, Jia ZW, Li HK, Liang ZG, Li KC, He Q. (2010). Multilevel binomial logistic prediction model for malignant pulmonary nodules based on texture features of CT image. European Journal of Radiology Vol.74(No.1): 124-129.

Wolfinger R, O'connell M. (1993). Generalized linear mixed models: a pseudolikelihood approach, Journal of Statistical Computation and Simulation Vol.488(No.3&4):233–243.

Ye X, Edwin J.R, Yu H, Guo JF, Geoffrey M, Eric AH. (2006). Computer-aided Classification of Interstitial Lung Diseases Via MDCT: 3D Adaptive Multiple Feature Method (3D AMFM), Academic Radiology Vol.13(No.8):969-978.

Yogesanl K, Jørgensen T, Albregtsen F, Tveter KJ, Danielsen HE. (1996). Entropy-Based Texture Analysis of Chromatin Structure in Advanced Prostate Cancer, Cytometry Vol.24(No.3):268-276.

Youngjoo L, Joon BS, June GL, Song SK, Namkug K, Suk HK. (2009). Performance testing of several classifiers for differentiating obstructive lung diseases based on texture analysis at high-resolution computerized tomography (HRCT), Computer Methods And Programs In Biomedicine. 206-215.

Huang YL, Chen DR. (2005). Support vector machines in sonography Application to decision making in the diagnosis of breast cancer, Journal of Clinical Imaging.179–184

Zhang J, Tong LZ, Lei W, Ning L. (2008). Texture analysis of multiple sclerosis: a comparative study, Magnetic Resonance Imaging. 1160–1166.

Zheng Z, Zhang YX, HU YX. (2007). Investigation of eye gaze based on independent component analysis and support vector machine[J], Journal of Optoelectronics.Laser Vol.18(No.7): 491-494.

Part 2

CT Image Analysis for Preoperational Planning

Liver Segmentation and Volume Estimation from Preoperative CT Images in Hepatic Surgical Planning: Application of a Semiautomatic Method Based on 3D Level Sets

Laura Fernandez-de-Manuel[1,5], Maria J. Ledesma-Carbayo[1,5], Daniel Jimenez-Carretero[1,5], Javier Pascau[2], Jose L. Rubio-Guivernau[1,5], Jose M. Tellado[3], Enrique Ramon[4], Manuel Desco[2] and Andres Santos[1,5]

[1]*Biomedical Image Technologies Lab, Universidad Politécnica de Madrid*
[2]*Medicina y Cirugía Experimental, Hospital General Universitario Gregorio Marañón*
[3] *Servicio de Cirugía General I, Hospital General Universitario Gregorio Marañón*
[4] *Servicio de Radiodiagnóstico, Hospital General Universitario Gregorio Marañón, Madrid*
[5]*Biomedical Research Center in Bioengineering, Biomaterials, and Nanomedicine (CIBER-BBN), Madrid*
Spain

1. Introduction

The advances in the understanding of the liver anatomy and physiology (Couinaud, 1999; Ryu & Cho, 2009), the improvement of medical imaging techniques (Radtke et al., 2007; Handels & Ehrhardt, 2009) and the progressive security of surgical instrumentation, allow surgeons to design complex liver resections more accurately and efficacious without jeopardizing patient safety. Pre-operative planning has become an essential task before undertake liver surgery, and requires mandatory mapping of both inflow and outflow hepatic vasculature, the assessment of the number and spatial relationships of the tumor(s), and frequently, an estimation of the future remnant liver volume (FRLV). Several determinants may modify threshold levels for a safe FRLV (for example, the presence and extension of cirrhosis, esteatosis or post-chemotherapy sinusoidal obstructive syndrome). Therefore, healthy functional liver volume estimation and functional performance analysis are tests further needed to make the final clinical decision before extensive hepatectomies.

Traditionally, FRLV has been extrapolated from preoperative computed tomography (CT) images using hepatic segmentation done manually in an otherwise time and labour-consuming process. Briefly, some commercial systems include tools that allow radiologists to manually segment 2D slices of a CT study in transverse (axial) views. Due to the high number of slices (usually ranging from 100 to 500 depending on the scanner), a sub-sampled version of the original CT is used in daily planning. However, even when using a sub-sampled version, the complete procedure takes longer than 30 minutes.

Many research groups work nowadays in the development of automatic and semiautomatic liver segmentation tools in order to help clinicians saving time and effort and increasing precision. Since the liver is located adjacent to other organs of similar CT gray values, and it presents a huge variability in size and shape among different patients, the development of segmentation tools has become a challenging problem with increasing interest in the last few years.

In this work we first present a summary of the state of the art in this field. Secondly, we propose the application of a semiautomatic tool to segment the healthy part of the liver and estimate the healthy liver volume from CT preoperative abdominal images, using techniques based on a sophisticated 3D Level Sets definition (Fernandez-de-Manuel et al., 2009) that combines intensity, gradient information and curvature restrictions extended with a morphological image pre-processing and a method to easily define 3D frontiers with adjacent regions. The algorithm has been developed to solve a specific request demanded by radiologists from the research team. The requirement in our work is that the segmentation should include only healthy parenchyma excluding tumors in order not to overestimate healthy liver volumes.

The proposed tool has been validated with several preoperative CT abdominal data sets. Resulting segmentations have been evaluated with respect to those obtained from radiologists' manual segmentations and supervised by clinicians.

2. State of the art

As it has been briefly introduced, the development of automatic and semiautomatic liver segmentation tools is particularly challenging due to liver's variability in size and shape and to the proximity to other organs of similar intensity values which generates blurred edges in CT images. Many works have been published in this field.

First attempts to perform automatic liver segmentation were based on gray-level statistics (Woodhouse et al., 1994; Gao et al., 1996). Liver gray levels can be estimated either by statistical analysis of manually segmented slices, either by histogram analysis with the aim of establishing an a priori knowledge about liver density. In most of the works based on gray-level statistics, a threshold is used to generate a binary volume that is later processed by morphological operators in order to separate desired organs. Recent gray-level methods have been presented by Soler et al. (Soler et al., 2001), Fujimoto et al. (Fujimoto et al., 2002), Liu et al. (Liu et al., 2005) and Lim et al. (Lim et al., 2004; Lim et al., 2005; Lim et al., 2006). However, the high variability among liver CT images due to the differences of intensity values in different kind of tumors and the different settings regarding contrast media, make difficult the optimal operation of the methods just based on gray-level statistics. Other approaches try to overcome the problem of liver's gray-level estimation by learning gray-level features corresponding to the liver from different CT images with methods based on neural networks. Tsai and Tanahashi (Tsai & Tanahashi, 1994) , Koss et al. (Koss et al., 1999) and Lee et al. (Lee & Chung, 2000; Lee et al., 2003) presented examples of automatic detection and labeling of abdominal organs with neural networks. A common difficulty of this kind of methods is that they usually need a big and highly varied training set to learn the variability among different patients.

Liver segmentation based on anatomical knowledge regarding size, position and shape of each abdominal organ includes several works that employ statistical shape models (SSM) and shape constrained deformable models. Montagnat and Delingette (Montagnat &

Delingette, 1997), Gao et al. (Gao et al., 1998) and Lamecker et al. (Lamecker et al., 2004) presented several of these techniques. The drawback of these methods is the model construction, which requires a huge quantity of training data properly collected in order to capture all the possible shapes; a really challenging task regarding the high amount of variable and complex liver shapes and sizes. Besides, these algorithms use to fail when processing not standard liver shapes and require too much computation time to achieve a good matching between model and image. Other works are based on the construction of probabilistic atlases. That is the case of the works presented in (Park et al., 2003; Zhou et al., 2005; Shimizu et al., 2006). First, a registration step of training CT images into a standard space defined by landmarks (manually or automatically chosen) is needed. The probabilistic atlas is generated by spatially averaging the registered surfaces. Then, it is used to compute the probability of belonging to a certain organ for each voxel in the image. Finally, the region that maximizes the posterior probability of being the desired organ is extracted by thresholding or using an iterative algorithm. This type of techniques carries several problems. Firstly, the huge amount of training images required. Secondly, the difficulty of finding an appropriate probability function. Finally, the high computation times required.

Some variants of region growing have been also applied to liver segmentation (Pohle & Toennies, 2001; Ruskó et al., 2007). However, for those cases, sophisticated restriction methods have to be taken into account in order to avoid over-flooding.

Live wire algorithms (Barrett & Mortensen, 1997) are the basis of several semiautomatic liver volume extraction tools currently used in clinical practice. An image is described as an undirected and weighted graph where pixels are represented by the vertexes, the edges connect neighboring pixels, and their weighs represent the cost of the connections computed from image features like gray value, gradient magnitude, gradient direction or Laplacian zero-crossing among others. Dijkstra's graph-search algorithm computes all possible minimum-cost paths between a starting seed point established by the user on the liver boundary and all the possible points in the image. After that, a desired boundary can be interactively chosen by selecting a free point with the mouse. Indeed, when the mouse pointer moves over the image, the previous boundary segment is deleted and the new minimal path between the seed point and the new position is displayed. When that minimal path is close to the desired boundary, the user can freeze it by adding a new seed point. It causes the reinitialization of the boundary detection. Thus, this process allows the user to have a full control over the segmentation. Many variants of this technique have been developed for years. In (Schenk et al., 2000; Schenk et al., 2001) the authors modified the original algorithm to reduce its computation time in order to extend it to 3D images. These methods speed up the work of radiologists manually drawing liver boundaries, but are highly dependent on the operator's skill.

Different approaches widely used in liver segmentation are Level Sets and snakes (Caselles et al., 1997; Pan & Dawant, 2001; Bekes et al., 2007; Garamendi et al., 2007; Lee et al., 2007; Platero et al., 2008), based on a speed function that controls the front propagation of an implicitly defined surface toward the liver boundary. Moreover, the propagation may be constrained by an a priori anatomic information or shape restrictions. The main problem of Level Sets is the definition of an appropriate speed function and its parameters.

Finding an efficient liver segmentation algorithm able to provide good segmentation results from CT liver images and avoiding the classical problems of standard segmentation methods (such as over-flooding, under or over-segmentation, long computing times and so on) is such a challenging and important task that a recent competition has faced this purpose. In October 2007, a contest whose aim was to compare different algorithms to segment the liver from clinical 3D CT scans was hold as part of the workshop *3D Segmentation in the Clinic: A Grand Challenge* in conjunction with MICCAI 2007 (Van Ginneken et al., 2007; Heimann et al., 2009). Teams that participated in the liver segmentation contest downloaded training and test data and submitted the results of their algorithms on test data both before and during the workshop. To evaluate the quality of a given segmentation, segmentations were compared to expert-generated references and rated according to detected deviations: Volumetric Overlap Error, Relative Volume Difference, Average Symmetric Surface Distance, Root Mean Square Symmetric Surface Distance and Maximum Symmetric Surface Distance. Some of the most successful proposals that got better punctuation were automatic methods based on statistical shape models with some additional free deformation (Heimann et al., 2007; Kainmueller et al., 2007; Saddi et al., 2007) and interactive segmentation methods requiring certain amount of user interaction such as manual refinement after a graph cut or a region growing method (Beck & Aurich, 2007; Beichel et al., 2007), two dimensional Level Sets with initialization (Dawant et al., 2007; Lee et al., 2007) and three dimensional Level Sets with initialization of 2D contours (Wimmer et al., 2007). However, in that workshop, the segmentation was defined as the entire liver tissue including all internal structures like big vessels systems, tumors, etc. Therefore, that segmentation definition does not exactly match the actual goal of our work (that is estimating healthy liver volumes).

Recently, most of new liver segmentation methods combine different techniques: statistical shape models, mathematical morphology and Level Set approaches. (Linguraru et al., 2010) present a clinical tool developed to segment liver and spleen based on probabilistic atlases. The atlases are created using manually segmented data from non contrast CT images. The organ locations are modeled in the physical space and normalized to the position of the xiphoid. The construction of the atlases enables the automated quantifications of liver and spleen volumes and heights, later improved by a geodesic active contour. In (Suzuki et al., 2010) a computerized liver extraction scheme based on geodesic active contour segmentation combined with level-set contour evolution and applied to liver donor images is presented. In (Jiang & Cheng, 2009) a threshold segmentation is combined with morphological image processing and active contour models in order to extract the initial contour and segment the liver slice by slice. In (Campadelli et al., 2010) a fully automatic, gray-level based segmentation framework based on a multiplanar fast marching method is proposed. Other sophisticated methods are based on Support Vector Machines (Luo et al., 2009).

3. Proposed method

In this work we propose the application of a tool based on Level Sets to segment the healthy part of the liver in CT preoperative abdominal images. The tool has been developed following the requirements demanded by radiologists inside the team: segmentation of healthy parenchyma excluding tumors in order not to overestimate healthy liver volumes. In this sense the proposed function allows to directly segment healthy parenchyma.

The tool combines a 3D active contour algorithm previously introduced in (Fernandez-de-Manuel et al., 2009) with morphological filtering and a fast manual frontier definition, in order to estimate healthy liver volumes. SSM models have been discarded due to the aim of segmenting a wide variety of shapes, sizes and liver pathologies with different kind of tumors and surgical stages. For this reason, a solution based on active contours with no "a prioris" has been approached. The proposed technique only requires the user to initialize a seed and different frontier points in the most common problematic regions before the automatic computation stage. In case that the first segmentation was not satisfactory, the user could redefine or add some other frontiers and repeat the automatic stage. Normally, the initial seed or frontiers do not need to be changed. Nevertheless, in clinical environment it is useful to give the opportunity to the radiologist of certain interaction that allows refining the segmentation having into account previous result. This is very useful in difficult and strange cases.

The proposed method has been validated with 5 preoperative CT abdominal data sets. Resulting segmentations have been numerically evaluated in terms of Overlap Error, Relative Volume Difference and Surface Distances with respect to radiologists' reference manual segmentations. The method has demonstrated good performance.

3.1 3D active contour algorithm

Active contour models are based on a curve (i.e. contour in 2D or surface in 3D) that evolves following different constraints given by the image. Traditionally, evolving constraints are based on the gradient of the image (Kass et al., 1987; Caselles et al., 1997), being suitable only for images with edges well defined by gradients. However, in 3D CT abdominal images, liver boundaries are not completely defined by a gradient. As we can observe in Fig. 1 the proximity of the liver to other organs of similar CT intensity values prevents from defining all the edges using only gradient information.

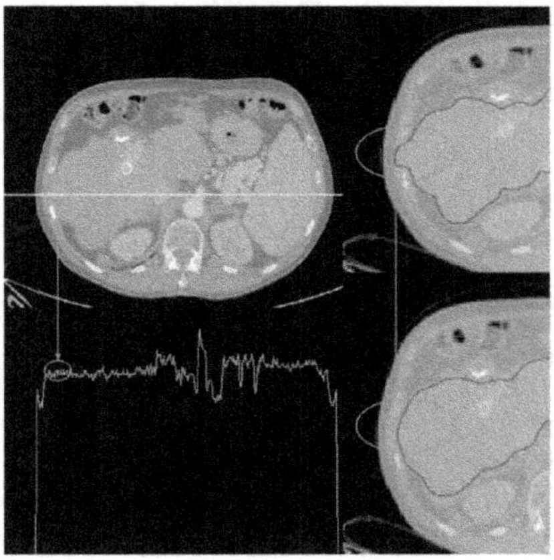

Fig. 1. *On the left*: transverse slice of an abdominal CT image and its profile of intensities along the yellow line showing the difficulty of establishing an intensity threshold between liver and adjacent intercostal muscles. *On the right*: active contour growing based on a classical gradient dependent definition *(above)* and the improvement introduced by the proposed method that avoids the contour to overflow among the intercostal space *(below)*.

In order to segment objects with boundaries not necessarily defined by a gradient, (Chan & Vese, 2001) proposed an active contour method consisting on the minimization of a force that depends on the image gray values inside and outside the curve at each iterative step. This method is based on Mumford-Shah segmentation techniques (Mumford & Shah, 1989):

$$F=\lambda_1 \int_{inside(C)} |u_0(x,y)-c_1|^2 dxdy + \lambda_2 \int_{outside(C)} |u_0(x,y)-c_2|^2 dxdy \quad (1)$$

where u_0 is a given image formed by two regions, C is an evolving contour, and the constants c_1 and c_2 are the averages of u_0 inside and outside C respectively.

This force can be formulated by Level Sets techniques as described in (Chan & Vese, 2001). Level Sets based active contour implementations have become very popular, due to their ability of handling discontinuities and the possibility of topological changes. For the Level Sets formulation, C is represented by a Lipschitz function ϕ:

$$\begin{aligned} C &= \partial\omega\{(x,y)\in\Omega:\phi(x,y)=0\} \\ inside(C) &= \omega = \{(x,y)\in\Omega:\phi(x,y)<0\} \\ outside(C) &= \Omega/\overline{\omega} = \{(x,y)\in\Omega:\phi(x,y)>0\} \end{aligned} \quad (2)$$

The function (1) can be expressed using ϕ and the Heaviside H and Dirac δ_0 functions. The associated Euler–Lagrange equation for ϕ is deduced by minimizing the function with respect to ϕ. Finally, a linear system is obtained that can be solved by an iterative method (for more details we refer the reader to (Chan & Vese, 2001)):

$$\begin{aligned} \frac{\phi_{i,j}^{n+1}-\phi_{i,j}^{n}}{\Delta t} &= \delta_h(\phi_{i,j}^{n})\left[\mu\cdot div\left(\frac{\nabla\phi^n}{|\nabla\phi^n|}\right)-\gamma\right. \\ &\left.+\lambda_1(u_{0,i,j}-c_1(\phi^n))^2-\lambda_2(u_{0,i,j}-c_2(\phi^n))^2\right] \end{aligned} \quad (3)$$

where $\mu\geq 0$, $\gamma\geq 0$, $\lambda 1$, $\lambda 2>0$ are fixed parameters and Δt and h are the time and space steps respectively, used to discretize the equation in ϕ with a finite difference implicit scheme. The term $div(\nabla\phi^n/|\nabla\phi^n|)$ is used to restrict the curvature of the contour. Subscripts i, j represent the position.

With parameters $\lambda 1=\lambda 2=1$ the equation produces a lineal force that is annulled in the mean value of intensity averages $c1$ and $c2$. With this definition the contour stops only when there is a notable difference between clear zones toward darker zones and not with sudden zones of very extreme intensities; so this method works properly only with those images that contain two homogenously well defined regions and textures. If there is a small area with an extreme intensity closer to $c1$ than to $c2$, it will be erroneously included into the segmentation, even when differing to $c1$ more than the absolute difference between $c1$ and $c2$. An example of this problem, hardly controlled by modifying $\lambda 1$ and $\lambda 2$ weights, can be appreciated in Fig. 2 (left) showing a contour based on the (Chan & Vese, 2001) equation growing into the ribs.

In order to solve this problem, some variations inside the function defined in (Chan & Vese, 2001) are proposed in (Fernandez-de-Manuel et al., 2009) to allow segmenting a homogenous region (liver) that is adjacent to other organs with higher or lower intensities in hepatic CT scans with a variable anatomy complexity. The proposed active contour method restricts the growth of the contour to a zone limited around the average gray value inside the liver. It combines both the modified energy function based on gray values, and a morphological gradient information in order to make the algorithm more robust. The Level Sets function derives from equation (1) and considerably improves the segmentation results on the hepatic images under study. The resulting linear system proposed in (Fernandez-de-Manuel et al., 2009), solved by iterative methods, is the following:

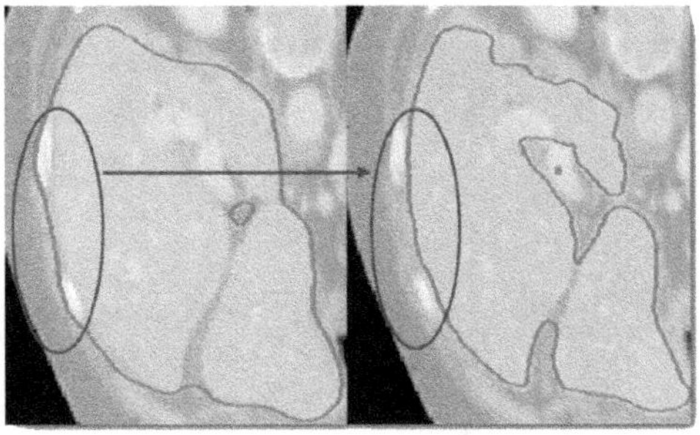

Fig. 2. *On the left*: 3D Active contour growing based on (Chan & Vese, 2001). *On the right*: 3D Active contour growing based on the redefinition of the force equation proposed in (Fernandez-de-Manuel et al., 2009). The growing of the contour into the ribs is successfully controlled in the right image.

$$\begin{aligned}\frac{\phi^{n+1}_{i,j,k}-\phi^{n}_{i,j,k}}{\Delta t} &= \delta_h(\phi^{n}_{i,j,k})\left[\mu\cdot div\left(\frac{\nabla\phi^n}{|\nabla\phi^n|}\right)-\gamma\right.\\ &\left.+\lambda_1\left|u_{0,i,j,k}-\rho\nabla u_{0,i,j,k}-c_1(\phi^n)\right|-\lambda_2\left|c_1(\phi^n)-c_2(\phi^n)\right|\right]\end{aligned} \tag{4}$$

where u_0 is a 3D image formed by two regions, one with almost constant intensity (liver), and the other one with different intensity organs. ϕ represents the evolving 3D contour. $\mu \geq 0$, $\gamma \geq 0$, ρ, $\lambda 1$, $\lambda 2 > 0$ are fixed parameters, the constants c_1 and c_2 depending on iteration n are the averages of u_0 inside and outside the contour respectively and Δt and h are the time and space steps respectively. The term $div(\nabla\phi^n/|\nabla\phi^n|)$ is used to restrict the curvature of the 3D contour. Subscripts i, j, k represent the position in the image. The algorithm starts with a small surface obtained from a seed point placed inside the healthy liver. The initial surface grows iteratively following the described linear system (4). The method has been implemented for 3D images inside a MATLAB framework limiting the force evaluation to a narrow band around the contour in order to reduce the complexity.

3.2 3D Multi-resolution strategy

Due to the large size of CT abdominal images, the method has been implemented following a multiresolution strategy in order to reduce computation time. Three pyramidal steps have been used (Fig. 3). In the first step, the resolution of the images is reduced by a factor of 4. This fast initial segmentation allows us to select the liver region and to get a first approximate surface. In the second step, the resolution is reduced by a factor of 2. A bicubic interpolation is applied in the resolution reduction process. At each step the growing surface begins with the previous step result and iterates to the actual surface of the liver. Finally, in the last step, the resolution of the image is the original one and it performs a final growing of the previous surface that segments properly the liver.

3.3 Pre-processing and definition of frontiers

The general active contour method is extended with a pre-processing step to address particular problems.

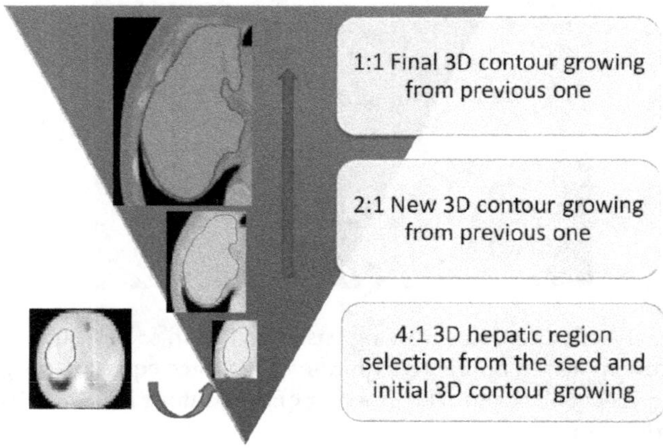

Fig. 3. Diagram of proposed pyramidal segmentation steps.

Firstly, in order to guarantee that the surface evolution properties are properly fitted to the data, an interpolation is applied to make images isotropic. Next, a median filter eliminates inhomogeneities inside the liver region. Kernel size is 3 in lowest resolution levels and no median filter is used in the higher resolution level.

In order to define 3D frontiers with conflictive regions, 6 points (3 segments) are selected. Each one of the segments is manually defined in each dimension (transverse, coronal and sagittal) using a multiplanar 3D viewer. These segments are integrated to reconstruct a parallelogram in the 3D space that approximates the restricted plane that separates the liver from the conflictive region. This approach allows the user to define 3D frontiers with minimal interaction. Then, a modification of the image gray values with an exponential function that grows from zero to the original gray image value around the 3D frontier is incorporated in order to restrict the surface growing around the selected area. Frontiers are typically needed for the cava vein, heart or kidney.

3.4 Post-processing

The active contour functional has been chosen carefully and its operation is convenient. However, a post-processing step is always essential in any kind of tool in order to smooth the results and fill-in small gaps. In the presented work, resulting segmentations are automatically refined with additional post-processing in order to recover original spatial representation, to smooth the surface and to eliminate unconnected zones. To complete this last step, a morphological erosion is applied to the resulting segmentation mask followed by a binary morphological reconstruction of the mask from the original seed point and a final morphological dilation.

4. Data and validation

The presented liver segmentation tool has been validated on five abdominal CT examinations (Table 1). The set includes cases of different liver size, shape, intensity and pathologic state. Studies 1, 2, 4 and 5 were acquired on a Philips Brilliance 16 slice CT scanner, and study 3 was acquired on a Philips AV Expander spiral CT. The pixel spacing varied between 0.69 and 0.84 mm, the inter-slice distance varied from 1 to 5 mm.

The images were segmented manually by radiologists, working slice-by-slice in transverse view. These manual segmentations were performed using all the slices of the study. The liver region was defined as the entire healthy parenchyma, excluding tumors and lesions in order to avoid overestimating the liver functional volume.

The semiautomatic segmentation has been carried out following steps described in Section 3. The Level-Sets function parameters (4) were fixed to $\gamma=0$, $\rho=1$, $\lambda 1=1$ *and* $\lambda 2= 1/5.5$ as these values were presented in (Fernandez-de-Manuel et al., 2009) as the ones with better results in CT scans.

The obtained segmentations have been evaluated by five metrics based on the ones described on (Heimann et al., 2009). This five metrics are as follows:

Volumetric Overlap Error (VOE), in percent:

$$VOE = \left(1 - \left(N_i / N_u\right)\right) \cdot 100 \tag{5}$$

where N_i is the number of voxels in the intersection of resulting segmentation and reference, and N_u is the number of voxels in the union of resulting segmentation and reference. This value is 0 for a perfect segmentation and 100 when there is no overlap.

Relative Volume Difference (RVD), in percent:

$$RVD = \left((V_s - V_r) / V_r\right) \cdot 100 \tag{6}$$

where V_s is the volume of the segmentation, and V_r is the volume of the reference. The best value is 0 (for exact volumes) and the worst one is 100.

Average Symmetric Surface Distance (ASSD), in mm:

$$d_i = dist(B_{s,i}, B_{r,i}),\ \forall i \quad \text{ASSD}=mean(d_i) \tag{7}$$

where $B_{s,i}$ is the edge voxel i of one of the images, and $B_{r,i}$ is the edge voxel i of the other (the closest voxel to $B_{s,i}$). Border voxels are those belonging to the segmented liver that have at least one of their 18 nearest neighbors not belonging to the segmented liver. *dist* represents the Euclidean distance, not signed, in mm and taking into account the different resolutions in the different scan directions. Distances between the two sets of border voxels (one set from each image) are stored. *mean* represents the mean value of distances. ASSD value is 0 for a perfect segmentation.

Root Mean Square Symmetric Surface Distance (RMSD), in mm:

$$d_i = dist(B_{s,i}, B_{r,i}),\ \forall i \quad RMSD = \sqrt{mean\left(\left(d_i\right)^2\right)} \tag{8}$$

This measure is similar to the previous one but in this case the squared distances between the two sets of border voxels are stored. RMSD value is 0 for a perfect segmentation.

Maximum Symmetric Surface Distance (MSSD), in mm:

$$d_i = dist(B_{s,i}, B_{r,i}),\ \forall i \quad \text{MSSD}=\max(d_i) \tag{9}$$

This measure is similar to the previous two, but in this case the maximum of all distance is taken instead of the average. MSSD is 0 for a perfect segmentation.

5. Results and discussion

Table 1 shows the experiment results including case descriptions, the number of required frontiers manually selected by the user, resulting metrics, and the computation time for each examination.

We can see that volume differences (absolute values of RVD) are smaller than 10% in all of the cases (Table 1). In all of them, the deviation is produced because of under-segmentation. Analyzing in detail the resulting images, we conclude that the region affected by these under-segmentations is, in the majority of the cases, the narrow end of the left liver lobe. This problem affects specially to the case 1 and the case 5, producing a Maximum Surface Distance bigger than 3 cm, which is exactly located in those narrow areas. Case 1 is probably the most difficult case presenting a very atypical shape and gray level distribution. In these narrow regions, the 3D contour finds difficulties to grow due to particularly restrictive curvature constraints. Further studies are warranted to correct the small misclassified areas by modifying curvature restrictions locally.

Most of the tumors were not included in the liver region, according to the requirements of the clinicians. In this sense, the proposed method works properly, as it excludes hyperintense and hypointense large tumors (Fig. 4). However, in some of the cases, small metastases completely surrounded by healthy parenchyma were not excluded during the process of contour growing, affecting considerable to the Surface Distance Errors (case 3). Nevertheless, this problem hardly modifies the final volume estimation, because of its small size.

Other segmentation minor errors were detected in the surroundings of the hepatic portal vein (case 2 and 4).

Case	Case description	# frontiers	VOE [%]	RVD [%]	ASSD [mm.]	RMSD [mm.]	MSSD [mm.]	Time [min.]
1	Hepatic carcinoma	13	13.13	-9.02	2.39	5.12	42.84	9.57
2	Liver after hepatectomy	0	10.80	-5.76	1.43	2.04	14.25	9.92
3	Portal embolization pre- right hepatectomy	4	10.48	-6.38	1.24	2.72	27.04	11.56
4	Metastasis	2	11.55	-4.46	1.79	3.09	21.91	3.67
5	Portal embolization pre- right hepatectomy	0	13.04	-9.41	2.13	3.67	33.44	3.82

Table 1. Cases descriptions, number of initial frontiers points, resulting metrics and computation times.

In general, resulting segmentations satisfied clinical requirements. Overlap errors, and volume errors were considered reasonable. Special attention will be made in further studies in order to solve problems affecting small areas. However, although Maximum Distance Errors (MSSD) were considerably high, the reasonable averages (ASSD and RMSD) show that these errors were produced in very punctual areas hardly modifying volumes. Most of the frontiers were defined in zones adjacent to the heart and cava vein. The number of frontiers needed to restrict forces in those areas depended on the image and varied from 0 to 13 frontiers in the most difficult case. Further studies are also warranted in order to reduce the user interaction.

The proposed method requires 7.7 minutes on average using a non optimized MATLAB code running on one core of a PC at 2.4 GHz with 4 GB memory.

Time refers to the time needed for the automated computation of the segmentation result after the seed point and frontiers have been set. Computation time depends on the image size, mainly on the inter-slice distance (that vary from 1 to 5 mm in our data) and this is the reason because it goes from 3 to 11 min. Note that the highest resolution level of the process employ all the slices of the original data and this is the more time-consuming step.

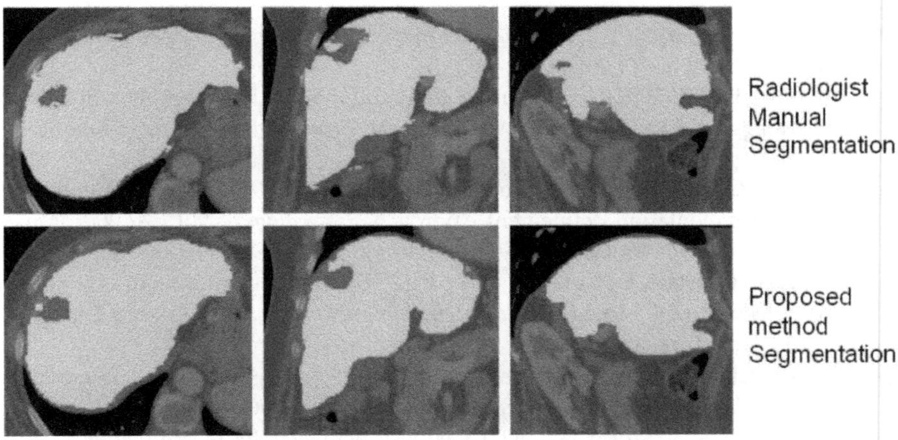

Fig. 4. Segmentation of healthy parenchyma in case 4. *Top*: radiologist manual segmentation. *Bottom*: resulting semiautomatic segmentation with presented method. Left to right: transverse, coronal and sagittal slices.

6. Conclusion

This chapter makes an especial effort in presenting, in a wide and complete context, the state of the art in the scope of the hepatic segmentation from CT images. It presents the newest and most sophisticated methods developed in this field in the last few years and notes the importance of hepatic volume estimation from CT scans for hepatic surgical planning. Moreover, the application of a semiautomatic liver 3D segmentation tool to segment and quantify the volume of the healthy parenchyma from CT preoperative abdominal images is presented. The tool combines a 3D active contour method implemented with Level Sets techniques with a multiresolution strategy, a morphological filtering post processing and a fast method to manually define specific frontiers. An initial seed point inside the healthy parenchyma manually selected by the user is required. If desired the user can also define several frontiers to delineate the separation with problematic regions like the kidney or the heart. The method has been validated with a set of five abdominal CT preoperative images with special difficulties. Further studies are needed in order to solve specific problems related with errors in narrow liver areas and reducing user interaction. Nevertheless, the proposed method has demonstrated good performance and a noticeable reduction of the time needed with respect to manual segmentations.

7. Acknowledgments

This study was partially supported by research projects TIN 2007-68048-C02, PI09/91058, PI09/91065, ENTEPRASE PS-300000-2009-5, AMIT-CDTI, TEC2010-21619-C04 and PRECISION IPT-300000-2010-3, from Spain's Ministry of Science & Innovation, the project ARTEMIS Comunidad de Madrid, and with assistance from the European Regional Development Fund (FEDER).

8. References

Barrett, W. A. & Mortensen, E. N. (1997). Interactive live-wire boundary extraction. *Med Image Anal,* Vol. 1, No. 4, pp. 331-41.

Beck, A. & Aurich, V. (2007). HepaTux–A Semiautomatic Liver Segmentation System. *Proceedings of MICCAI 2007 Workshop: 3D Segmentation in the Clinic-A Grand Challenge,* pp. 225–233.

Beichel, R.; Bauer, C.; Bornik, A.; Sorantin, E. & Bischof, H. (2007). Liver Segmentation in CT Data: A Segmentation Refinement Approach. *Proceedings of MICCAI 2007 Workshop: 3D Segmentation in the Clinic-A Grand Challenge,* pp. 235–245.

Bekes, G.; Nyül, L. G.; Máté, E.; Kuba, A. & M., F. (2007). 3D Segmentation of Liver, Kidneys and Spleen from CT Images. *International Journal of Computer Assisted Radiology and Surgery,* Vol. 2, pp. 45-46.

Campadelli, P.; Casiraghi, E. & Pratissoli, S. (2010). A segmentation framework for abdominal organs from CT scans. *Artif Intell Med,* Vol. 50, No. 1, pp. 3-11.

Caselles, V.; Kimmel, R. & Sapiro, G. (1997). Geodesic active contours. *International Journal of Computer Vision,* Vol. 22, No. 1, pp. 61-79.

Couinaud, C. (1999). Liver anatomy: portal (and suprahepatic) or biliary segmentation. *Digestive Surgery,* Vol. 16, No. 6, pp. 459-467.

Chan, T. F. & Vese, L. A. (2001). Active contours without edges. *IEEE Transactions on Image Processing,* Vol. 10, No. 2, pp. 266-277.

Dawant, B. M.; Li, R.; Lennon, B. & Li, S. (2007). Semi-automatic segmentation of the liver and its evaluation on the MICCAI 2007 grand challenge data set. *Proceedings of MICCAI 2007 Workshop: 3D Segmentation in the Clinic-A Grand Challenge,* pp. 215–221.

Fernandez-De-Manuel, L.; Rubio, J. L.; Ledesma-Carbayo, M. J.; Pascau, J.; Tellado, J. M.; Ramón, E.; Desco, M. & Santos, A. (2009). 3D Liver Segmentation in Preoperative CT Images using a Level-Sets Active Surface Method. *Proceedings of IEEE Engineering in Medicine and Biology Society (EMBC 2009),* pp. 3625-3628.

Fujimoto, H.; Gu, L. & Kaneko, T. (2002). Recognition of abdominal organs using 3D mathematical morphology. *Systems and Computers in Japan,* Vol. 33, No. 8, pp. 75-83.

Gao, L. M.; Heath, D. G. & Fishman, E. K. (1998). Abdominal image segmentation using three-dimensional deformable models. *Investigative Radiology,* Vol. 33, No. 6, pp. 348-355.

Gao, L. M.; Heath, D. G.; Kuszyk, B. S. & Fishman, E. K. (1996). Automatic liver segmentation technique for three-dimensional visualisation of CT data. *Radiology,* Vol. 201, No. 2, pp. 359-364.

Garamendi, J. F.; Malpica, N.; Martel, J. & Schiavi, E. (2007). Automatic segmentation of the liver in CT using level sets without edges. *Proceedings of Iberian Conference on Pattern Recognition and Image Analysis,* pp. 161-168.

Handels, H. & Ehrhardt, J. (2009). Medical Image Computing for Computer-supported Diagnostics and Therapy Advances and Perspectives. *Methods of Information in Medicine,* Vol. 48, No. 1, pp. 11-17.

Heimann, T.; Meinzer, H. P. & Wolf, I. (2007). A statistical deformable model for the segmentation of liver CT volumes. *Proceedings of MICCAI 2007 Workshop: 3D Segmentation in the Clinic-A Grand Challenge,* pp. 161–166.

Heimann, T.; Van Ginneken, B.; Styner, M. A.; Arzhaeva, Y.; Aurich, V.; Bauer, C.; Beck, A.; Becker, C.; Beichel, R.; Bekes, G.; Bello, F.; Binnig, G.; Bischof, H.; Bornik, A.; Cashman, P. M. M.; Chi, Y.; Cordova, A.; Dawant, B. M.; Fidrich, M.; Furst, J. D.; Furukawa, D.; Grenacher, L.; Hornegger, J.; Kainmuller, D.; Kitney, R. I.; Kobatake, H.; Lamecker, H.; Lange, T.; Lee, J.; Lennon, B.; Li, R.; Li, S.; Meinzer, H. P.; Nemeth, G.; Raicu, D. S.; Rau, A. M.; Van Rikxoort, E. M.; Rousson, M.; Rusko, L.; Saddi, K. A.; Schmidt, G.; Seghers, D.; Shimizu, A.; Slagmolen, P.; Sorantin, E.; Soza, G.; Susomboon, R.; Waite, J. M.; Wimmer, A. & Wolf, I. (2009). Comparison and Evaluation of Methods for Liver Segmentation From CT Datasets. *IEEE Transactions on Medical Imaging,* Vol. 28, No. 8, pp. 1251-1265.

Jiang, H. Y. & Cheng, Q. S. (2009) Automatic 3D Segmentation of CT Images Based on Active Contour Models. IN Thalmann, D.;Shah, J. J. & Peng, Q. S. (Eds.) *2009 11th IEEE International Conference on Computer-Aided Design and Computer Graphics, Proceedings.* pp. 540-543.

Kainmueller, D.; Lange, T. & Lamecker, H. (2007). Shape constrained automatic segmentation of the liver based on a heuristic intensity model. *Proceedings of MICCAI 2007 Workshop: 3D Segmentation in the Clinic-A Grand Challenge,* pp. 109-116.

Kass, M.; Witkin, A. & Terzopoulos, D. (1987). Snakes-Active Contour Models. *International Journal of Computer Vision,* Vol. 1, No. 4, pp. 321-331.

Koss, J. E.; Newman, F. D.; Johnson, T. K. & Kirch, D. L. (1999). Abdominal organ segmentation using texture transforms and a Hopfield neural network. *IEEE Transactions on Medical Imaging,* Vol. 18, No. 7, pp. 640-648.

Lamecker, H.; Lange, T. & Seebass, M. (2004) Segmentation of the liver using a 3d statistical shape model. *Technical report, Zuse Institute Berlin.*

Lee, C. C. & Chung, P. C. (2000). Recognizing abdominal organs in CT images using contextual neural network and fuzzy rules. *Proceedings of 22nd Annual International Conference of the IEEE Engineering in Medicine and Biology Society,* pp. 1745-1748.

Lee, C. C.; Chung, P. C. & Tsai, H. M. (2003). Identifying multiple abdominal organs from CT image series using a multimodule contextual neural network and spatial fuzzy rules. *IEEE Transactions on Information Technology in Biomedicine,* Vol. 7, No. 3, pp. 208-217.

Lee, J.; Kim, N.; Lee, H.; Seo, J. B.; Won, H. J.; Shin, Y. M. & Shin, Y. G. (2007). Efficient liver segmentation exploiting level-set speed images with 2.5 D shape propagation. *Proceedings of MICCAI 2007 Workshop: 3D Segmentation in the Clinic-A Grand Challenge,* pp. 189–196.

Lim, S. J.; Jeong, Y. Y. & Ho, Y. S. (2005). Segmentation of the liver using the deformable contour method on CT images. *Proceedings of SPIE,* pp. 570-581.

Lim, S. J.; Jeong, Y. Y. & Ho, Y. S. (2006). Automatic liver segmentation for volume measurement in CT images. *Journal of Visual Communication and Image Representation,* Vol. 17, No. 4, pp. 860-875.

Lim, S. J.; Jeong, Y. Y.; Lee, C. W. & Ho, Y. S. (2004). Automatic segmentation of the liver in CT images using the watershed algorithm based on morphological filtering. *Proceedings of SPIE,* pp. 1658.

Linguraru, M. G.; Sandberg, J. K.; Li, Z. X.; Shah, F. & Summers, R. M. (2010). Automated segmentation and quantification of liver and spleen from CT images using normalized probabilistic atlases and enhancement estimation. *Medical Physics,* Vol. 37, No. 2, pp. 771-783.

Liu, F.; Zhao, B. S.; Kijewski, P. K.; Wang, L. & Schwartz, L. H. (2005). Liver segmentation for CT images using GVF snake. *Medical Physics,* Vol. 32, No. 12, pp. 3699-3706.

Luo, S. H.; Hu, Q. M.; He, X. J.; Li, J. M.; Jin, J. S. & Park, M. (2009). Automatic Liver Parenchyma Segmentation from Abdominal CT Images Using Support Vector Machines. *Proceedings of 2009 Icme International Conference on Complex Medical Engineering,* pp. 522-526.

Montagnat, J. & Delingette, H. (1997). Volumetric medical images segmentation using shape constrained deformable models. *Proceedings of First Joint Conference CVRMED-MRCAS'97,* pp. 13-22.

Mumford, D. & Shah, J. (1989). Optimal approximations by piecewise smooth functions and associated variational problems. *Comm. Pure Appl. Math,* Vol. 42, No. 5, pp. 577-685.

Pan, S. Y. & Dawant, B. M. (2001). Automatic 3D segmentation of the liver from abdominal CT images: a level-set approach. *Medical Imaging: 2001: Image Processing, Pts 1-3,* Vol. 2, No. 27, pp. 128-138.

Park, H.; Bland, P. H. & Meyer, C. R. (2003). Construction of an abdominal Probabilistic atlas and its application in segmentation. *IEEE Transactions on Medical Imaging,* Vol. 22, No. 4, pp. 483-492.

Platero, C.; Poncela, J. M.; Gonzalez, P.; Tobar, M. C.; Sanguino, J.; Asensio, G. & Santos, E. (2008). Liver segmentation for hepatic lesions detection and characterisation. *Proceedings of IEEE International Symposium on Biomedical Imaging: from Nano to Macro*, pp. 13-16.

Pohle, R. & Toennies, K. D. (2001). Segmentation of medical images using adaptive region growing. *Medical Imaging: 2001: Image Processing, Pts 1-3,* Vol. 2, No. 27, pp. 1337-1346.

Radtke, A.; Nadalin, S.; Sotiropoulos, G. C.; Molmenti, E. P.; Schroeder, T.; Valentin-Gamazo, C.; Lang, H.; Bockhorn, M.; Peitgen, H. O.; Broelsch, C. E. & Malago, M. (2007). Computer-assisted operative planning in adult living donor liver transplantation: A new way to resolve the dilemma of the middle hepatic vein. *World Journal of Surgery,* Vol. 31, No. 1, pp. 175-185.

Ruskó, L.; Bekes, G.; Németh, G. & M., F. (2007). Fully Automatic Liver Segmentation for Contrast-enhanced CT Images. . *Proceedings of MICCAI 2007 Workshop: 3D Segmentation in the Clinic-A Grand Challenge,* pp. 143-150.

Ryu, M. & Cho, A. (Eds.) (2009) *The New Liver Anatomy: Portal Segmentation and the Drainage Vein,* Springer, ISBN 978-4-431-95992-2, New York.

Saddi, K.; Rousson, M.; Chefd'hotel, C. & Cheriet, F. (2007). Global-to-Local Shape Matching for Liver Segmentation in CT Imaging. *Proceedings of MICCAI 2007 Workshop: 3D Segmentation in the Clinic-A Grand Challenge,* pp. 207-214.

Schenk, A.; Prause, G. & Peitgen, H. O. (2000). Efficient semiautomatic segmentation of 3D objects in medical images. *Proceedings of Medical Image Computing and Computer-Assisted Intervention - MICCAI 2000,* pp. 186-195.

Schenk, A.; Prause, G. & Peitgen, H. O. (2001). Local cost computation for efficient segmentation of 3D objects with live wire. *Medical Imaging: 2001: Image Processing, Pts 1-3,* Vol. 2, No. 27, pp. 1357-1364.

Shimizu, A.; Ohno, R.; Ikegami, T.; Kobatake, H.; Nawano, S. & Smutek, D. (2006). Multi-organ segmentation in three dimensional abdominal CT images. *International Journal of Computer Assisted Radiology and Surgery (CARS 2006)* Vol. 1, No. 7, pp. 76-78.

Soler, L.; Delingette, H.; Malandain, G.; Montagnat, J.; Ayache, N.; Koehl, C.; Dourthe, O.; Malassagne, B.; Smith, M.; Mutter, D. & Marescaux, J. (2001). Fully automatic anatomical, pathological, and functional segmentation from CT scans for hepatic surgery. *Comput Aided Surg,* Vol. 6, No. 3, pp. 131-42.

Suzuki, K.; Kohlbrenner, R.; Epstein, M. L.; Obajuluwa, A. M.; Xu, J. W. & Hori, M. (2010). Computer-aided measurement of liver volumes in CT by means of geodesic active contour segmentation coupled with level-set algorithms. *Medical Physics,* Vol. 37, No. 5, pp. 2159-2166.

Tsai, D. Y. & Tanahashi, N. (1994). Neural-Network-Based Boundary Detection of Liver Structure in Ct Images for 3-D Visualization. *1994 Ieee International Conference on Neural Networks, Vol 1-7,* Vol., 3484-3489.

Van Ginneken, B.; Heimann, T. & Styner, M. (2007). 3D segmentation in the clinic: A grand challenge. *Proceedings of MICCAI 2007 Workshop: 3D Segmentation in the Clinic-A Grand Challenge,* pp. 7.

Wimmer, A.; Soza, G. & Hornegger, J. (2007). Two-stage semi-automatic organ segmentation framework using radial basis functions and level sets. *Proceedings of MICCAI 2007 Workshop: 3D Segmentation in the Clinic-A Grand Challenge,* pp. 179–188.

Woodhouse, C. E.; Ney, D. R.; Sitzmann, J. V. & Fishman, E. K. (1994). Spiral Computed-Tomography Arterial Portography with 3-Dimensional Volumetric Rendering for Oncologic Surgery Planning - a Retrospective Analysis. *Investigative Radiology,* Vol. 29, No. 12, pp. 1031-1037.

Zhou, X.; Kitagawa, T.; Okuo, K.; Hara, T.; Fujita, H.; Yokoyam, R.; Kanematsu, M. & Hoshi, H. (2005). Construction of a probabilistic atlas for automated liver segmentation in non-contrast torso CT images. *Proceedings of CARS 2005: Computer Assisted Radiology and Surgery*, pp. 1169-1174.

6

Functional Assessment of Individual Lung Lobes with MDCT Images

Syoji Kobashi, Kei Kuramoto and Yutaka Hata
University of Hyogo
Japan

1. Introduction

CT is an effective modality for evaluating the structure inside the body and the 3-D shape of organs of interest because of ability of high spatial resolution and of high acquisition speed. However, CT is weak to evaluate a function of organs because CT only maps X-ray absorption coefficients of materials constructing human body. Therefore, study of functional imaging of organs by using CT images will be a breakthrough of image diagnosis. This chapter introduces a novel method for estimating pulmonary function using MDCT.

The human lung is composed of five anatomical compartments called "lung lobes." The right lung is segmented into three lung lobes (the upper, middle and lower lobes), and the left lung is segmented into two lung lobes (the upper and lower lobes). Thoracic surgeries such as a living-donor lobar lung transplantation (LDLLT) (Date et al., 2003a) and the lobectomy (Kirby et al., 1993) often operate by a lung lobe. LDLLT is an operation that transplants the right and left lower lobes of two living donors to a recipient. In this surgery, predicting the postoperative forced vital capacity (FVC) of a recipient is necessary to select the adequate donors. The lobectomy is a treatment that extirpates lung lobe. This surgery excises the diseased region such as lung or improves breathing function by reducing the lung capacity that overexpands by emphysema. In this surgery, predicting the postoperative FVC is necessary to investigate the effectiveness of the surgery, too. Since these surgeries treatment lobe by lobe, the prediction should be based on individual lung lobes. Although a spirometry, which is widely used in a clinical field, enables us to measure the FVC of whole lung, it is not available for the FVCs of the individual lung lobes.

Date et al. have proposed a method for approximating FVCs of individual lung lobes by determining the contribution ratio to FVC of the whole lung (Date et al., 2003b). The contribution ratio is determined from the number of lung segments occupied in the lung lobe. The FVC of recipients that underwent the LDLLT measured at 6 months was correlated well with the grafts FVCs of donors estimated by their method ($r = 0.802$). However, the method does not consider the variation of the lobar function among subjects. To consider such variation, a tracheal tube can measure the FVCs of the right and the left lung respectively. However, the method is invasive due to the use of anesthesia and the tracheal tube, and it still cannot measure the FVCs of the individual lung lobes.

This chapter proposes a novel method for measuring the FVCs of individual lung lobes by using volume data acquired from CT scanner. This approach is based on an assumption that the FVC of whole lung can be expressed as the change of lung lobe volumes between inspiratory and expiratory. Thus, the contribution ratio of lung lobes can be obtained by measuring the volumes of lung lobes for each of inspiratory lung and of expiratory lung. Because of the use of MDCT images, the proposed method is less invasive in comparison with the use of the tracheal tube. The proposed method can consider the variation of the lobar function among subjects.

There are several segmentation methods of lung lobes from MDCT images. Zhou et al. (Zhou et al., 2004) and Saita et al. (Saita et al., 2004) extract the lobar fissures in MDCT images to determine the boundary surface between lung lobes. They are called LFB (lobar fissure based) method. Because lobar fissure indicates right boundary surface of lung lobe, this approach is high accuracy. However, this approach has two limitations; (1) it is limited to apply the method by a lack of the lobar fissures, and (2) false positive (FP) regions of lobar fissures will be extracted.

To overcome the difficulty of lacked lobar fissures, we proposed a new method (Kobashi et al., 2010) that estimates the boundary surface between the lung lobes with the tubular tissue density, which is called TTB (tubular tissue density based). The tubular tissues consist of the peripheral blood vessels and peripheral bronchus. Because the tubular tissues do not cross over the boundary surface between the lung lobes, this method defines the boundary surface as the region where the tubular tissue density is low. Therefore, this approach can be applied to MDCT images that have a lack of lobar fissures.

2. Method

2.1 Image acquisition and forced vital capacity measurement of the whole lung

MDCT images were acquired from an MDCT scanner (LightSpeed Ultra16, GE Medical Systems, WI, USA). The acquisition parameters for the chest MDCT images were: the tube voltage was 120 kV; the tube current was 440 mA; the field of view (FOV) was 360 mm; the matrix size was 512 × 512 pixels; the slice thickness was 0.625 mm and was with no gap. Each sliced image included volumetric data, and a volume dataset from the apex of the lung to the diaphragmatic surface was composed of over 450 contiguous axial planes. Given these conditions, the acquisition time requiring breath holding was about 10 sec. Fig. 1 shows raw MDCT images of the chest.

Two sets of MDCT image were acquired with inspiratory condition and with expiratory condition. For each dataset, the proposed method segmentes the lung lobes, and measrues

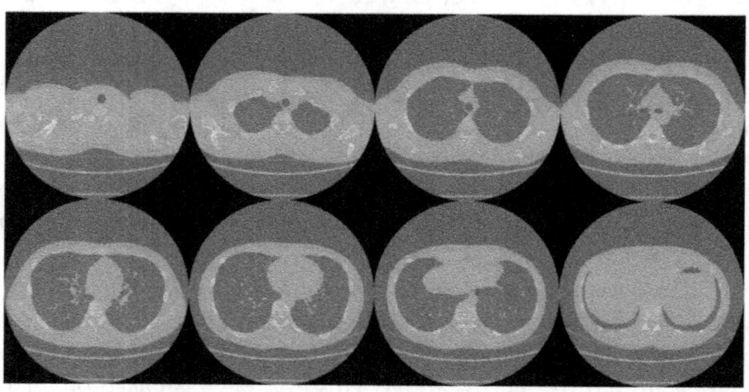

Fig. 1. Raw MDCT images of the chest. Upper-left to lower-right are superior to inferior.

the individual volumes. Thus, we can estimate the change of lung lobe volumes between the inspiratory and the expiratory conditions. The contribution rate for the whole lung capacity can be estaimated. By using the whole lung FVC measured by a spirometer, the individual lung FVCs are estimated.

2.2 Image analysis

This study defines tubular tissues as a set of peripheral blood vessels and peripheral bronchi. Because the tubular tissues do not exist on the boundary between the lung lobes, the method determines the boundary by finding a 3-D continuous space where few tubular tissues exist. Therefore, the method does not depend on detection accuracy of the lobar fissures from MDCT images. The finding process is automatically performed with a fuzzy control (Kobashi et al., 2010), and is composed from the following steps. They are applied to both of MDCT datasets with inspiratory and with expiratory conditions.

Step 1. Segment the lung region from MDCT images.

The lung region is segmented by 3-D region growing (RG) and morphological operation which consists of 3-D erosion and dilation methods. The bronchial region is removed from the segmented region by extracting the air region inside the bronchial walls using 3-D RG according to the method proposed by Mori et al. (2000).

Step 2. Extract the tubular tissues.

The peripheral blood vessels have higher CT values than the surrounding parenchyma, and the peripheral bronchi also have high CT values. In summary, tubular tissues have high CT values in the lung region. Thus, the peripheral blood vessels and peripheral bronchi are collectively extracted and are called tubular tissues. They are extracted by an adaptive thresholding using mean of a local window. Fig. 2 shows an example of the extracted tubular tissues. Then, tubular tissue density is calculated for each voxel in the lung region.

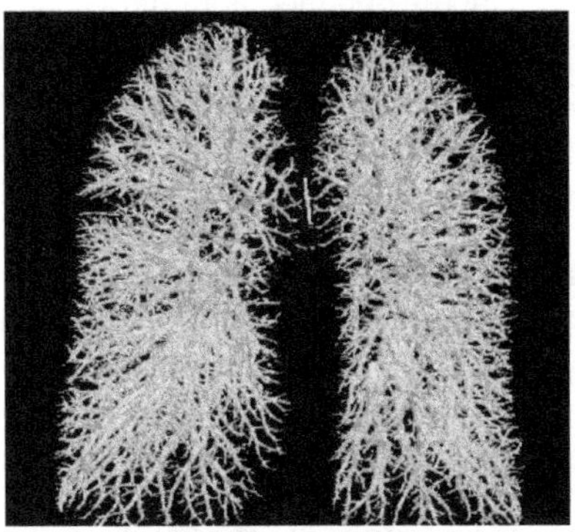

Fig. 2. 3-D rendering image of the extracted tubular tissues.

Step 3. Determine the initial surface.

An examiner gives a plane, which runs a space where few tubular tissues using a configured graphical user interface (GUI). The GUI displays the 3-D rendering images of the extracted tubular tissues. The examiner rotates the rendering image to find a space with few tubular tissues. As shown in Fig. 3, by giving a straight line on the rendering image, a plane forwarding to the view angle is obtained as the initial surface of the boundary between the lung lobes.

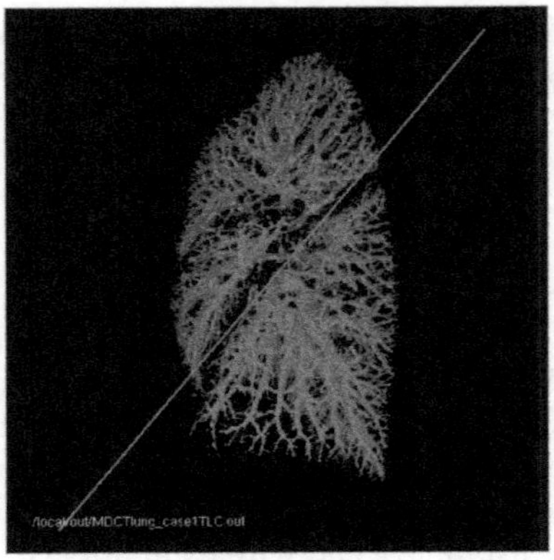

Fig. 3. Manual determination of initial surface using the configured GUI. This figure shows the rendering image of tubular tissues in the right lung. Two cracks of tubular tissues corresponding to the major and minor fissures can be found. The examiner rotates the rendering image and gives a straight line on the rendering image.

Step 4. Deform the curved surfaces and obtain the boundaries.
The initial surface is converted into trapezoidal mesh. By moving the vertexes of the mesh, the surface can be deformed. The movement of the vertexes is automatically performed with fuzzy control system, which evaluates the anatomical knowledge on the lobar boundaries: (1) the moving vertex moves toward a space with low tissue density, and (2) the deforming surface model maintains a smoothed surface. The anatomical knowledge is described by fuzzy IF-THEN rules (e.g., Han et al., 2007), and the vertexes are moved to a position with the higher fuzzy degree belonging to the lobar boundaries.
Step 5. Segment the lung lobes by the obtained boundaries.
Step 3 and step 4 are applied to determine one boundary for the left lung, and to determine two boundaries for the right lung. Using the boundaries, the left lung is decomposed into the upper and the lower lung lobes, and the right lung is decomposed into the upper, the middle, and the lower lung lobes.

2.3 Estimation of individual forced vital capacity

This approach is based on an assumption that the FVC of whole lung is collerated with the differences of volumes between inspiratory and expiratory. The proposed method can calculate volumes of the individual lung lobes from a set of MDCT images on inspiratory and expiratory of the same subject. Therefore, by using the volumes of the segmented lung lobe region, it is possible to estimate the FVCs of individual lung lobes.

We consider that the FVC of whole lung is the sum of the FVCs of individual lung lobes. If we can calculate the ratios that each lung lobe can contribute to the FVC of whole lung, the FVCs of individual lung lobes are predicted. The contribution ratios are associated with the volume differences of the segmented lung lobe region between inspiratory and expiratory. Therefore, the FVCs of individual lung lobes are estimated by using the FVC of whole lung measured by the spirometry and the contribution ratios.

The proposed method defines the contribution ratio of the lung lobe of interest R(t) (t = {the right upper lobe, right middle lobe, right lower lobe, left upper lobe, and left lower lobe}) through the following equation,

$$R(t) = \frac{V_i(t) - V_e(t)}{\sum_{q \in t} V_i(q) - V_e(q)} \quad (1)$$

where Vi and Ve are the inspiratory and expiratory volume of the segmented lung lobe region, respectively. In consequently, the FVCs of individual lung lobes FVC(t) are predicted in the following equation,

$$FVC(t) = R(t) \cdot FVC_{lung} \quad (2)$$

where FVC_{lung} denotes the FVC of whole lung measured by the spirometry, and sum of contribution ratios equals to 1. Therefore, the sum of $FVC(t)$ equals FVC_{lung}. Because of the use of the image information (*i.e.*, chest MDCT images), $R(t)$ can reflect the variation of the respiratory function among subjects in comparison with the conventional method that fixes the contribution ratio (Date et al., 2003b).

4. Experimental results

The proposed method was applied to four normal subjects who were recruited in our institute. Table I shows the profiles of the subjects. All the subjects provided written informed consent according to a guideline approved by the local Ethics Committee. In the eight collected MDCT datasets, there were partial lacks in the delineation of the lobar fissure.

Subjects	Sex	Age (YO)	Height (cm)	Smoking History	VCP (cc)	FVC (cc)	FEV1% (%)
A	Male	23	175	No	4380	3440	87
B	Male	23	172	No	4300	3780	91
C	Male	22	173	No	4350	2890	99
D	Male	21	178	Yes	4490	3980	91

Table I. Subject profiles; YO means years old, VCP means vital capacity predicted, and FEV1% means ratio of FEV1 (forced expiratory volume in one second) to FVC.

Fig. 3 shows raw MDCT images, the experimental results with the proposed method, and lobar fissures extracted by conventional method for comparison. In raw MDCT image, lobar fissures appear with the higher CT values than the surrounding region. However, over-extraction and under-extraction tend to be occurred. In contrast, the proposed method determines the lobar boundaries for the lacked fissures.

To evaluate the determined boundaries with the proposed method, they were compared with boundaries manually delineated by a physician. Because the proposed method requires an interaction to determine the initial surface, for each dataset, the proposed method was applied 10 times. Table II shows the comparison results for each boundary; the left major fissure, the right major fissure, and the right minor fissure. The accuracy was evaluated by measuring the shortest distance between the automatically determined boundary and the manually delineated boundary. The mean ± standard deviation (SD) of detecting accuracy was 3.20 ± 1.72 [mm].

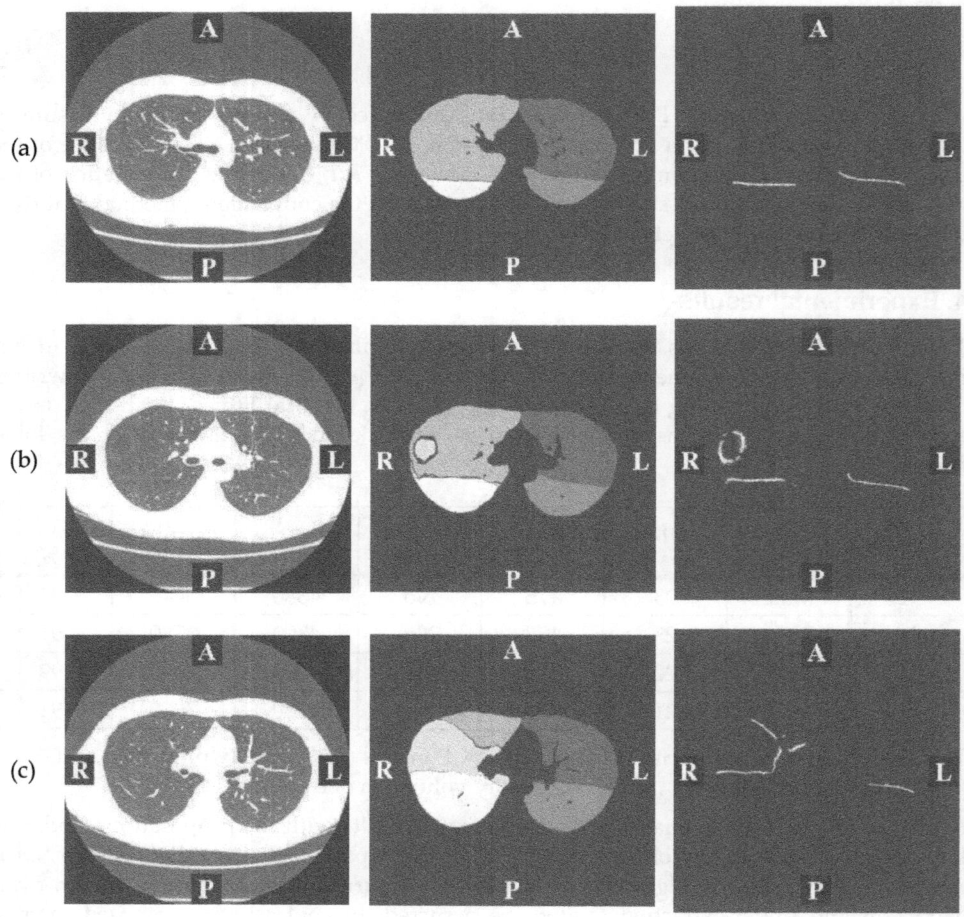

Fig. 3. 2-D segmentation results of subject A. (a) 170th slice, (b) 186th slice, and (c) 212th slice; (left) raw MDCT images, (middle) lung lobes segmented with the proposed method, (right) extracted lobar fissures with the conventional method.

		Left Major	Right Major	Right Minor
Subject A	Inspiratory	3.29±1.83	3.62±1.69	2.87±1.78
	Expiratory	3.34±1.75	3.43±1.68	2.60±1.62
Subject B	Inspiratory	3.29±1.68	3.54±1.69	3.62±1.72
	Expiratory	3.16±1.76	3.39±1.67	3.33±1.68
Subject C	Inspiratory	2.71±1.79	3.37±1.75	3.19±1.80
	Expiratory	3.09±1.63	3.33±1.68	2.69±1.71
Subject D	Inspiratory	3.65±1.65	3.06±1.79	3.49±1.76
	Expiratory	3.05±1.71	2.94±1.75	2.83±1.82

Table II. Accuracy of detecting lobar boundaries with the proposed method (mean ± standard deviation [mm]).

Fig. 4 shows the surface shaded display (SSD) images of the segmented lung lobes. For any subject, and for any condition of inspiratory or expiratory, the lung lobes were segmented well. The comparison of lung lobes between the conditions of inspiratory and expiratory demonstrates that the lobes deform largely by inspiration. Next, by counting the number of voxels for each lung lobe, the volumes can be measured. Table III shows the lung lobe volumes estimated by the proposed method. To validate the proposed method, lung lobe volumes were measured manually by delineating the lung lobe boundaries with physicians. Error ratio is computed by $\frac{truth - estimated}{truth}$. The absolute mean error ratio across the lung lobes on the inspiratoy condition was 0.9 % and on the expiratory condition was 1.2 %, and the mean was 1.1 %. As shown in this table, there are no differences of segmentation accuracy among subjects, lung lobes, and inspiratory/expiratory conditions.

Using the estimated lung lobe volumes shown in Table III, contribution ratio was calculated by Eq. (1). The contribution ratios calculated with the present method, and the fixed contribution ratios introduced by Data et al. (2003b) are shown in Table IV. There are slight differences between the estimated contribution ratios and the fixed parameters: e.g., the contribution ratio of the right middle lobe was lower than the fixed one, and the right lower lobe was higher than the fixed one. In addition, we can show the differences of contribution ratios among the subjects.

Finally, FVCs of lung lobes were estimated by using Eq. (2). Table V shows the estimated FVCs of the individual lung lobes for all subjects. By using this table, we may predict FVC after LDLLT. For example, assume the left lower lobe of subject A and the right lower lobe of subject B are transplanted into a recipient. In this case, after LDLLT, FVC of the recipient can be predicted as 2217.4 cc (=1026.2 cc + 1191.1 cc), and FVC of two donors, subject A and subject B, will be 2413.8 cc (=3440 cc - 1026.2 cc) and 2588.9 cc (=3780cc -1191.1 cc), respectively. In the similar way, FVC after LDLLT with the other combination of donors can be predicted. Thus, by using this technique, we might choose the better donors for the recipient. Of course, FVC after LDLLT will be affected by the other factors. Therefore, we should validate this technique in the future.

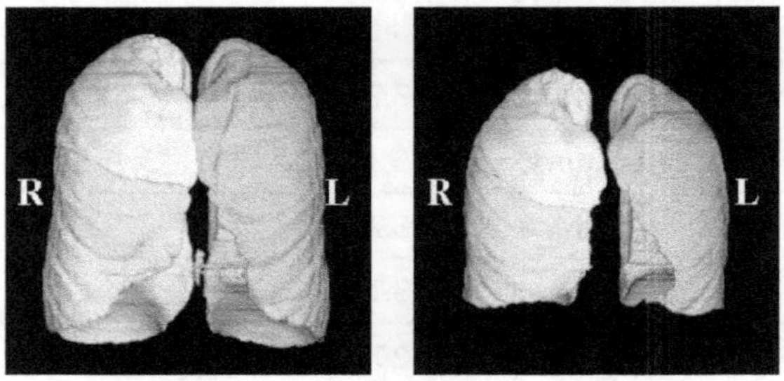

(a) Subject A.

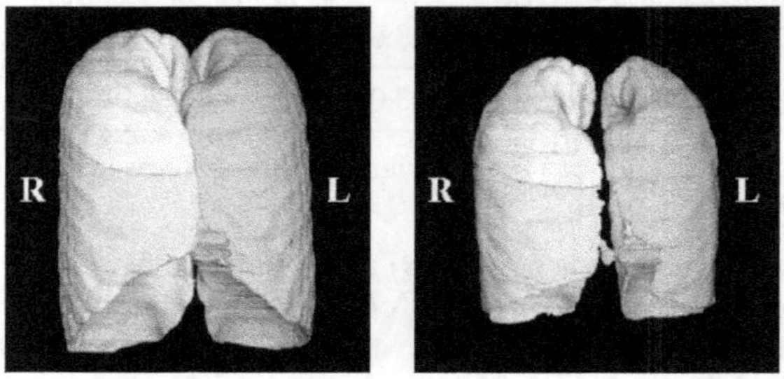

(b) Subject B.

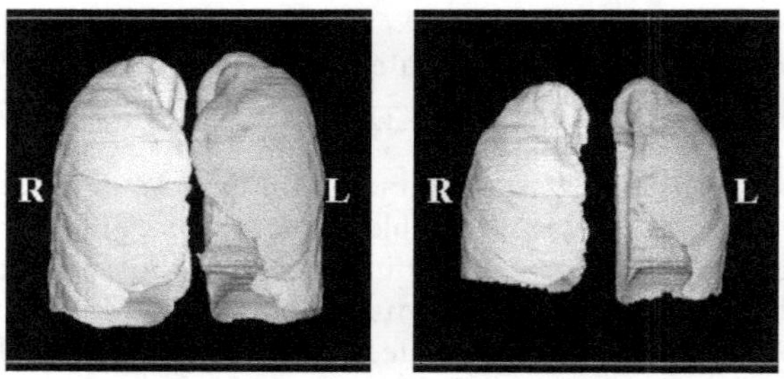

(c) Subject C.

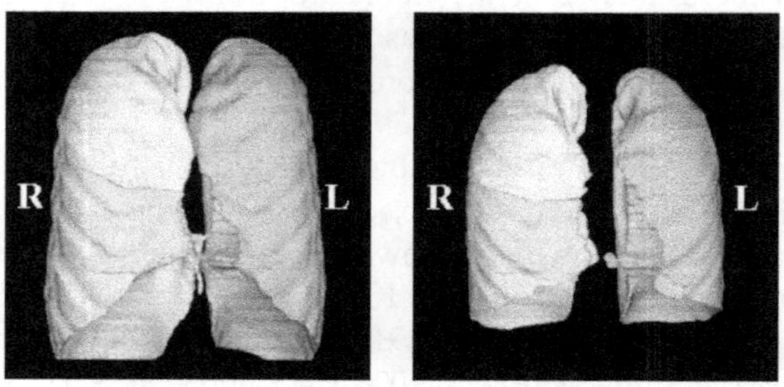

(d) Subject D.

Fig. 4. SSD images of segmentation results; left and right; the segmentation results of a subject with inspiratory and expiratory, respectively. Different lung lobes are displayed with the different colours.

			Left Upper	Left Lower	Right Upper	Right Middle	Right Lower
A	Inspiratory	Truth	1157	1408	938	451	1604
		Estimated	1169	1396	937	452	1604
		error ratio	1.0%	-0.9%	-0.1%	0.2%	0.0%
	Expiratory	Truth	683	645	565	298	883
		Estimated	673	655	571	294	881
		error ratio	-1.5%	1.6%	1.1%	-1.3%	-0.2%
B	Inspiratory	Truth	1207	1709	937	496	1814
		Estimated	1213	1703	942	493	1811
		error ratio	0.5%	-0.4%	0.5%	-0.6%	-0.2%
	Expiratory	Truth	740	834	561	338	945
		Estimated	744	830	571	326	946
		error ratio	0.5%	-0.5%	1.8%	-3.6%	0.1%
C	Inspiratory	Truth	1058	1111	779	362	1266
		Estimated	1039	1130	771	348	1288
		error ratio	-1.8%	1.7%	-1.0%	-3.9%	1.7%
	Expiratory	Truth	584	479	440	205	636
		Estimated	575	487	426	210	644
		error ratio	-1.5%	1.7%	-3.2%	2.4%	1.3%
D	Inspiratory	Truth	1150	1486	999	454	1661
		Estimated	1168	1469	993	458	1665
		error ratio	1.6%	-1.1%	-0.6%	0.9%	0.2%
	Expiratory	Truth	623	684	530	277	817
		Estimated	623	684	535	275	812
		error ratio	0.0%	0.0%	0.9%	-0.7%	-0.6%
Inspiratory		absolute mean	1.2%	1.0%	0.6%	1.4%	0.5%
Expiratory		absolute mean	0.9%	0.9%	1.7%	2.0%	0.6%
Total		absolute mean	1.1%	1.0%	1.2%	1.7%	0.5%

Table III. Estimated lung lobe volumes with the proposed method (cc).

Subject	Left Upper	Left Lower	Right Upper	Right Middle	Right Lower
A	20.0%	29.8%	14.7%	6.4%	29.1%
B	17.1%	31.8%	13.5%	6.1%	31.5%
C	20.8%	28.8%	15.4%	6.2%	28.8%
D	19.3%	27.8%	16.2%	6.5%	30.2%
Mean	19.3%	29.6%	15.0%	6.3%	29.9%
Conv. fixed parameter	21.1% (=4/19)	26.3% (=5/19)	15.8% (=3/19)	10.5% (=2/19)	26.3% (=5/19)

Table IV. Estimated contribution ratios of the individual lung lobes. "Conv. fixed parameters" are parameters introduced by Data et al (2003b).

Subject	Whole lung	Left Upper	Left Lower	Right Upper	Right Middle	Right Lower
A	3440	686.9	1026.2	506.9	218.8	1001.3
B	3780	645.8	1202.2	510.9	230.0	1191.1
C	2890	600.3	831.8	446.3	178.5	833.1
D	3980	768.1	1106.3	645.5	257.9	1202.2

Table V. Estimated FVCs of lung lobes with the proposed method (cc). The whole lung FVC was measured by spirometry, and the others were estimated by the proposed method.

7. Conclusion

This chapter presents a novel method for estimating individual lung lobe FVC with MDCT images. The new method can be applied to chest MDCT images with lacked fissures. Moreover, this will be the first attempt to estimate the individual lung lobe FVC. In the future, we should validate the estimated individual lung lobe FVC. In addition, the effectiveness of this technique will be discussed through future clinical studies.

8. References

Date, H.; Aoe, M.; Nagahiro, I.; Sano, Y.; Andou, A.; Matsubara, H.; Goto, K.; Tedoriya, T. & Shimizu, N. (2003). Living-donor lobar lung transplantation for various lung diseases, *The Journal of Thoracic and Cardiovascular Surgery*, Vol. 126, No. 2, pp. 476-481.

Date, H.; Aoe, M.; Sano, Y.; Nagahiro, I.; Andou, A.; Matsubara, H.; Goto, K.; Tedoriya, T. & Shimizu, N. (2003). How to predict forced vital capacity of the recipient after living-donor lobar lung transplantation, *The Journal of Heart and Lung Transplantation*, Vol. 22, No. 1, pp. S181-S181.

Han, H. & Ikuta, A. (2007) Returning to the Starting Point of the "Fuzzy Control", *Int. J. Innovative Computing, Information and Control*, vol.3, no.2, pp.319-333.

Kirby, T. J. & Rice, T. W. (1993). Thoracoscopic lobectomy, *The Annals of Thoracic Surgery*, Vol. 56, pp.784-786.

Kobashi, S. & Hata, Y. (2010). Lung Lobar Segmentation Using Tubular Tissue Density from Multidetector-row CT images, *International Journal of Innovative Computing, Information and Control*, Vol. 6, No. 3(A), pp. 829-842.

Mori, K.; Hasegawa, J.; Suenaga Y. & Toriwaki, J. (2000). Automated anatomical labeling of the bronchial branch and its application to the virtual bronchoscopy system, *IEEE Trans. on Medical Imaging*, Vol.19, No.2, pp.103-114.

Saita, S.; Yasutomo, M.; Kubo, M.; Kawata, Y.; Niki, N.; Eguchi, K.; Ohmatsu, H.; Kakinuma, R.; Kaneko, M.; Kusumoto, M.; Moriyama, N. & Sasagawa, M. (2004). An extraction algorithm of pulmonary fissures from multi-slice CT image, *Proc. SPIE Conf. Medical Imaging*, Vol. 5370, pp. 1590–1597.

Zhou, X.; Hayashi, T.; Hara, T.; Fujita, H.; Yokoyama, R.; Kiryu, T. & Hoshi, H. (2004). Automatic recognition of lung lobes and fissures from multi-slice CT images, *Proc. SPIE Conf. Medical Imaging*, Vol. 5370, pp. 1629–1633.

7

AutoCAD for Quantitative Measurement of Cervical MPR CT Images Reconstructed in ImageViewer Interface

Hou Lisheng, Ruan Dike, Cui Hongpeng and Bai Xuedong
Orthopaedic Department, Navy General Hospital, Beijing
The People's Republic of China

1. Introduction

As surgical skills develop in spinal field, transpedicular screw fixation of the lower thoracic, thoracolumbar, and lumbar spines have already been performed successfully, even using freehand technique by trained surgeons. The benefits of transpedicular screw fixation are widely accepted in the thoracolumbar spinal region for very stable fixation effect. Abumi et al first introduced transpedicular screw fixation in the subaxial cervical spinal region in 1991 and reported their initial clinical results in 1994 [1]. Since then, some other spinal surgeons began to accept transpedicular screw fixation in the subaxial cervical region as one choice [5]. But whether this fixation method can be accepted widely as a routine choice has been disputed till now. The main concern comes from the potential violation of the pedicle cortices and following damages to adjacent neurovascular structures [6][12]. To diminish subaxial cervical pedicle (SCP) screw malposition ratio as low as possible and to ensure successful clinical results, the complex morphologic features and projections of subaxial cervical pedicles should be clearly understood. That is, the exact diameter, inclinations at transverse and sagittal plane, cortical thicknesses at different orientations, and cortical thicknesses adjacent to pedicle entrance should be determined before any transpedicular screw fixation was performed, even by experienced surgeons using meticulous surgical techniques[Fig.1]. Although morphologic studies of the cervical spine have been reported as a way to evaluate the feasibility and safety of the technique, many have focused on transverse diameter of the pedicles, which is far from enough [3].Thorough understanding of the subaxial cervical spinal pedicle anatomy is mandatory to avoid injury to the vertebral artery, spinal cord or a nerve root [8][11][14].

Because of their inherent ability to render bony anatomy in three dimensions, CT scans can provide the best osseous detail of subaxial cervical pedicles. Volumetric CT could reconstruct multiplanar CT images based on raw sequential transaxial CT images [7]. Multiple planar reconstruction (MPR) CT images could provide vivid anatomic data of subaxial cervical pedicles at different planes and different orientations for further detailed study. MPR CT images can be reconstructed using the CT-machine attached Advantage Workstation. If time permitted, quantitative measurement of MPR CT images can be fulfilled using the measurement tools of the CT machine-attached Advantage Workstation. But in clinical practice, large clinical CT scanning tasks are under schedule , the Advantage

Workstation could only fulfil routine MPR reconstruction and measurement work; it is not realistic to reconstruct wanted subaxial cervical MPR CT images and to finish quantitative measurement using the measurement tools of the Workstation at every time (Fig. 2) . Also, one could not expect that a CT-machine operator could reconstruct satisfied MPR CT images and finish relative measurement as a spinal surgeon really needed. If primary MPR CT images are not qualified, reviewing or reconstructing more MPR images based on raw CT data for further observation and quantitative measurement becomes more difficult. One feasible substitute choice is to develop other software which is free of CT-machine and could fulfil reconstructing satisfied MPR CT images and quantitative measurement based on raw transaxial CT images at a free computer.

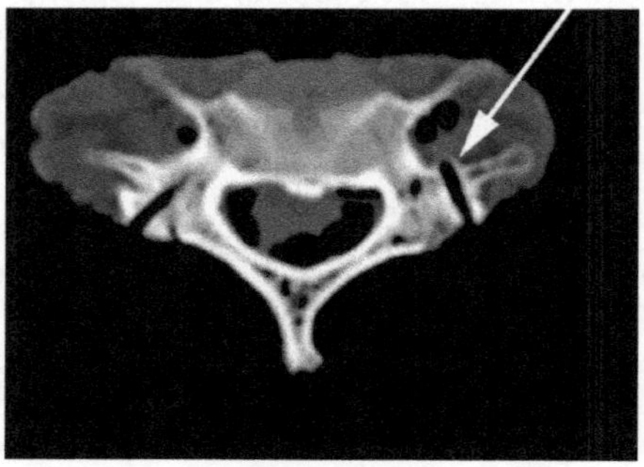

Fig. 1. Lateral wall violation of mispositioned screw trajectory

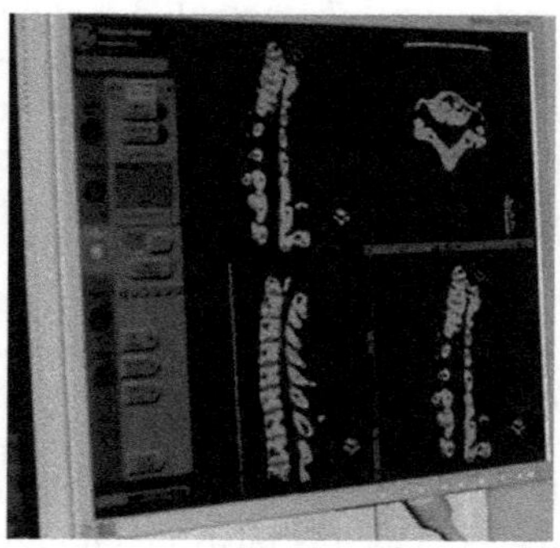

Fig. 2. It is not realistic to finish quantitative measurement using the measurement tools of the CT machine-attached Advantage workstation at every time

To some extent, we found ImageViewer software could fulfil this requirement. The software is one sharestation of Silver picture archiving and communication system (PACS) which was developed by Beijing Silver medical information Technical Corporation Limited of People's Republic of China (webdress: http://www. minipacs. com). The software could provide qualified electronic MPR CT images with reference ruler present based on sequential raw transaxial CT images (Fig.3). However this software also has some defects; for example, it could not finish electronic measurements on reconstructed MPR CT images. Later we found this defect could be compensated by AutoCAD software with the help of Adobe Photoshop software.

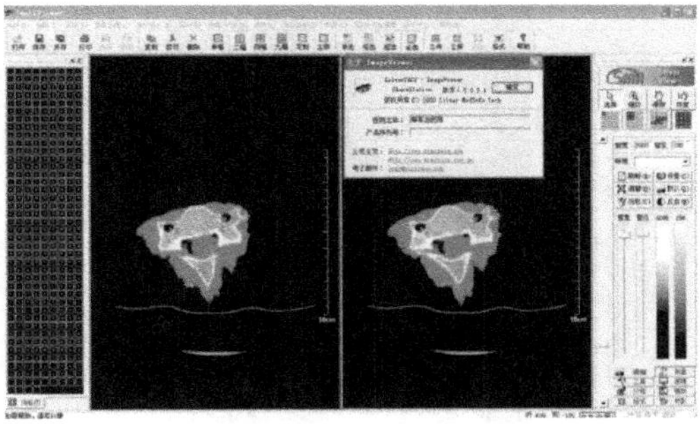

Fig. 3. Raw CT image opened in ImageViewer interface (Chinese Version)

In this chapter we describe the technique of using AutoCAD2010 software to perform quantitative electronic measurement on subaxial cervical MPR CT images which were reconstructed with Imageviewer interface of Silver PACS software at the basis of sequential raw tranaxial CT images. As the morphology of SCP and quantitative anatomical data were got, unsuitable pedicles were rejected; successful subaxial cervical transpedicular screw fixation could be finished.

2. Important

To ensure accuracy of subaxial cervical transpedicular fixation, the pedicle's morphology and orientation must be clearly understood preoperatively. Multiple planar reconstructed (MPR) CT images can provide vivid MPR images for detailed observation (Fig.4). Meanwhile, quantitative electronic measurement of these images can be fulfilled using the measurement tools of the CT machine-attached Advantage Workstation. Theoretically, all needed quantitative data could be easily obtained at Advantage Workstation. But as large routine clinical CT scanning tasks and multiple planar reconstruction works are under schedule every day, it is not realistic to do extra MPR reconstructions and quantitative electronic measurement of subaxial cervical pedicles at Advantage Workstation every time as one spinal surgeon really needs. If there exists some other software which can fulfil the multiple reconstruction work meanwhile fulfil quantitative measurement which is free of CT machine, that would be a good substitute solution method. ImageViewer software is one sharestation of Silver picture archiving and communication system (PACS), it was developed by Beijing Silver medical information Technical Corporation Limited and has been authorized to our hospital. Primarily the software was developed to provide online command dashboard screen observation of raw CT images at remote terminal computers; meanwhile it also could reconstruct qualified electronic MPR CT images with reference ruler present by reformatted method based on sequential raw transaxial CT images (Fig.2). Also the software could finish some primary linear and angular measurement on raw digital images, although not accurate. To our great pity, it could not finish electronic measurements on reconstructed MPR CT images.
To compensate this defect, we used the computer's PrtSc key to capture a snapshot of the computer screen which was exhibiting the electronic MPR CT images with reference ruler present at ImageViewer interface, and pasted it to a new opened file which was created in Adobe Photoshop CS software and used the *crop* tool to crop the needed image region and saved it as in JPG format [2]. The JPG format image was then inserted to opened AutoCAD file as raster image to finish electronic quantitative measurement. By such steps, the morphology of SCP and quantitative anatomical data could be gotten successfully.

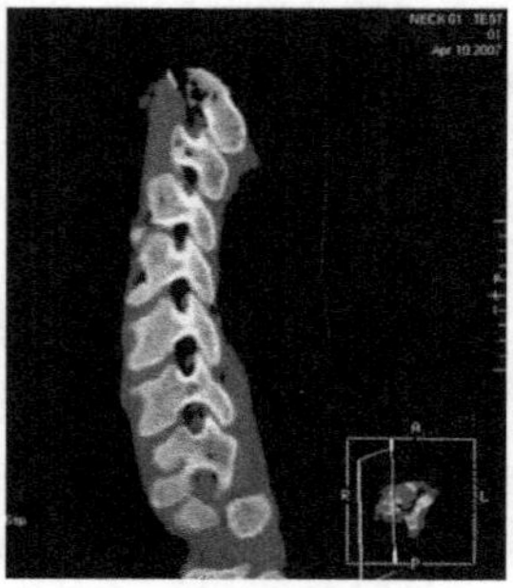

Fig. 4. Reconstructed sagittal CT images at CT machine-attached Advantage Workstation

Based on these data, we fulfilled successful subaxial cervical transpedicular screw fixation manipulation. In this chapter, we introduce the details of using AutoCAD2010 software[3] to perform quantitative electronic measurement on subaxial cervical MPR CT images which were reconstructed with ImageViewer interface of Silver PACS software at the basis of sequential raw transaxial CT images.
As the raster images opened in AutoCAD program were not real digitized images but JPG format ones. The precision is still limited, to some extent. Also, the procedures were tedious. In the near future, we hope new version of ImageViewer software can be developed to fulfil electronic quantitative measurement on MPR CT images.

3. Content

3.1 Getting raw transaxial CT images

Volumetric CT ((GE, LightSpeed 16) scanning was performed on cervical spine samples with the samples on prone position one by one. We made sure the samples' longitudinal axes were parallel to the CT machine's longitudinal axis. The scan length was kept constant as 5-mm thickness. The entire subaxial cervical region was enrolled within the scanning region (Fig. 5).

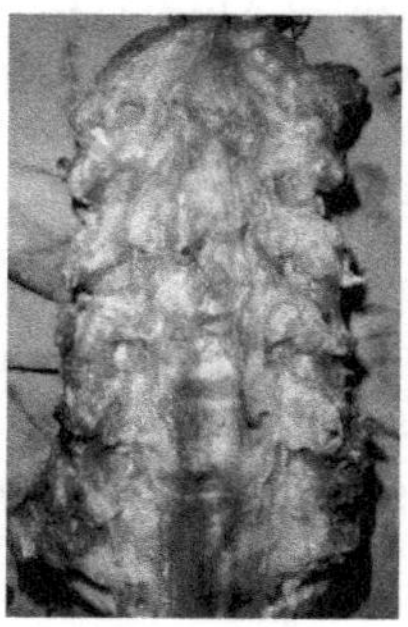

Fig. 5. Cervical spine sample

Sequential raw transaxial CT image data of each sample were then generated by interpolation reconstruction method for a 0.625-mm thickness at 0.625 mm reconstruction intervals and saved as digital imaging and communication in medicine (Dicom) format documents using the CT machine-attached Advantage Workstation software. These image data could be stored in Disk array machine, so that they could be observed online at a remote terminal computer or downloaded to hard disc of a terminal computer through Picture Archiving and Communication System (PACS)[6]. These data could also be directly burned to a compact disc or saved to a USB (Universal Serial Bus) flash disk. Here chose to burn the data to a compact disc.

3.2 Reconstructing MPR CT images using the post-processing function of ImageViewer software

Installed Imageviewer software to its default location on our personal computer. The software could also be installed to any other location.

(1). Starting ImageViewer

ImageViewer is a very good Windows program, we could make the program window appear on-screen in numerous ways.

1. On the Windows *taskbar*, click *Start*, point to *All Programs*, point to *ImageViewer* button, then click;
2. Open the ImageViewer folder, double-click the ImageViewer program icon
3. During installing process, we chose to create an ImageViewer shortcut icon on our computer desktop. So, double-clicking the shortcut icon also could start the program.

The running ImageViewer program window was shown as Fig.6

Fig. 6. The ImageViewer Interface Window

The *title bar* locates at the top of the screen, a *menu* bar just below it, a *standard* toolbar is below the *menu* bar, and a floating *integrated toolbox* pane on the right, which are very like those found in Microsoft Office System program window. If you have installed this softare, what you see on your screen might not match the graphics in Fig.5 exactly. That depends whether toolbars are chosen *hide* or *show*. The settings could be toggled by clicking their relative buttons on *View* menu's subcommands.

(2). Opening raw sequential CT images

1. On the *Standard* toolbar of the ImageViewer , click the *Open* button. Or press Ctrl +O to open *the Open dialog box*.
2. In *the Open dialog box*, navigate to the folder that contains the sequential raw CT images.
3. Chose the sequential images that we want to open, then press Alt+O , or click the *Open* button, the chosen images will display (Fig.7). The image numbers displayed in the work area may vary. This depends on what display pattern we chose. Click relative *display settings* buttons on the *standard* toolbar, then the display pattern would change to fulfil our request (Fig. 8).

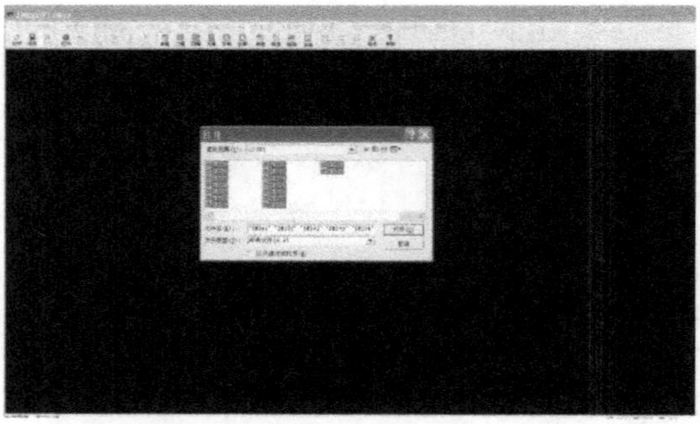

Fig. 7. To navigate to the folder which contains the raw CT images

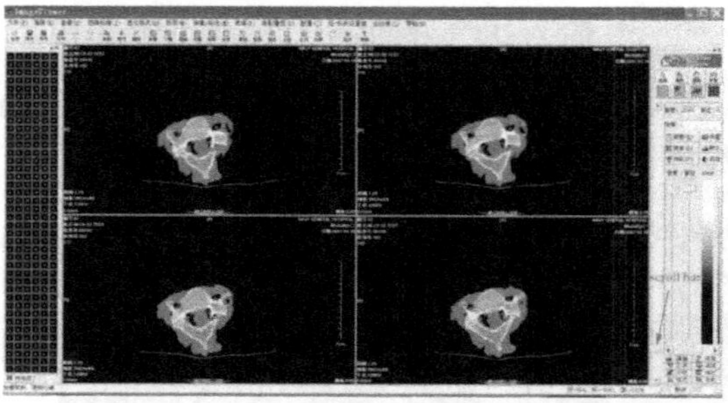

Fig. 8. Raw transaxial CT images opened at ImageViewer interface in sequence (four images in one work area).

Only a few of the images can be displayed on the screen. We could choose to display other images by clicking their relative thumbnails on the left, or by dragging the *Scroll bar* just right to the *work area.*

4. Deleting unnecessary images.

Following observation and identification, delete those raw images which are not belonged to the subaxial cervical spinal region from the folder (Fig.9~10).

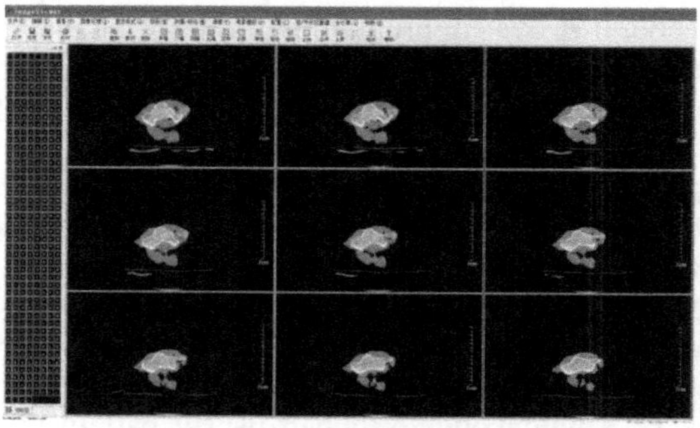

Fig. 9. Proximal transaxial images should be deleted(C1~2 spinal region, nine images in one work area)

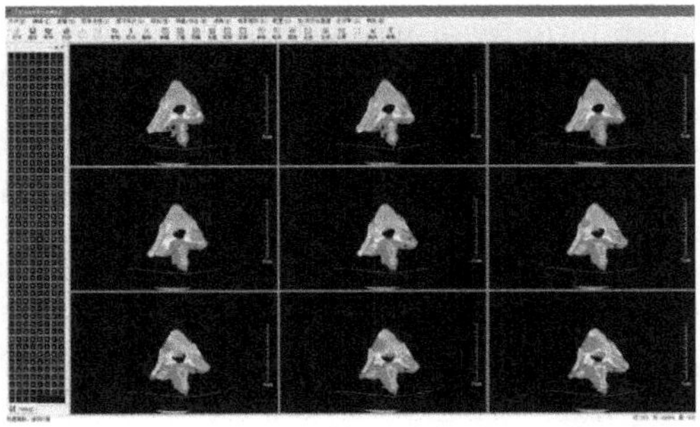

Fig. 10. Distal images should be deleted (upper thoracic spinal region)

5. Reconstructing MPR CT images

Click *delete* button on the *standard* toolbar to delete all the displayed images at the work area (the original images still exist in the folder). Then open all the images which should be included in the reconstruction region from the folder again, then clicked the *coronal/sagittal reconstruction* menu and scroll down to choose *begin reconstructing* icon and click (Fig.11). The MPR CT images with reference ruler then appear (Fig. 12). At this step, the raw axial images are used for guiding as a reference.

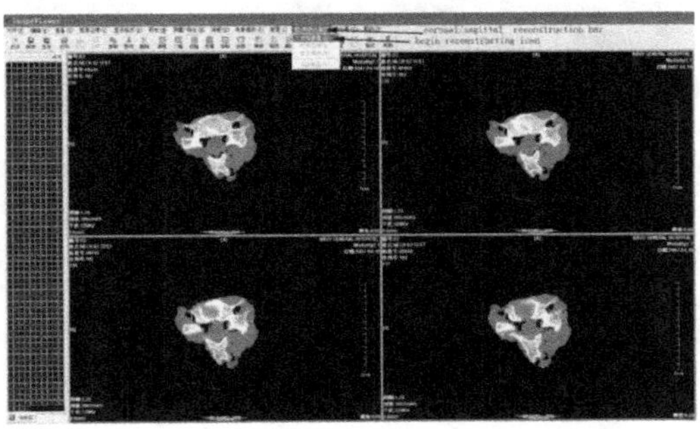

Fig. 11. To click *begin reconstructing* icon

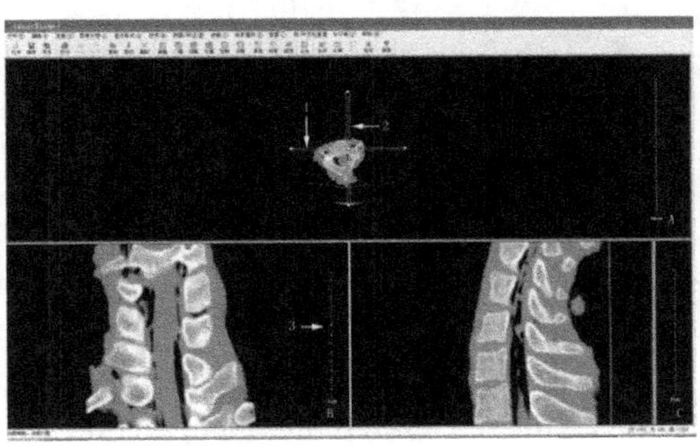

Fig. 12. Reconstructed MPR CT images at ImageViewer interface. A: Raw transverse CT image (act as localizer); B: Reconstructed coronal CT image ;C: Reconstructed sagittal CT image. 1.Localizer indicates coronal reconstructing plane; 2.Localizer indicates sagittal reconstructing plane;3.Reference ruler at coronal reconstructed CT image interface

The raw CT images chosen for reconstruction must be in sequence, neither repeated, nor interrupted images are permitted. Or the reconstruction couldn't be fulfilled.

6. Adjusting required MPR images

Mov the mouse cursor to the raw axial CT image(Fig. 13A), and choose the coronal reconstructing plane localizer (Fig.12,arrow1) then drag the coronal localizer to proper position and inclination. During this process, the reconstructed coronal CT image will change simultaneously. The same can be done to sagittal reconstructing plane localizer (Fig. 13, arrow3). By such process, the real coronal MPR image which was perpendicular to the longitudinal axis of the pedicle and sagittal MPR image which just bisects the pedicle along its longitudinal axis are reconstructed. The lateral cortex is confirmed to be the thinnest (Fig.13-B).

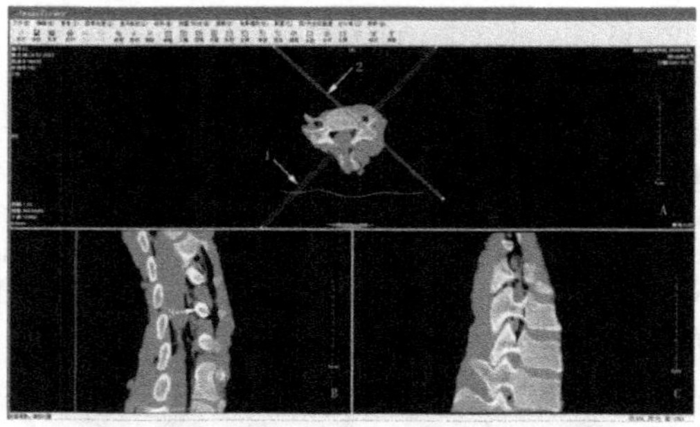

Fig. 13. To drag the localizers to suitable position and angulation to recontruct satisfied MPR images. A: Raw transverse CT image (acted as localizer); B: Reconstructed requierd coronal CT image; C: Reconstructed required sagittal CT image. 1.Localizer indicates coronal reconstructing plane;2.Localizer indicates sagittal reconstructing plane.3.Recontructed coronal image of subaxial cervical pedicle; 4.Reconstructed sagittal image of subaxial cervical pedicle

7. Adjusting the size of MPR images

Select the *zoom* tool from the floating *integrated toolbox* pane on the far right side of the work area, or click the *"image"* menu and scroll down to choose *"zoom"* subcommand icon and

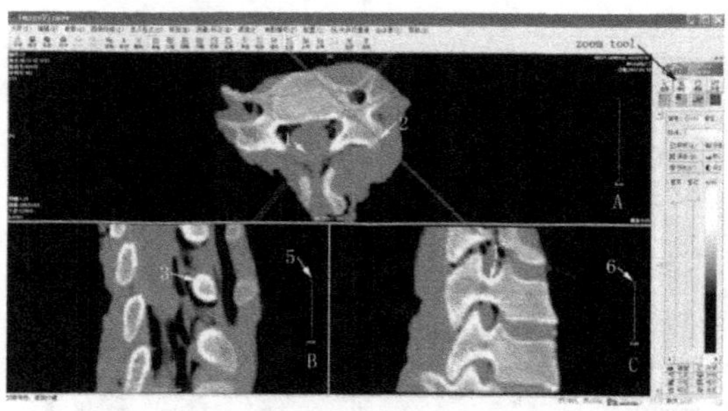

Fig. 14. To Select the zoom tool to magnify the raw CT image, the reconstructed MPR images maginfied simultaneously with the reference rulers changing too.A:Magnified raw transaxial CT image;B:Reconstructed coronal CT image(magnified);C: Reconstructed sagittal CT imgage(magnified). 1.Localizer indicated coronal reconstructing plane;2.Localizer indicated sagittal reconstructing plane;3.Recontructed coronal image of subaxial cervical pedicle; 4.Reconstructed sagittal image of subaxial cervical pedicle;5.Changed reference ruler at coronal MPR image interface;6.Changed reference ruler at sagittal MPR image.

click. Then move the cursor over the raw transaxial CT image area (Fig.14-A), the cursor would look like a tiny magnifying glass with a plus sign (+) in the center. Presse the left key of the mouse and drag the cursor downwards or rightwards, the raw image can be enlarged. Meanwhile, the reconstructed coronal and sagittal MPR images will enlarge with the reference rulers changing simultaneously. If we drag the cursor upwards or leftwards, the raw and reconstructed images would diminish simultaneouly.

8. To reconstruct MPR images from only one vertebral raw transaxial CT images

We could also choose part of sequential raw transaxial CT images which mainly come from only real vertebra, thus the reconstructed MPR images only displayed the proper CT images of one vertebral structure (Fig.15).

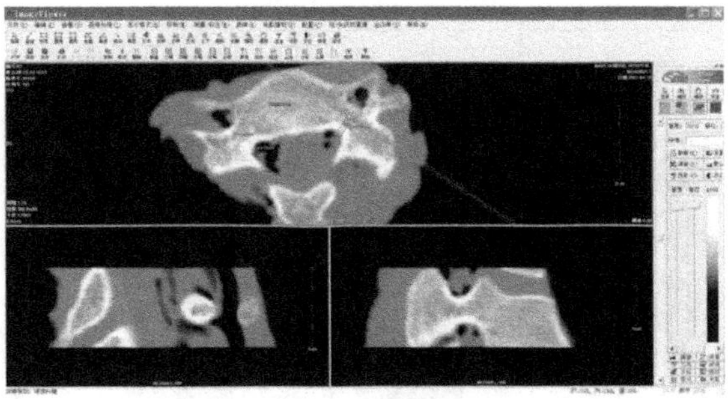

Fig. 15. Reformatted MPR CT imges from sequential raw transaxial CT images of only one cervical vertebra

(3). Simple and rough linear and angular measurement of raw transaxial CT image.

Chose *line* icon at the *measure* toolbar (Tip: we could click *View* button on the *standard* menu and then click the *measure toolbar* subcommand button to show the toolbar if it was hidden). We could finish rough linear measurement at raw transaxial CT image. If we chose *angular* icon, the angular measurement could be finished on raw CT images. But linear or angular measurement could not be fulfilled at reconstructed MPR image (Fig 15). The linear measurement precision is limited as 0mm. Angular measurement precision is 0.0^0. Compared to the measurement precision that AutoCAD could provide, the values are rougher.

3.3 Creating .JPG documents of MPR CT images with Adobe Photoshop CS

(1). Capturing a snapshot of the computer screen

First press *Windows Print Screen* Key to capture a snapshot of the computer screen which exhibits the ImageViewer interface with the raw CT and reformatted CT images and copy the snapshot to the clipboard

(2). Creating a new image document with Adobe Photoshop CS.

Firstly, start Adobe Photoshop CS program to open the Photoshop interface, then press Ctrl+N to create a new image document. After this, the *New* Dialog Box appears. On the *New* dialog box, choose *resolution* as 300 pixels/inch, *color mode* as RGB color, *background contents* as white, then click *OK*(Fig. 16). The new document work area appears.

Following , press Ctrl+V, the snapshot will be pasted to the new created document as a new layer (Fig. 17).

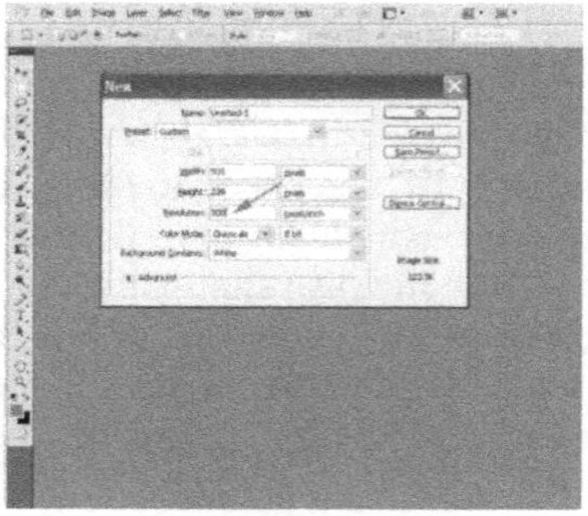

Fig. 16. To create a new document with Adobe Photoshop

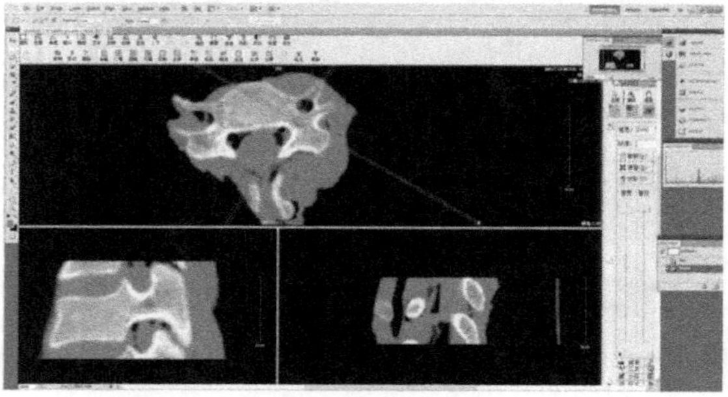

Fig. 17. To paste the snapshot in the new created document opened in Adobe Photoshop

(3). Editing image

Choose *rectangular marquee tool* at the toolbox (locate at the left side of the work area). Then move the cursor over the image window, drag the cursor to draw a rectangule around the required image area and then release the mouse button. An animated dashed line indicates that the area inside it is selected.

Click the *Image* menu and drag down to select the *crop* icon, and then click. Only the selected image is left (Fig. 18).

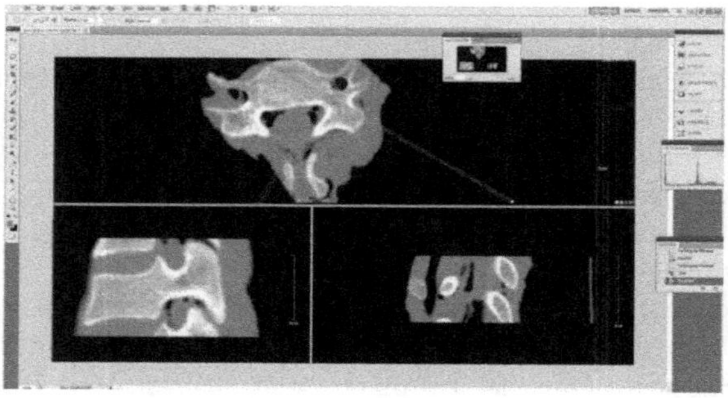

Fig. 18. Only selected area is left after clicking Crop icon

Following , click the *layer* menu and drag down to select the *merge layer* icon to merge the two layers together.

(4). Saving the merged image document as .JPG image
Click the *File* menu and drag down to select *save as* icon, the *Save As* dialog box appears, saved the image as .JPG document to destined folder for further use[3] (Fig.19).

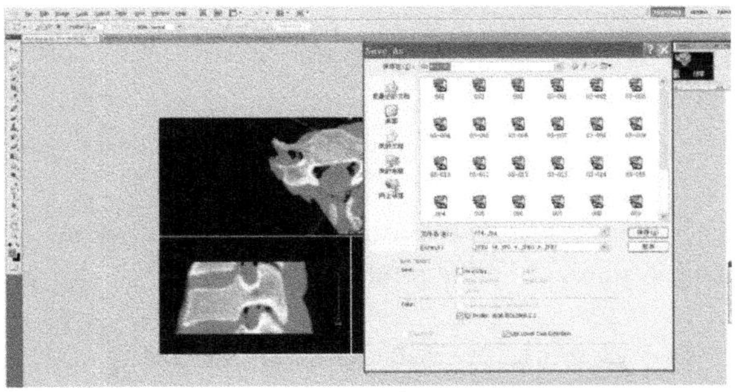

Fig. 19. To save the selected area as .JPG document

3.4 Finishing electronic quantitative measurement of MPR CT images using AutoCAD 2010

(1). Starting AutoCAD 2010
We can select one of the following to start AutoCAD:

1. Double-click the AutoCAD shortcut icon on the desktop.
2. Click the Start button→(All) Programs→Autodesk→AutoCAD 2010→ AutoCAD2010 icon, then clicked.

After this step, the *New Features Workshop* box appears, select the *Maybe Later* option on the left and click *OK* (Fig.20). The AutoCAD program window will appear.

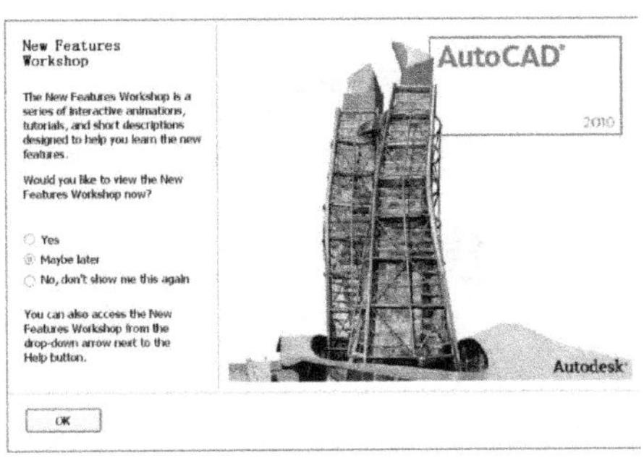

Fig. 20. To select *Maybe later* option when encounter the *New Features Workshop*

(2). (2)Inserting MPR CT image as raster image
We did the followings:

1. On the ribbon, click the *Insert* tab.
2. On the *Reference* panel, click the *attach* button (Fig. 21), the *Select Reference File* box will appear (Fig .22).

On the "*Select Reference File*" box, navigate to the folder that contains the MPR CT images. Then browse to the raster image file (.JPG format) that we want to attach (the image we want to fulfil quantitative measurement in AutoCAD) and select it, then click *Open* (Fig.22).

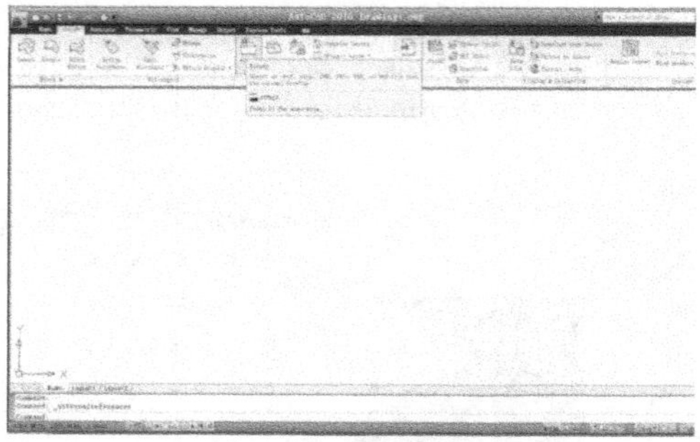

Fig. 21. To access attach command on the reference panel

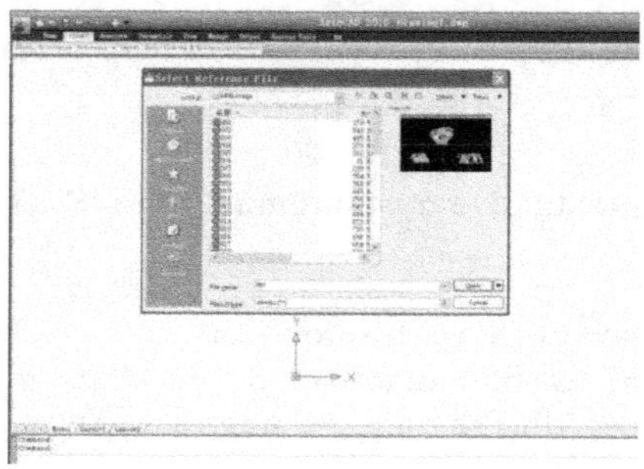

Fig. 22. To choose the image that we wanted to measure

The *Select Image File* dialog box closes, and the *Attach Image dialog* box appears. Click *Details* button to display additional information about the selected image (Fig. 23).

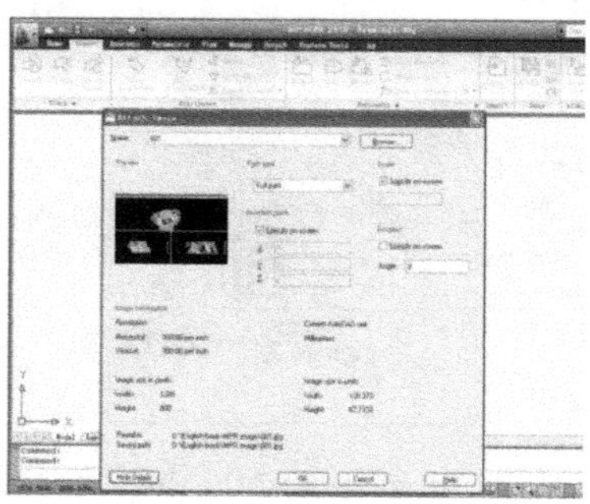

Fig. 23. To attach a raster image reference

The path to and the name of the file we selected appear in the *Found In* and *Saved Path* fields, respectively. The *Name drop-down list* allows us to select a previously attached raster image file, and *Browse* allows us to specify a different raster image file to reference. The *Image Information* area provides feedback on how the image would be scaled when it is inserted. We could also click *Hide Details* button to hide the additional information.

In the Path Type area, we specify the path format as full path. In the Insertion Point area, choose <0,0,0>,in the *Scale* area, choose <1>, in the *Rotation* area, choose <0>, then press *OK* button (we could also choose other choices). The selected MPR image appears at AutoCAD work area.

(3). Adjusting the image to proper location and proper magnified extent.

Move the cursor to work area, then right-clicked the mouse to display shortcut menu and chose *zoom* button (Fig.24).

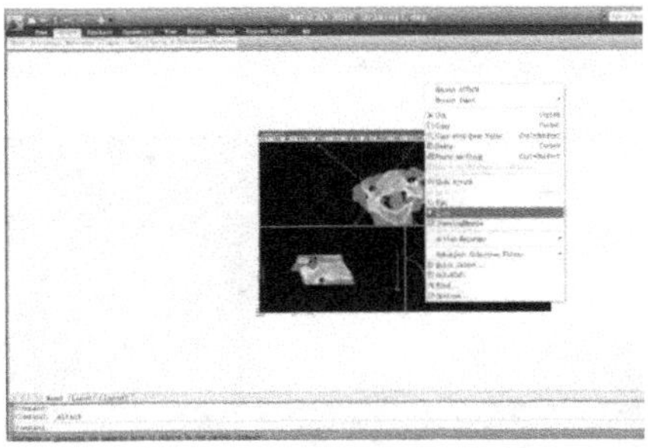

Fig. 24. To choose *zoom* shortcut

We then right-clicked the mouse again to display *zoom* menu shortcut and chose *zoom extends* button, the inserted image fitted the whole window (Fig.25).

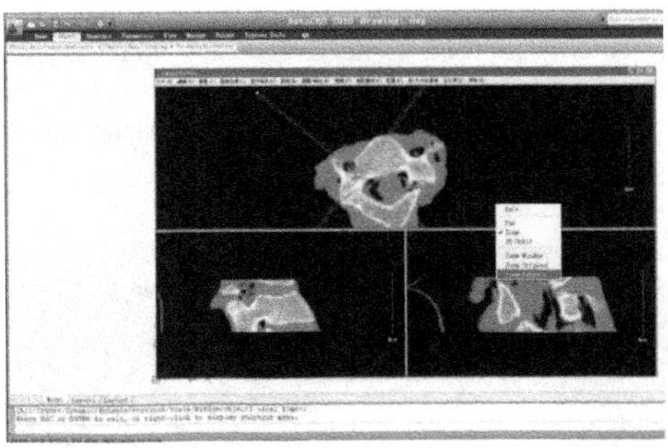

Fig. 25. To choose *zoom extents* to make the image occupy the whole active window area.

Then we moved the portion that we wanted to measure to the center of the window screen and adjusted it to suitable size by using *pan* and *zoom* icons' functions alternatively (Fig.26).

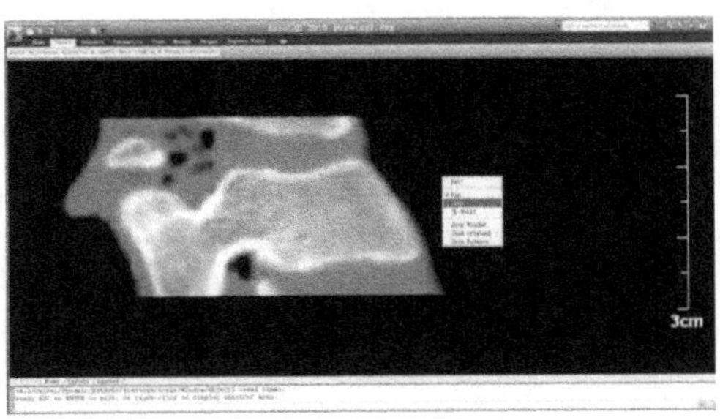

Fig. 26. To move the measured portion to the center of the active window screen by *pan* and *zoom* buttons alternatively.

(4). Adjusting reference factor for accurate measurement

1. On the ribbon, click the *Home* tab.
2. On the *Draw* panel, click the *point* button.
3. Then draw *point* objects at the start point and end point of the reference ruler of the MPR image, respectively. Later, they are chosen as specified node points for the origins of dimensions (Fig .27).

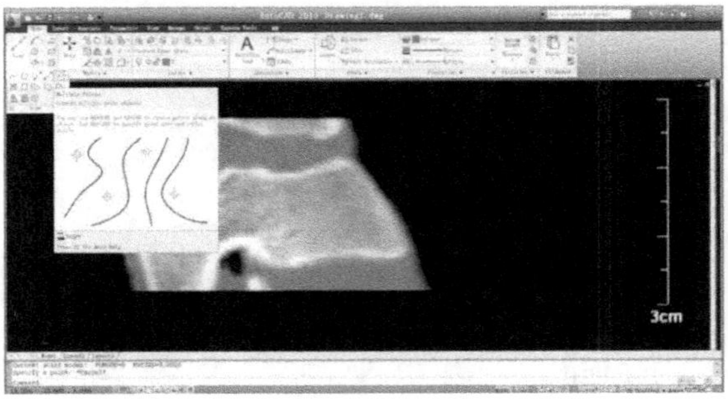

Fig. 27. To draw point objects for the origins of dimensions

4. Toggling the *Object Snaps* on for correct measurement.

Object snaps let one pick a precise point. We use *object snaps* to make sure that the dimensions are created with the correct measurement. *Node* objects are chosen as specified points. Clicking the *Object Snap* button toggles the *Object Snap* on if it is off, then right-click the *Object Snap* (OSNAP) button on the *Status Bar* and toggle the *Node* object snaps on from the shortcut menu (Fig.28).

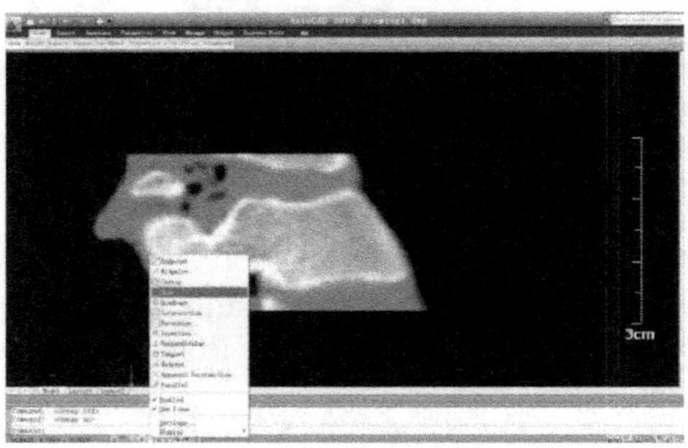

Fig. 28. To turn the *Node* object snap on from the shortcut menu.

5. Creating a new dimension style

Type *dimstyle* on the *command* line to display the *Dimension Style Manager* dialog box, then click *New* button. The *Create New Dimension Style* dialog box is displayed.

In the *New Style Name* text box, enter *reference* as the new name for the dimension style. In the *Start With* drop-down list, select *standard*. After this, click *continue* button. The *New Dimension Style* dialog box then is displayed. Click *OK* button to return to the *Dimension Style Manager* dialog box. Then click *Set Current* button to set the *reference* dimension style to current. Following click *Close* button to close the dialog box. The *reference* dimension style is applied to dimensions we created.

6. Creating a linear dimension

On the ribbon, click the *Annotate* tab. Then on the *Dimensions* panel, click the dimension flyout button and chosoe *linear* icon (Fig.29).

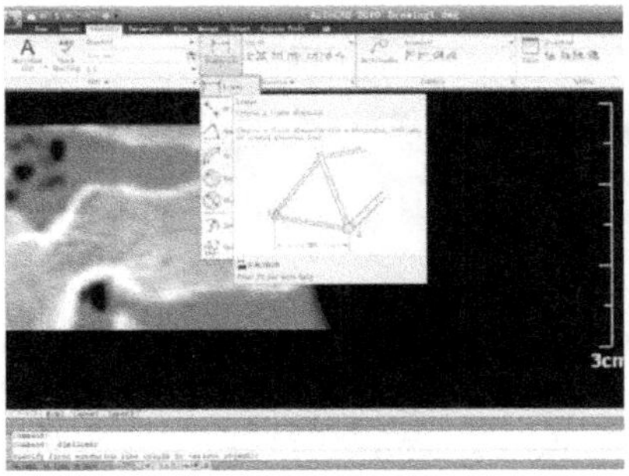

Fig. 29. To choose liner dimension

At the prompt, pick the node which had been drawn at the start location of the reference ruler for the first origin point of the dimension. After this, the prompt *Specify second extension line origin* is displayed. Then move the cursor to the second node which has been drawn at the end point of the reference ruler for the second origin point of the dimension and click. As the prompt *Specify dimension line location* is displayed, pick a point to place the dimension, the linear dimension will display. But the value is not identical to real reference ruler length (Fig.30).

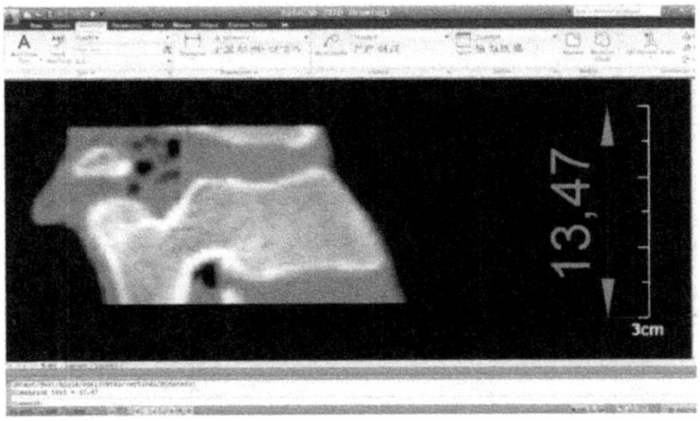

Fig. 30. Original vertical linear dimension is displayed

7. Displaying correct reference value by modifying the dimension style in use.

Type *dimstyle* on the *command* line to display the *Dimension style Manager* dialog box again. In the *Styles list* box, select reference, then click *Modify* button to display the *Modify Dimension Style* dialog box. In the *Modify Dimension Style dialog* box, click *Symbols and Arrows* tab, change the *arrow size* to desired size; click *Text* tab, chang the text height to desired height; click *Primary Units* tab, specified *Precision* as 0.0, *suffix* as mm, specify *measurement Scale factor* to a proper value, then click *OK* to save the changes to the *reference* dimension style and to close the *Modify Dimension Style* dialog box. Any dimensions using the modified style (reference) are automatically updated to reflect the changes. Here when we modify the *measurement Scale factor* to 2.2240, the vertical linear dimension value is identical to the real reference ruler length (30.0mm). By changing other styles proper value, the dimensions created are shown clearly on the computer screen (Fig.31).

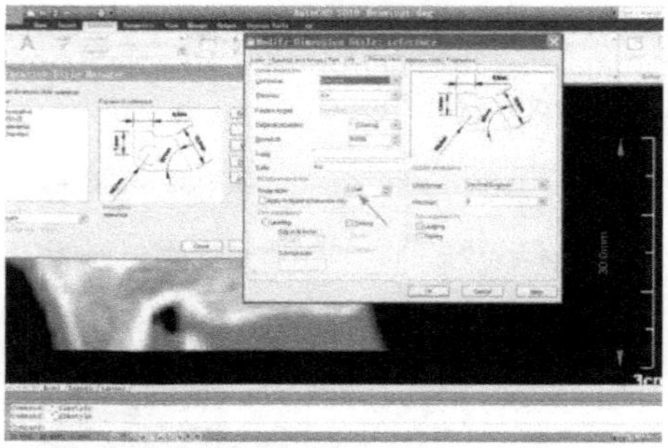

Fig. 31. To adjust *Scale factor* till the vertical linear dimension value changes identical to the reference ruler value the dimensions created can be observed clearly.

(5). Correct electronic quantitative measurement of the MPR CT images
To get correct linear distance values, operate as the followings:

1. On the ribbon, click the *Home* tab.
2. On the *Draw* panel, click the *point* button
3. Draw point objects at the MPR CT image's proper positions to identify the start point and end point for relative linear dimension display.
4. On the Dimensions panel, choose the aligned linear dimension button
5. Pick the *start* node and then the *end* node. Then relative aligned distance value displays (Fig.32). The value is just the one we want to get. Here the value's precision is 0.0mm. We could choose to change precision setting on the *Modify Dimension Style* dialog box as we like; Toggling *Object* snaps on and turning on the *Node* object snaps guarantee correct and precise measurement if the positions of point objects are positioned correct. As the start and end nodes are fixed, the aligned linear dimension value is determined identical, no matter what time we do the measurement.

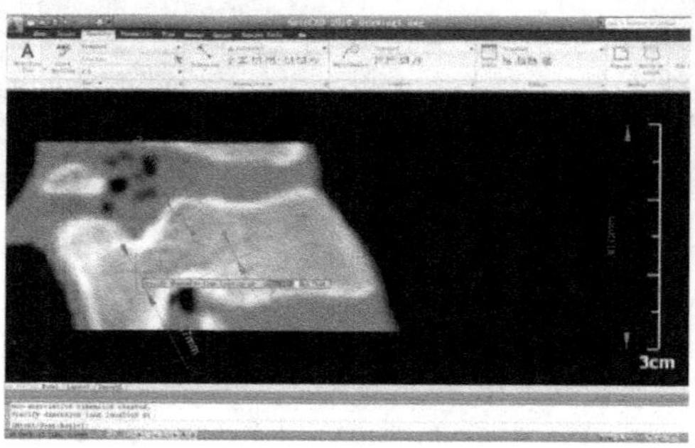

Fig. 32. Electronic quantitative measurement of the MPR sagittal CT image.

The reference ruler length at sagittal image is not identical to that at coronal image. We 'd first made correct reference value on coronal MPR CT image by modifying *scale factor* value at *Primary Units* tab in the *Modify Dimension Style* dialogue box, then repeat the same steps, the electronic quantitative measurement of the coronal CT image could be achieved successfully (Fig. 33).

Chose *Angular Dimension*, then the superior and medial angles of the pedicle can be displayed (Fig.34).

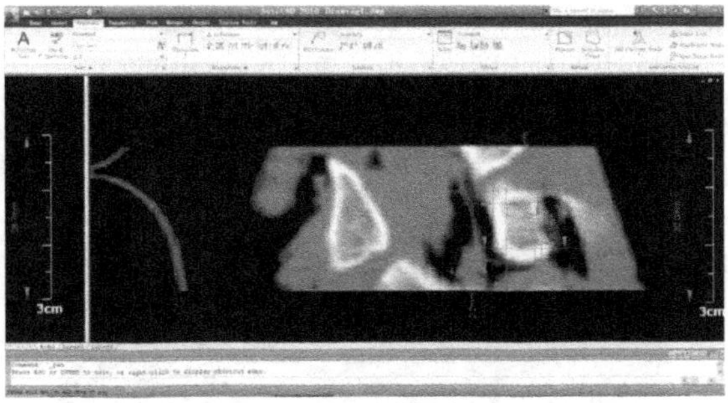

Fig. 33. To finish electronic quantitative measurement of the MPR coronal CT image

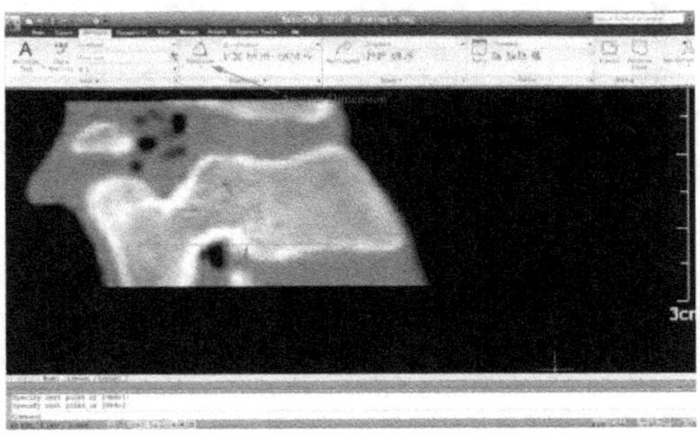

Fig. 34. To finish electronic quantitative angular measurement of the MPR sagittal CT image

We could also make correct electronic quantitative measurement of the raw Transaxial CT images if we are not satisfied with the values measured in ImageViewer software.
Repeat the above-mentioned steps, each pedicle's linear and angular quantitative data could be gotten precisely as desired.
The following table is some linear value data we got in eight subaxial cervical samples.

	MCP	LCP	SCP	ICP	ACL	ACS	ACI	PCT
C3	1.9±0.3 (1.3~2.1)	0.8±0.4 (0.3~1.2)	2.1±0.5 (1.5~2.7)	2.3±0.6 (1.9~3.2)	2.3±0.5 (1.6~2.9)	1.9±0.4 (1.6~2.7)	1.9±0.3 (1.5~2.2)	0.9±0.2 (0.8~1.2)
C4	2.3±0.7 (1.8~3.5)	1.4±0.4 (0.9~2.0)	2.4±0.5 (1.8~2.8)	2.2±0.4 (1.9~2.8)	2.2±0.3 (1.9~2.7)	2.1±0.3 (1.7~2.4)	2.5±0.6 (1.8~3.2)	0.9±0.4 (0.5~1.4)
C5	2.3±0.2 (2~2.6)	1.5±0.3 (1.1~1.8)	2.5±0.8 (1.8~3.6)	2.3±0.6 (1.9~3.3)	2.0±0.3 (1.7~2.5)	1.8±0.7 (1.3~3.3)	2.8±0.6 (1.8~3.8)	1.2±0.4 (0.8~1.8)
C6	1.9±0.2 (1.5~2.2)	1.2±0.2 (0.8~1.3)	2.4±0.6 (2.0~3.6)	2.3±0.5 (1.9~3.1)	1.7±0.2 (1.3~1.9)	1.8±0.3 (1.3~2.0)	2.8±0.4 (2.4~3.5)	1.0±0.3 (0.8~1.4)
C7	2.0±0.5 (1.5~2.8)	0.9±0.3 (0.5~1.3)	2.0±0.3 (1.6~2.5)	2.2±0.4 (1.6~2.7)	1.8±0.2 (1.6~2.2)	1.8±0.3 (1.5~2.2)	2.1±0.4 (1.6~2.5)	0.9±0.3 (0.6~1.3)

* MCP: medial cortex of pedicle. LCP:lateral cortex of pedicle SCP:superior cortex of pedicle. ICP: inferior cortex of pedicle ACL:anterior cortex of lamina ACS:anterior cortex of superior articularis ACI:anterior cortex of inferior articularis PCT posterior cortex of transverse foramen

Table 1. Cortex thickness measurement of subaxial pedicle and its adjacent structures

The results confirmed that the lateral cortex of the subaxial cervical pedicles was significantly thinner than medial, superior, and inferior counterparts.
Based on above-mentioned and other relative linear and angular values, we tried some new techniques to perform subaxial cervical transpedicular manipulation by hand. All suitable pedicles were performed successfully (Fig .35).

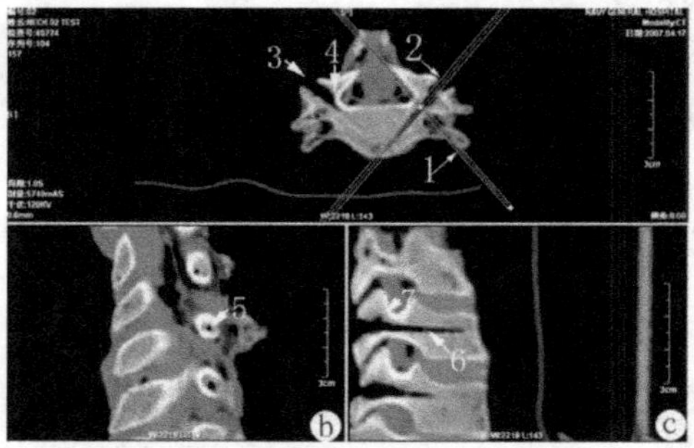

Fig. 35. Successful subaxial transpedicular manipulation

Although it seems tedious and troublesome from the above-mentioned steps description, but if one is familiar with AutoCAD, it is very easy to finish the steps mentioned-above. What we need to do is just translating the MPR image into JPG-format image and inserted it into AutoCAD interface as raster image. Other measurement steps are very simple and easy to do.

4. Conclusion

To make successful transpedicular screw fixation in subaxial cervical spinal region, the anatomical characteristics of subaxial cervical spine must be thoroughly understood. Many previous morphologic studies based on cadaveric specimens and CT images have mainly focused on transverse diameter of the pedicles [15]. Realizing the complex morphologic features of the subaxial cervical pedicles in spatial orientation and vital neurovascular structures adjacent, these studies are far from enough. To get successful subaxial cervical transpedicular screw insertion, surgeons must make in mind the anatomical features in three dimensions clearly. Volumetric CT scanning could reconstruct multiplanar CT images needed at CT-machine attached Advantage Workstation. But it is not realistic to reconstruct wanted subaxial cervical MPR CT images and to finish quantitative measurement using the measurement tools of the Workstation at every time, while a spinal surgeon who is interested in subaxial cervical transpedicular screw insertion study may not allowed to manipulate the Advantage Workstation. Even the surgeon is allowed to manipulate at rare condition, he may not familiar with the sophisticated operating procedures. ImageViewer software is a very good and easy-to-learn Windows program and has been authorized to our hospital. Every terminal computer has been installed this program. The software could reconstruct qualified MPR CT images with reference ruler present based on sequential raw CT images to fulfil primary and qualitative observation. AutoCAD program is developed primary to create accurate 2D and 3D designs, to do much more complex things that were not possible with board drafting, and the new-emerged versions are able to be installed on personal computers, have become into something that we could take on-site with us. AutoCAD program has been introduced into medical field to realize precise quantitative measurement in recent years [7]. But using AutoCAD to realize quantitative measurement of MPR CT images are rarely reported. By selecting proper MRP CT images reconstructed using ImageViewer program and saving them as .JPG images using Adobe Photoshop program, we got raster images for further quantitative measurement with AutoCAD program. When these images were inserted into opened AutoCAD document, and proper nodes were drawn at special locations of the images, we could get precise linear and angular values, which guaranteed our entrance point and direction determination of transpedicular screw fixation. With these quantitative data in mind, we successfully finished subaxial cervical pedicle screw fixation manipulation on suitable pedicles.

There are two kinds of images: bitmap and vectorgram images [13] .Vectorgram images are essentially presentation of computer programming language based on mathematical expressions, no matter simple or sophisticated, their qualities are not influenced by magnifying or decreasing the image. While the qualities of bitmap images are determined by image size dimensions and resolution. The images in JPG format are belonged to bitmap kind. Realizing JPEG compressed images would produce some artifacts, the visualization of details of MPR CT images inserted in AutoCAD program for quantitative measurement is determined by raw .JPG image size. So determining the specified points for measurement is mainly estimated by the observers, what we introduced here is just the very likelihood estimation of special points' determination. Thus the measurement data got were non-rigid. But we think they are satisfied enough to guide the pedicle screw insertion.

It seems tedious and troublesome from the description above, but if one is familiar with AutoCAD, it is very easy to finish the steps mentioned-above. In fact, what we need to do is just translating the MPR image into JPG-format image and inserted it into AutoCAD interface as raster image. Other measurement steps are very simple and easy to do.

5. References

[1] Abumi K, Itoh H, Taneichi H, et al. (1994). Transpedicular screw fixation for traumatic lesions of the middle and lower cervical spine: description of the techniques and preliminary report.J Spinal Disord. 7(1):19-28.

[2] Carvalho FB, Gonçalves M, Tanomaru-Filho M.(2007).Evaluation of chronic periapical lesions by digital subtraction radiography by using Adobe Photoshop CS: a technical report. *J Endod*.33(4):493-497.

[3] Eising EG, Jentzen W, Görges R,et al.[2007].Economic image compression of output documentation of the most frequent examinations in nuclear medicine. *Acad Radiol*.14(8):967-973.

[4] Hussein KW, Rajion ZA, Hassan R, et al.(2009). Variations in tooth size and arch dimensions in Malay school children. *Aust Orthod J*. 25(2):163-8.

[5] Ishikawa Y, Kanemura T, Yoshida G,et al.(2010). Clinical accuracy of three-dimensional fluoroscopy-based computer-assisted cervical pedicle screw placement: a retrospective comparative study of conventional versus computer-assisted cervical pedicle screw placement.*J Neurosurg Spine*. 13(5):606-611.

[6] Kast E, Mohr K, Richter HP, et al. (2006). Complications of transpedicular screw fixation in the cervical spine. *Eur Spine J*. 15(3):327-334.

[7] Le AH, Liu B, Huang HK.(2009). Integration of computer-aided diagnosis/detection (CAD) results in a PACS environment using CAD-PACS toolkit and DICOM SR.*Int J Comput Assist Radiol Surg*. 4(4):317-329.

[8] Minn KW, Hong KY, Lee SW.(2010).Preoperative TRAM free flap volume estimation for breast reconstruction in lean patients. *Ann Plast Surg*.64(4):397-401.

[9] Miyazaki M, Takita C, Yoshiiwa T,et al.(2010). Morphological analysis of the cervical pedicles, lateral masses, and laminae in developmental canal stenosis.*Spine (Phila Pa 1976)*. 2010;35(24):E1381- E1385.

[10] Reinhold M, Magerl F, Rieger M, et al. (2007). Cervical pedicle screw placement: feasibility and accuracy of two new insertion techniques based on morphometric data.*Eur Spine J*. 16(1):47-56.

[11] Tan J, Lim Joon D, Fitt G, et al.(2010).The utility of multimodality imaging with CT and MRI in defining rectal tumour volumes for radiotherapy treatment planning: a pilot study.*J Med Imaging Radiat Oncol*.54(6):562-568.

[12] Tomasino A, Parikh K, Koller H, et al. (2010). The vertebral artery and the cervical pedicle: morphometric analysis of a critical neighborhood.*J Neurosurg Spine*. 13(1):52-60.

[13] Woo HS, Lee JM.(2009).Using Adobe Acrobat to create high-resolution line art images.*AJR Am J Roentgenol*. 193(2):W112- W117.

[14] Yukawa Y, Kato F, Yoshihara H, et al. (2006). Cervical pedicle screw fixation in 100 cases of unstable cervical injuries:pedicle axis views obtained using fluoroscopy. *J Neurosurg Spine*. 5(6):488-493

[15] Yusof MI, Ming LK, Abdullah MS, Yusof AH(2006). Computerized tomographic measurement of the cervical pedicles diameter in a Malaysian population and the feasibility for transpedicular fixation. *Spine (Phila Pa 1976)*. 31(8):E221- E224.

Part 3

CT Image Analysis for Radiotherapy

8

Image Processing Methods in CT for Radiotherapy Applications

Boussion Nicolas[1,2], Fayad Hadi[2], Le Pogam Adrien[2], Pradier Oliver[1,2] and Visvikis Dimitris[1,2]
[1]*CHU de Brest, Hôpital Morvan, Service de radiothérapie*
[2]*INSERM U650 LaTIM, Brest*
France

1. Introduction

X-ray computed tomography images (CT) are widely used in radiotherapy planning because they provide electronic densities of tissues of interest which are mandatory to a correct dose computation. Furthermore, the good spatial resolution and soft/hard tissues contrast allow precise target delineation. In this context of dose calculation and delivery, two challenging problems regarding CT images and radiotherapy are adressed here.

First, we present a new automated approach to respiratory motion prediction. Respiratory motion leads to artifacts in the lower part of the lungs and blurs contours of tissues especially in thoracic and upper abdominal cases. Four-dimensional acquisitions allow accounting for this difficulty but at the expense of dosimetric considerations. On the other hand, the knowledge of the organs' motion during radiotherapy treatment is necessary (a) to a good conformation of the isodoses to the target contours and (b) to a sufficient protection of the organs at risk. In this study, we present a model-based method able to predict the internal movement of organs from CT images and external respiratory signals. A promising objective could be the improvement of dose computation and of real-time target tracking during treatment delivery.

In the second part of this work, we present state-of-the-art image combination algorithms able to provide superior information when determining target contours from CT images. The aim is to extract pertinent information from both worlds of medical imaging, morphology and function, and to present them in a single image.

2. Respiratory monitoring using predictive models based on 4D CT

2.1 Four-dimensional image-based motion management

In external radiotherapy, respiratory-induced organ and tumor motion limits the accuracy of the treatment delivery. This is because, under breathing, the photon beam may from one hand hit on normal tissues while on the other it may miss some of the tumor volume. A solution to this problem is the gating approach (Veda *et al* 2001; Keall *et al* 2002) : the beam is delivered only at a given phase of the breathing cycle, according to an external respiratory signal (pressure belt around the thorax, optical system, active breath-holding). Although this could potentially reduce tumor motion, most patients (especially with lung cancer) have usually trouble in holding or controlling their breathing. Furthermore the method is rather time consuming. Actually, there is a very interesting alternative to gating which consists of a continuous irradiation of the target during its movement. It is generally referred to as "tumour tracking" and the principle relies on a real-time adjustment of the beam according to a respiratory signal. A number of articles are currently published about this domain of research, but one of the challenging points is the ability to adapt the beam in real-time. Electronic devices, computer methods, and mechanical movements of the LINAC are not sufficiently rapid to allow actual real-time delivery. In this context, we have developped a model which is able to continuously predict the movement of the thorax and the abdomen from a four-dimensional CT exam (4D CT). This approach could help compensating the dead-time problems described previously, just by incorporating reliable tumour position estimates.

The use of 4D CT images reduces the problems caused by respiratory motion and can improve the quality of the radiation therapy (Rietzel et al, 2005). However, 4D CT images correspond to given positions in the respiratory cycle and are not continuous in time. In addition, respiratory cycle irregularities limit the efficiency of 4D CT. To resolve this issue, McClelland et al (McClelland et al, 2006, 2008) worked on the generation of a patient specific model of the motion of the target tumor and the adjacent anatomy. This model provides displacements over the respiratory cycle for any point in the CT volume and is continuous over the respiratory cycle. However this model describes an average respiratory cycle and as such the predictability of the model is limited to the information given by that average respiratory cycle and not the acquired, potentially irregular, respiratory signal. In the study presented in this chapter, we propose an approach based on the creation of a continuous patient specific model that takes into account respiratory signal irregularities while describing, in the same time, respiration induced organ motion. The acquired CT data in cine mode were examined to form continuous CT volumes using a combined phase and amplitude binning procedure based on the information given by a registered respiratory signal (Real-time Position Management: RPM). A B-spline elastic registration is used to spatially register the obtained CT volumes. Finally, the patient specific motion model is reconstructed by performing a 2D fitting for the displacement of every registration control point separately, i.e. every displacement is fitted against the amplitude and the phase values extracted from the acquired respiratory signal. The assumption behind the use of the external respiratory measurements is that a correlation between the acquired respiratory signal and the internal motion exists (Kanoulas et al 2007, Gierga et al 2005). As a result, the issues associated with the non continuous volumes caused by 4D CT acquisitions, and the respiratory signal irregularities, are resolved. This model can hence create a CT volume corresponding to any position in the respiratory cycle using a given respiratory phase and corresponding amplitude.

2.2 Description of the methodology

2.2.1 Dataset

The clinical data were acquired on a multislice CT (MSCT) and on a combined PET/CT scanner with a cine CT scan capability. A cine CT scan consists of the continuous acquisition of projections over many gantry rotation cycles while the imaging table remains stationary. As a consequence the X rays do not stop between two continuous axial scans. Each CT scan covers 2cm (8×2.5mm) on an 8-slice MSCT. The duration of each cine CT is normally 1s longer than the average breath cycle, and 19 to 23 images are acquired per slice location. A 0.5s gantry rotation is used for high temporal resolution. The interval between each cine image is 0.45s, and the total reconstruction angle is 360°. Fourteen different slice locations were acquired for every patient. During the whole acquisition, the time, as well as the amplitude and phase of the patient breathing were recorded. The Realtime Position Management (RPM) system records in addition to the patient respiratory trace, a flag indicating when the CT X-ray tube was on, allowing therefore the time-sampling of the CT data with respect to the respiration phase. A software was developed to examine these acquired 8-slice volumes in order to form 19 (or 23 depending on patient acquisition time) 8 ×14 volumes (512×512×112 voxels, with dimensions 0.97×0.97×2.5 mm^3). The obtained CT volume corresponding to the full expiration will be referred to from here onwards as the "reference volume". Moreover, this software removes 8-slice volumes that correspond to irregular breathing (Pan et al, 2007) and then, based on the phase extracted from the respiratory signal and a spline amplitude based interpolation, all CT volumes are reconstructed. The present study includes the analysis of three patients, who were asked to breathe normally and regularly.

2.2.2 Elastic registration method

Elastic registration of reconstructed CT volumes is performed using a spatio-temporal algorithm for motion reconstruction from a series of images. This method uses a semi-local spatio-temporal parametric model for the deformation using B-splines and reformulates the registration task as a global optimization problem (Ledesma-Carbayo et al, 2006). The obtained transformation Dt(x) between the frame f(x,t) at time t and the reference frame f(x,0) was defined as a linear combination of B-spline basis functions, located in a rectangular grid (Seungyong et al, 1997):

$$D_t(x) = x + \sum_{j \in Z^N} c_j \beta_r(x / h - j) \tag{1}$$

where $\beta_r(x)$ is a tensor product of centered B-splines of degree r, and j are the indices of the grid locations. Many different transformation grid spacings were tested and finally cubic B-splines with grid spacing set to 5×5×5 pixels provided the best results and were used to represent the deformation.

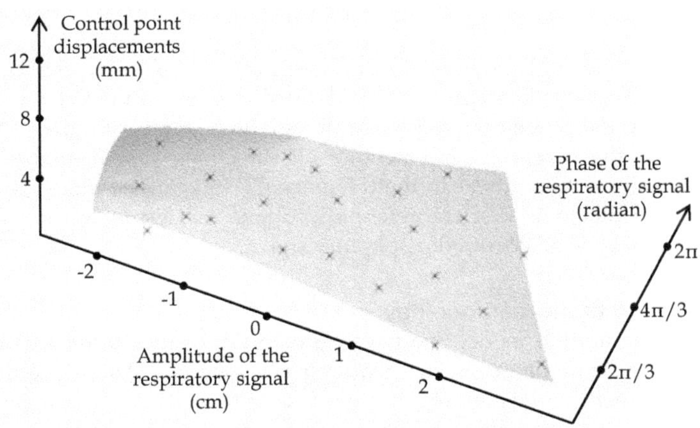

Fig. 1. A 2D-Bspline fitting for one displacement in one direction. The displacement are fitted in function of the phase and amplitude extracted from the respiratory signal.

2.2.3 Patient specific motion model

The patient specific motion model is reconstructed by performing a 2D fitting for the x, y and z displacement for every registration control point separately. The value of every displacement is effectively plotted against the amplitude and the phase of the corresponding CT volume and a 2D-Bspline is then fitted to the data. Figure 1 shows an example of this process in the case of a unique displacement in one direction.

Let $\Omega = \{(x,y), 0 \le x < m, 0 \le y < n\}$ be a rectangular domain in the xy-plane. The approximation 2D-Bspline function f is defined by a control lattice Φ in the domain Ω. Let $\phi_{i,j}$ be the value of the ij-th control point on the control lattice Φ located at (i,j) for $i = \{-1,0,\ldots,(m+1)\}$ and $j = \{-1,0,\ldots,(n+1)\}$. Finally f is defined in terms of these control points by:

$$f(x,y) = \sum_{k=0}^{3}\sum_{l=0}^{3} \beta_k(s)\beta_l(t)\phi_{(i+k)(j+l)} \tag{2}$$

where $i = |x| - 1$, $j = |y| - 1$, $s = x - |x|$, $t = y - |y|$ and βk, βl are uniform cubic b-spline basis function defined as :

$$\beta_0(t) = \frac{1-t^3}{6} \tag{3}$$

$$\beta_1(t) = \frac{3t^3 - 6t^2 + 4}{6} \tag{4}$$

$$\beta_2(t) = \frac{-3t^3 + 3t^2 + 3t + 1}{6} \tag{5}$$

$$\beta_3(t) = \frac{t^3}{6} \tag{6}$$

The patient specific model thus consists of a series of control points that correspond to every displacement in every direction. As a consequence, one can predict the corresponding CT image based on the phase and amplitude of a given respiratory signal. This is simply done by calculating the pixels displacement in all directions based on the different B-spline coefficients and applying them to the reference CT image. The model leads to a non rigid transformation that will alter the reference volume and estimate the CT volume for any position according to an acquired respiratory signal.

2.2.4 Evaluation of the methodology

To evaluate the motion model, we have derived CT images using this model having the same amplitude and phase as the acquired CT volumes. These predicted volumes are compared to their corresponding acquired volumes. At each comparison, one of the acquired CT volumes was not included in the motion model creation and was used as a ground truth for comparison purpose only. The correlation coefficient is used for that purpose. It measures a linear affine relation between the intensity of the compared images. The correlation coefficient between two images A and B is given by:

$$\rho(A,B)=\sum_i\sum_j\frac{(i-m_A)(j-m_B)}{\sqrt{\sigma_A}\sqrt{\sigma_B}}pij$$

where i and j are the voxel intensities of images A and B respectively, m_A is the mean of the image intensities, σ_A is the standard deviation and pij is the joint probability. A correlation of 1 indicates a perfect matching of the two compared images. In addition to the correlation coefficients, pixel-to-pixel image differences were used to provide global CT image comparisons. Finally, local profiles served to perform local image comparisons between the CT volumes.

2.3 First results

In this study results for three patients are presented and for each patient three CT volumes corresponding to different amplitudes and phases were derived using the model. At each prediction step, four different CT volumes were compared; namely the acquired CT (original data: not used in the model creation step), the predicted CT volume using our model, the predicted CT volume using the model based on the use of the phase parameter (phase based model, McClelland et al, 2006) and that derived using the model based on the amplitude parameter (amplitude based model).
Figure 2 shows the coronal view of an original CT image (fig. 2(a)), and the corresponding slices from the derived CT volumes using the new developed model, as well as the phase only and amplitude only based models. The profile results show little advantage from the 2D model in comparison to the 1D amplitude based model, while a more important difference is seen with respect to the 1D phase based model. Figure 3 shows the difference image between the original acquired CT and the predicted image using the 2D model as well as the 1D phase and amplitude based models. Finally, figure 4 shows the analysis on the correlation coefficient results for all three patients between the original and the corresponding model derived CT volumes. The results of both figures 3 and 4 demonstrate a closer matching and better correlation between the original CT volume and the one derived using the 2D model, rather than the 1D phase or amplitude models.

2.4 Future work

It is very important to monitor the respiratory movements when delivering radiotherapy treatments in the thorax or in the upper abdomen. Gating and tracking are techniques that lead to a better conformation of the dose to the target, while preserving organs at risk in the same time. In this context, 4D CT images with concomitant recording of the respiratory movements are very useful tools. For this reason we have proposed a patient specific continuous respiratory motion model from such 4D CT acquisitions. The first results show that including both phase and amplitude for the model construction is better than including only one of the two parameters. The demonstration of the efficacy of a 2D model over previous 1D models relies especially on the management of respiratory signal irregularities and on a signal continuity guaranteed during the whole respiratory cycle. The developed model is accurate in describing organ and tumor motion. It is useful for improving the quality of the dose delivery, and it could be of interest also for improving the accuracy of dose calculation. Potential limitations are cases where the correlation between the external acquired respiratory signal and the internal motion is not guaranteed. Numerous studies are currently performed to find the best way to estimate the organ movements from external signals (skin surface etc...). This knowledge will contribute to improve the tumour tracking approaches which are based on personalized predictive models as the one we presented here.

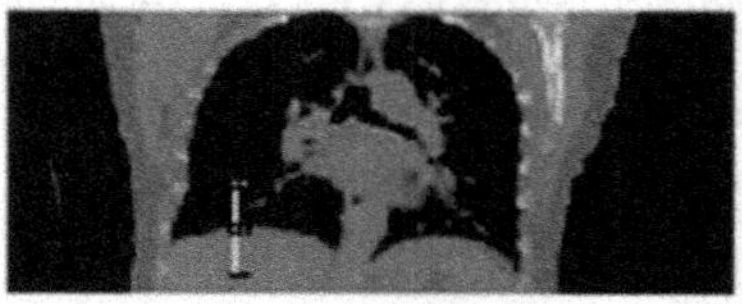

(a) CT images

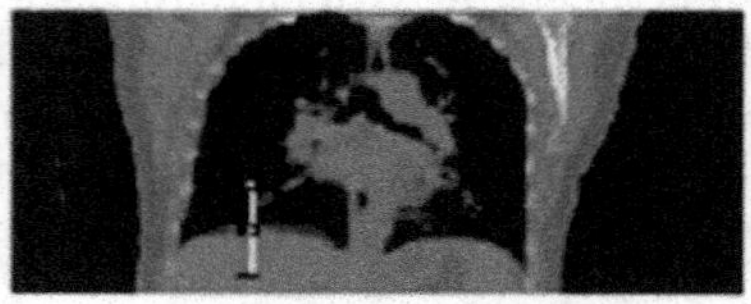

(b) 2D Spline Fitting

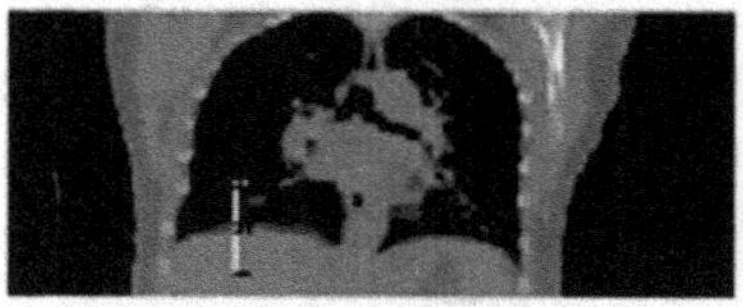

(c)1D Amplitude Fitting

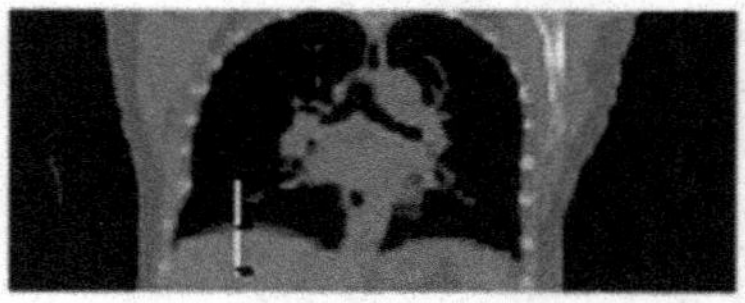

(d) 1D Phase Fitting

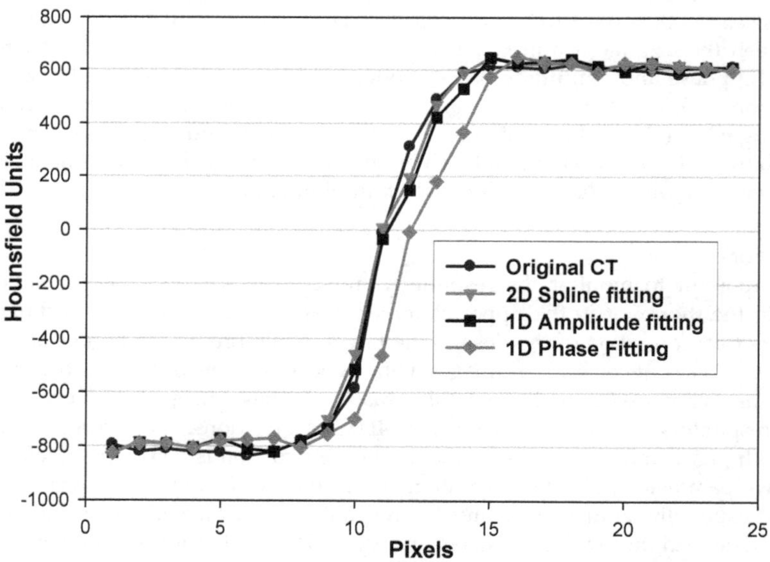

Fig. 2. Coronal view of (a) an original CT image, the same slice from the CT derived from (b) using our 2D model, (c) the phase based model, and (d) using the amplitude based model. In the bottom of the figure we can see the corresponding HU profiles drawn in (a), (b), (c) and (d).

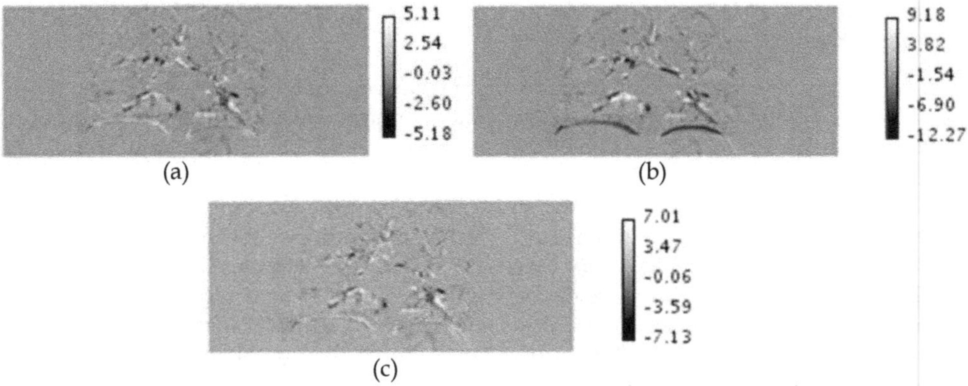

Fig. 3. Coronal view of the difference image between the original CT and the corresponding derived image using (a) our 2D model, (b) the 1D phase only model, and (c) the 1D amplitude only model. Gray pixels indicate areas where images are very similar, while black and white pixels show areas where images differ significantly.

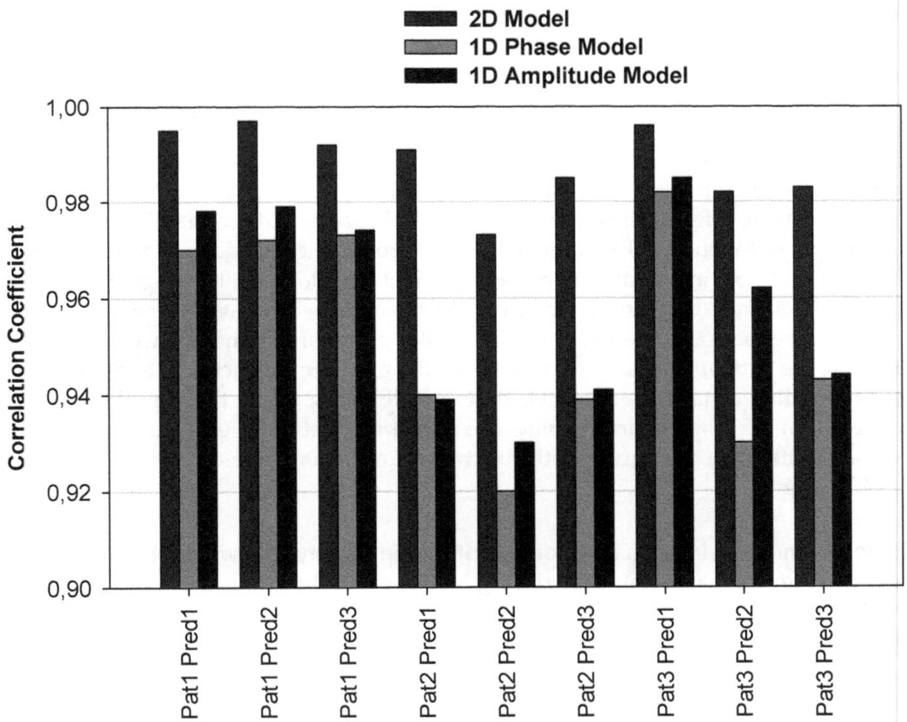

Fig. 4. Comparison of the correlation coefficients derived using the 2D model as well as the 1D phase and amplitude models, for all three patients and for different predicted volume amplitudes and phases.

3. Combination of CT with functional images for better delineation of targets in radiotherapy

In radiotherapy, the accurate delineation of the tumours and the organs at risk (OAR) remains a critical step of the treatment planning phase. In a first step, the physician manually or semi-automatically draws regions of interest in the CT images of the patient (target, OAR). Then, the treatment planning system (TPS) is used to compute the dose received by the target and the OAR, the aim being to give the maximum dose to the target while preserving OAR in the same time. During this process, the images obtained by computed tomography are mandatory because they give access to the electronic densities of the tissues, which allows dose calculation by the TPS. CT images also provide valuable anatomical data with good spatial resolution and hard/soft tissues contrast. However, it has been shown that discrepancies often appear between morphological size and shape of the tumor seen in CT, and its functional activity seen in positron emission tomography (PET). The glucose metabolism is for instance obtained in whole-body PET after injection of ^{18}FDG. In this case, necrotic parts of a tumor may be visible on ^{18}FDG PET images but not in the CT images. This point is of importance since a higher dose should be delivered to the active part of a tumour than to the necrotic parts. This dose delivery scheme is sometimes referred to as dose painting, i.e. the ability to deliver different levels of dose to different parts of a single target. This dose escalation process leads to a better efficacy especially in prostate cancer for example.

The main difficulty in dose painting is the definition of the target and the delineation of its inner active parts. As already stated, computed tomography gives precise but uniform images while PET is able to segment active/necrotic sub-parts of a given tumour, but with a significantly lower spatial resolution. Images appear more blurred and contours of the different organs are difficult to delineate. These effects are included in what is often referred to as partial volume effects. These latter have several aspects but are mainly caused by the wide point spread function of PET imaging devices from which we define spatial resolution. The full width at half maximum of the point spread function eventually gives the spatial resolution, which may be seen as the ability to separate two points on the reconstructed image. More precisely the spatial resolution is the minimal distance between two actual points inside the patient necessary to separate them on the reconstructed image. If the points are closer than that distance, it is practically impossible to separate them on the image and they appear as a big single blurred point. The aim of the method presented now is to build an enhanced image incorporating both functional and anatomical data from the CT and ^{18}FDG PET images.

3.1 Fusion of medical images in a context of multimodality: the wavelet framework

The enhanced image that we are introducing here is computed using a 3D wavelet analysis where details of two images are extracted at different levels of spatial resolution. Considering that the level of resolution of the initial CT image is q, (referred to as CTq) and that of the initial PET image is r = q + p, (referred to as PETr), we can perform the extraction of the spatial frequencies at a level of resolution common to CT and PET (q+p+1), using the "à trous" algorithm. This discrete wavelet transform algorithm was introduced by Dutilleux (Dutilleux, 1987), developed by Holdschneider (Holdschneider et al, 1989) and detailed by Starck (Starck et al, 1998). The process gives an image sequence of coarser and coarser spatial resolution by performing successive convolutions with a low-pass filter h (Boussion et al, 2006).

Practically, at each iteration j, the spatial resolution of the degraded image deg_{j-1} is degraded to give the degraded image deg_j according to :

$$\deg_j(k,l) = \sum_{m,n} h(m,n)\deg_{j-1}(k + m2^{j-1}, l + n2^{j-1}) \tag{7}$$

The first approximation image deg0 is taken as I, the original image. The difference $deg_{j-1} - deg_j$ is the wavelet coefficients w_j containing the details (edges, texture) at a resolution level between deg_{j-1} and deg_j. The procedure that reconstructs the original image from its layers of details wk is called synthesis and is given by:

$$\deg_0 = I = I_N + \sum_{k=1}^{k=N} w_k \tag{8}$$

with N the number of iterations from the initial image I to the final degraded image I_N of spatial resolution decreased by 2^N. The algorithm can be easily implemented by performing the following steps:

1. Initialize j to 0: start with the original image I = deg0 (deg stands for degraded image).
2. Increment j and carry out a convolution of deg_{j-1} with a low-pass filter h in order to obtain deg_j (the distance between the central voxel and the adjacent ones is 2j−1).
3. The wavelet coefficients w(j) at this level of resolution are given by $deg_{j-1} - deg_j$.
4. If j is less than the required number N of resolutions go to step 2.
5. The set W = $\{w(1), w(2), \ldots, w(N), \deg_N\}$ is the wavelet transform of I.

In a practical point of vue, zeros are inserted between lines and columns of the filter h at each iteration j of the process. This particularity gives its name to the algorithm "à trous" which in French means "with holes". In the present study, we have chosen a low pass filter corresponding to a B-spline interpolation implemented sequentially according to:

$$h(x,y) = h(x) \otimes h(y) \tag{9}$$

with:

$$h(0) = 3/8, h(\pm 1) = 1/4\ h(\pm 2) = 1/16 \text{ and } h(n) = 0 \text{ if } |n| > 2 \tag{10}$$

The initial image can always be perfectly reconstructed by adding the different layers and the final degraded image of the wavelet decomposition on a voxel-to-voxel basis. As a consequence, we have the two following equations:

$$PET_r = PET_{q+p}(x,y,z) = PET_{q+p+1}(x,y,z) + w_{q+p+1}^{PET}(x,y,z) \tag{11}$$

$$CT_q = CT_{q+p+1}(x,y,z) + \sum_{k=1}^{k=p+1} w_{q+k}^{CT}(x,y,z) \tag{12}$$

with w^{PET} and w^{CT} the wavelet coefficients from the wavelet decomposition of respectively (i) the functional PET image of "low" spatial resolution and (ii) the anatomical CT image of "high" spatial resolution. The final enhanced image, or fused image, is then given straightforwardly by:

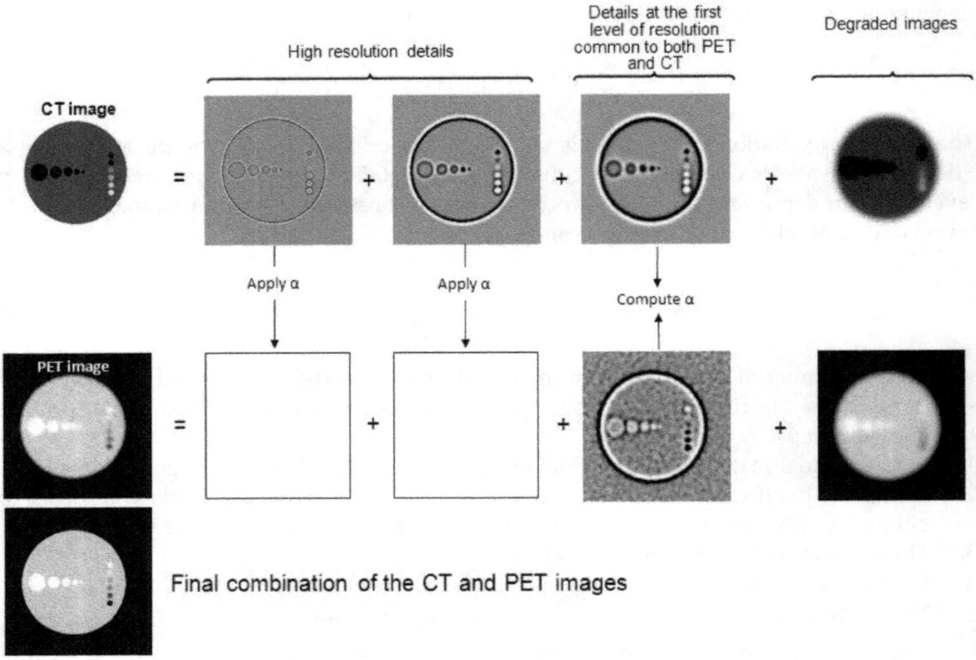

Fig. 5. Illustration of the CT-PET combination process on simulated images. (a) wavelet transform of the original simulated CT image (three iterations were arbitrarily chosen in this example); (b) wavelet transform of the original simulated PET image; the lacking details of the PET image are retrieved from the existing details of the CT images which are modified according to the α model; (c) the fused CT-PET image is the pixel-to-pixel addition of the original PET image with the retrieved details coming from CT.

$$ENH_p(x,y,z) = PET_{q+p+1}(x,y,z) + w_{q+p+1}^{PET}(x,y,z) + \alpha(x,y,z)\sum_{k=1}^{k=p} W_{q+k}^{CT}(x,y,z) \qquad (13)$$

where the parameter α is just the mean voxel-to-voxel ratio of wavelet coefficients at resolution q+p+1:

$$\alpha = mean(\frac{W_{q+p+1}^{PET}}{W_{q+p+1}^{CT}}) \qquad (14)$$

In equation (9), each pixel is processed individually and the parameter α is computed locally using a 3D moving cube, simultaneously applied within the PET and CT wavelet layers. For the sake of clarity, the whole process is illustrated on fig. 5 where synthetic images are used in order to facilitate the understanding of the method.

3.2 Examples of fused images

Some examples are given on fig. 6 and fig.7 where one can see the transverse view of a CT image, of the corresponding [18]FDG PET image, and of the final fused image.

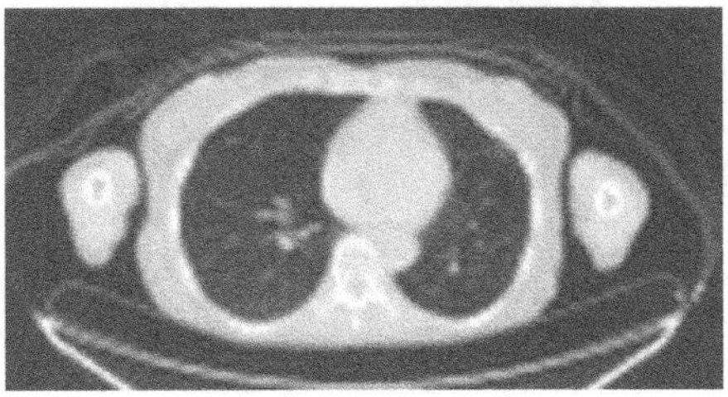

(a)

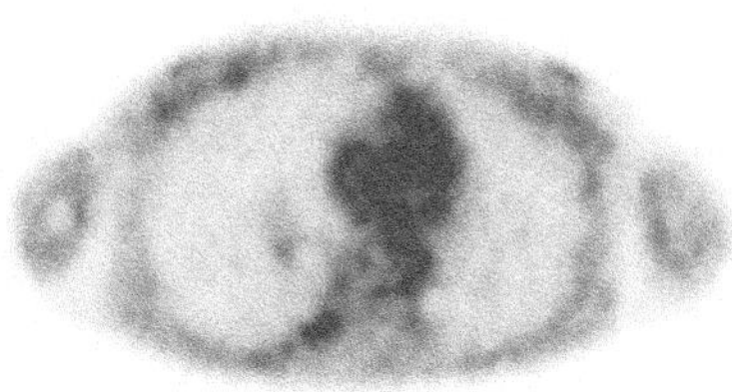

(b)

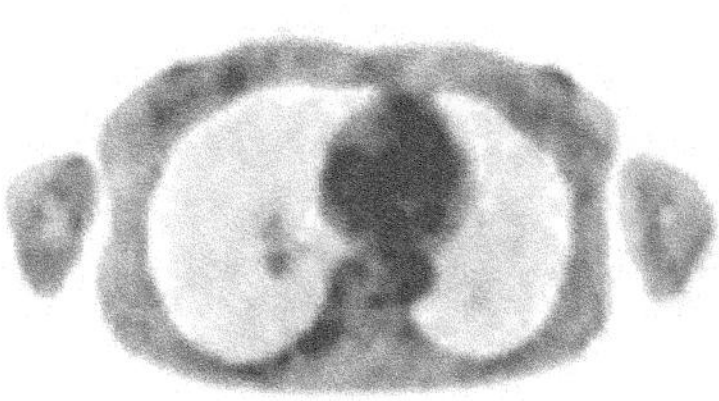

(c)

Fig. 6. Example of CT-PET fusion using wavelet-based decomposition. (a) CT image, (b) PET image and (c) fused CT-PET image, where the contours of the pulmonary lesion become more visible.

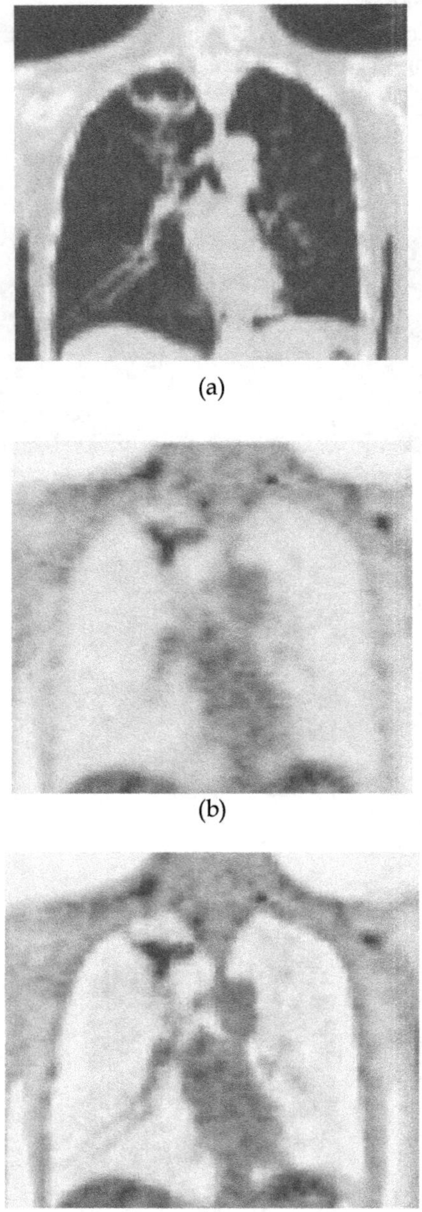

(a)

(b)

(c)

Fig. 7. This example is another pertinent illustration of what fusion permits to obtain. In the fused image (c), both anatomical details coming from CT and functional information coming from PET are visible at the same time.

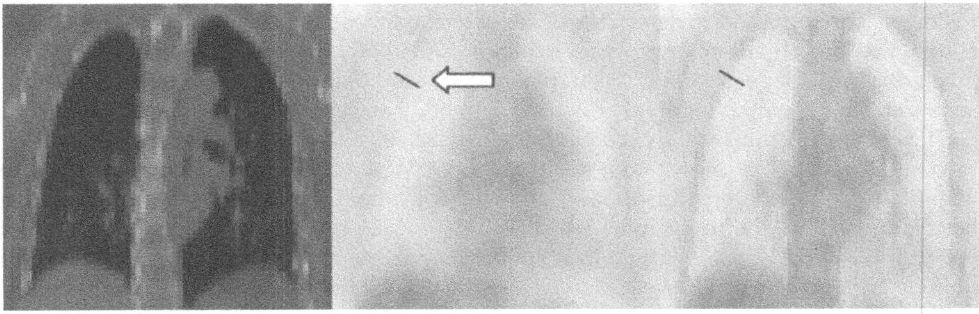

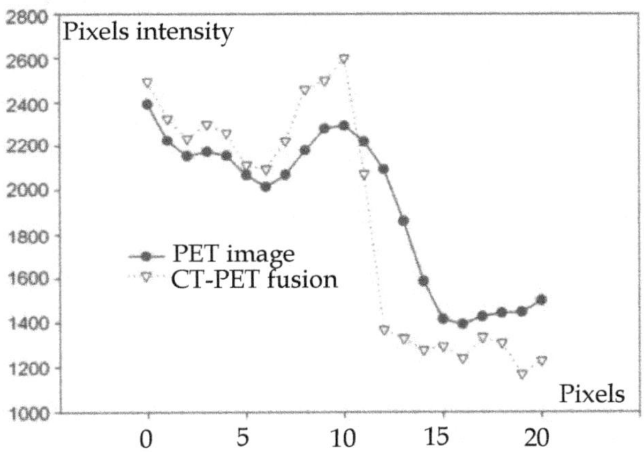

Fig. 8. In this case, we illustrate the fusion with a quantitative analysis of the pixels values along a given profile (see arrow for location). The two curves clearly demonstrate the gain in contrast given by the fusion process. The slope of the curve corresponding to the fused image is sharper than the one corresponding to the original PET image. This improvement if directly coming from the incorporation of high resolution details of the CT image.

3.4 Potential improvements

In this part of the study a new approach to CT/PET image fusion has been proposed for whole-body imaging. Contrary to the great majority of existing methods, the aim of the presented work was to provide the user with a fused image preserving both anatomical and functional data. The objective is therefore different from simply presenting two images in a visually convenient fusion display in the sense that quantitative analysis is also here considered as a possible step. In the proposed methodology the anatomical information is present in terms of improved contrast while the intensity in the organs is comparable with the functional information presented by the PET. This is of paramount importance in cancer staging and treatment follow-up for instance, where quantitative assessment of activity uptake is necessary. Furthermore, for applications in radiotherapy, the efficient image fusion proposed in this article may be of key interest. Indeed, when considering day-to-day clinical use, this algorithm appears user-friendly and allows physicians to gain a lot of time when making diagnosis and when planning radiotherapy treatment on a dedicated software. However, the model that is used to modify the detail layers (images of wavelet coefficient) obtained in the CT decomposition may be considered too simplistic (mean voxel-to-voxel division). A more sophisticated model would be preferable when absolute quantitation is mandatory, for tumour follow-up for example. For this specific purpose we have designed an alternate model which is able to take into account local discrepancies between CT and PET. Adopting a local model may be more appropriate, in particular for limiting artifacts coming from structures present in the CT only. The methodology itself is of course not restricted to whole-body imaging in the oncology domain. Provided two co-registered images are available, one functional and the other anatomical, the process can be applied in a wide range of clinical areas. The main difference with the initial model relies on the definition of the α parameter. In the first method, α is just the global mean of the wavelet ratios (equation 14). In this improved approach (Le Pogam et al, 2008), α is in particular computed locally as a median value instead of a mean value. This point allows improving the quantitative correction of PET images without incorporating artifacts in the final fused image. This original approach is quantitatively relevant in the sense that it leads to a direct correction of partial volume effects.

As an illustration we give an example of partial volume correction in the PET image of a lung lesion (fig.10). In this case, the high resolution details provided by the CT image not only improve the visual aspect of the PET image, but it also corrects the image for the partial volume effect. As a consequence, the direct segmentation of the target for radiotherapy treatment becomes possible.

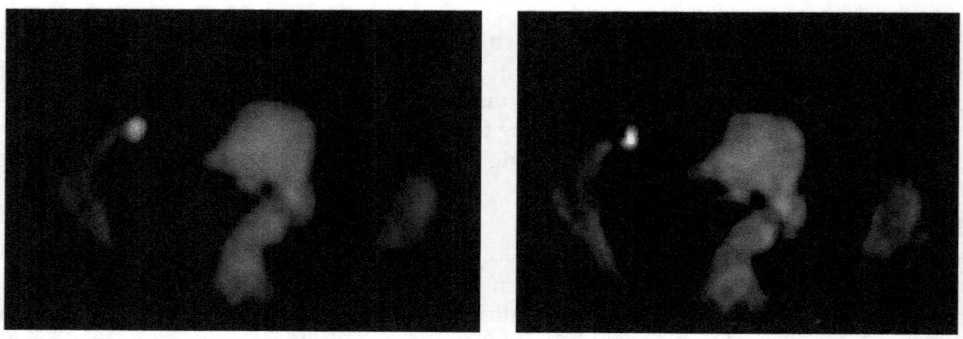

Fig. 10. Original PET image before (left) and after (right) fusion with a corresponding CT image, by using a local model instead of a global one.

4. Conclusion

In this chapter we have presented two CT image processing methods dedicated to radiotherapy. X-ray computed tomography is indeed the only image modality mandatory to classical radiotherapy treatment planning. It permits to visualize the anatomy of the patient and in particular to delineate targets and organs at risk. The link between Hounsfield Units and electronic densities also leads to the pre-treatment computation of the dose delivered to the patient. However, new treatment technologies like intensity modulated radiotherapy require more and more data to improve the precision and the efficacy of the treatment delivery. In this context, the monitoring of the respiratory signal and the incorporation of functional imaging in the treatment process are of significant interest. One of the objectives of this chapter was thus to underline the increasing synergy between CT images and others medical signals. The presented studies also illustrated the multi-disciplinary features of modern radiotherapy.

5. References

Boussion, N.; Hatt, M.; Lamare, F.; Bizais, Y.; Turzo, A.; Cheze-Le Rest C. & Visvikis, D. (2006). A multiresolution image based approach for correction of partial volume effects in emission tomography. *Phys Med Biol.* Vol 7;51(7), pp 1857-76.

Dutilleux, P. An Implementation of the Algorithme "à trous" to compute the wavelet transform, Proceedings of Congrès ondelettes et méthodes temps-fréquence et espace des phases, Marseille, France, Springer–Verlag, 1987, pp. 298–304.

Gierga D.; Brewer, J.; Sharp, G.; Betke, M.; Willet, C. & Chen, G. (2005) The correlation between external and internal markers for abdominal tumors: implications for respiratory gating. *Int. J. Radiat. Oncol. Biol. Phys,* vol. 61, pp. 1551–1558.

Holdschneider, R.; Kronland-Martinet, R.; Morlet, J. & Tchamitchian, P. (1989). A real time algorithm for signal analysis with the help of the wavelet transform, in: J.M. Combes, et al. (Eds.), Wavelets, Springer–Verlag, Berlin.

Kanoulas, E.; Aslam, J.; Sharp, G.; Berbeco, R.; Nishioka, S.; Shirato H, & Jiang, S. (2007) Derivation of the tumor position from external respiratory surrogates with periodical updating of the internal/external correlation, *Phys. Med. Biol.,* vol. 52, pp. 5443–5456.

Keall, JJ.; Kini, VR.; Vedam, SS. & Mohan R. (2002) Potential radiotherapy improvements with respiratory gating. *Australas. Phys. Eng. Sci. Med.,* vol. 25(1), pp.1–6.

Ledesma-Carbayo, MJ.; Mahia-Casado, P.; Santos, A.; Perez-David, E.; Garcia-Fernandez, MA.; & M Desco. (2006) "Cardiac motion analysis from ultrasound sequences using nonrigid registration: validation against doppler tissue velocity," *Ultrasound Med. Biol.,* vol. 32, pp. 483–490.

Le Pogam, A.; Boussion, N.; Hatt, M.; Turkheimer, F.E.; Prunier-Aesch, C.; Guilloteau, D.; Baulieu, J.L. & Visvikis, D. (2008). A 3D multi resolution local analysis approach for correction of partial volume effects in emission tomography. *Proceedings of Nuclear Science Symposium Conference Record.*pp 5300-5303.

McClelland, JR.; Blackall, JM.; Tarte, S.; Chandler, AC.; Hughes, S.; Ahmad, S. Landau, DB.; Hawkes, DJ. (2006) A continuous 4d motion model from multiple respiratory cycles for use in lung radiotherapy. *Med. Phys.,* vol. 33, pp. 3348–3358.

McClelland, JR.; Gao, G.; Tarte, S.; Blackall, JM.; Hughes, S.; Chandler, AC.; Ahmad, S. Landau, DB.; Hawkes, DJ. (2008) Removing artifacts from 4dct volumes acquired in cine mode using b-spline non-rigid registrations. 50th Annual Meeting AAPM, Med. Phys, vol. 35, p. 2992.

Pan, T.; Sun, X.; & Luo, D. (2007). Improvement of the cinect based 4d-ct imaging. *Med. Phys.*, vol. 34(11), pp. 4499–4503.

Rietzel E, Chen GTY, Choi NC, & Willet CG. (2005) Four-dimensional image-based treatment planning: target volume segmentation and dose calculation in the presence of respiratory motion. *Int J Radiat Oncol*, vol. 61, pp. 1535–1550.

Seungyong, L.; Wolberg, G. & Shin, SY. (1997). Scattered data interpolation with multilevel b-splines, *IEEE Trans. Vis. Comput. Graph.*, vol. 3(3), pp. 228–244.

Starck, JL.;, Murtagh, F.; Bijaoui, A. (1998). *Image processing and data analysis: the multiscale approach*, Cambridge University Press, Cambridge, UK.

Vedam, SS.; Keall PJ.; Kini VR. & Mohan R. (2001). Determining parameters for respiration-gated radiotherapy. *Med. Phys.*, vol. 28, pp. 2139–2146.

9

CT-Image Guided Brachytherapy

Janusz Skowronek, MD, PhD, Ass. Prof.
Brachytherapy Department, Greater Poland Cancer Centre, Poznań
Poland

1. Introduction

The name "Brachytherapy" is derived from ancient Greek words for short distance (*brachios*) and treatment (*therapy*) and refers to the therapeutic use of encapsulated radionuclides placed within or close to the tumor. Brachytherapy (BT), used as an integral part of cancer treatment for almost a century, developed in last three decades a rapid growth with the development of afterloading devices and the introduction of artificial radionuclides. The impressive progress of three dimensional (3D) imaging, the rapidly increasing speed and capacity of computers, and the sophisticated techniques developed for the treatment planning, opened a new era.
Brachytherapy plays a crucial role in the curative treatment of many tumors. CT and/or MRI compatible applicators allow a sectional image based approach with a better assessment of GTV (Gross Tumor Volume) and CTV (Clinical Target Volume) compared to traditional approaches. Accurate and reproducible delineation of GTV and CTV, as well as healthy (critical) organs, has a direct impact on treatment planning, especially it is possible to optimize the reference isodoses to the target.
A two-film typical localization technique does not allow the definition of the three-dimensional (3D) extensions of the planning target volume (PTV) and organs at risk (OARs). Furthermore, using traditional dosimetry systems the dose report is related to the geometry of the implant and not to the target volume. In modern BT both treatment planning and plan evaluation have to be based on real 3D volume of the PTV and OARs.

2. Rationale for CT- Image Guided Brachytherapy

Utilization of 3D sectional imaging in brachytherapy (BT) planning of different tumor sites allows for a clinically meaningful dose escalation in the target, while respecting normal tissue tolerance. 3D treatment planning has made promising progress in the last decade of radiotherapy. Currently, the conformal 3D external beam radiation therapy (EBRT) is the permanent part of routine clinical work in most of the radiotherapy departments. Moreover, the 3D brachytherapy treatment planning has just become the center of interest.
As far as the method of sectional imaging is concerned, there are some important advantages afforded by CT compared to other imaging modalities (Barrett et al., 2009). CT scanning provides detailed cross-sectional anatomy of the normal organs, as well as 3D tumor information. These images provide density data for radiation dose calculations by conversion of CT Hounsfield units into relative electron densities using calibration curves. Compton scattering is the main process of tissue interaction for megavoltage beams and is

directly proportional to electron density. Hence CT provides ideal density information for dose corrections for tissue inhomogeneity, such as occurs in lung tissue. Clinical studies have shown that 30%-80% of patients undergoing radiotherapy benefit from the increased accuracy of target volume delineation with CT scanning compared with conventional simulation. It has been estimated that the use of CT improves overall 5-year survival rates by around 3.5%, with the greatest impact on small volume treatments (Barrett et al., 2009).

CT scans taken for brachytherapy treatment planning usually differ from those taken for diagnostic use. Ideally, planning CT scans are taken on a dedicated brachytherapy CT scanner by a therapy trained radiographer. Protocols for CT scanning are developed with the radiologist to optimize tumor information, to ensure full body contour in the reconstruction circle and scanning of relevant whole organs for DVHs. CT scans are transferred digitally to the target volume localization console using an electronic network system. The CTV, PTV, body contour and normal organs (OARs) are outlined by a team of radiation oncologist and physicist (Barrett et al., 2009).

The rationale behind CT guidance in BT is twofold: (1) to assure an optimal position of BT catheters within the target volume by controlling their insertion and (2) to assist the process of detection and contouring of the target volume and organs at risk (OARs). CT guidance of insertion can be accomplished preoperatively or during an intraoperative procedure. Standard preoperative strategy is based on integration of initial CT findings and clinical and/or ultrasound findings at BT. CT-guided treatment planning is in this case most commonly performed only after the procedure, limiting the ability to correct an eventually suboptimal implantation. Obtaining an additional pre-planning CT just a few days before the application can facilitate the ability for an accurate insertion. An overview of the current approaches in CT guided BT is presented in this chapter.

One of the best approaches for CT-guided brachytherapy was made by Kolotas and al. (Kolotas et al., 1999). They described development of a CT-based brachytherapy catheter application and treatment planning procedure which is focused on anatomy (PTV and healthy tissues) based optimization, and with evaluation using the conformal index COIN of the 3D dose distribution. The clinical feasibility of this new method, which is essentially a new philosophy in the practice of interstitial brachytherapy, has been proved for several tumor sites (Kolotas et al., 1999). Catheter implantation using CT imaging is first performed to localize the tumor and the surrounding critical tissues. Then, CT-guided catheter implantation is performed in the CT room and, if necessary, contrast enhanced, cross-sectional images are made. This imaging procedure determines the choice of the application technique including the type of catheters to be used. Aluminum skin markers and painting can also be used for this localization procedure. The CT table top drive mechanism and the markers are then used to navigate between the CT slices and the patient. In cases where a template can be used this offers an additional navigation possibility for catheter insertion through the numbered holes of the template which are also visible on the CT slices. Based on the pre-implantation imaging and clinical information, and after local anesthesia and sedation, catheter insertion is commenced with the patient remaining on the CT table. The maximum insertion depth and direction as well as position (in case of template the whole number) of the catheter can be estimated from the CT information. This information is displayed on a monitor within the CT room and therefore is immediately available to the physician. This is a real advantage for the physician when implanting the catheters since this provides rapid and effective control of catheter position and geometry and ensures avoidance of injuries to neighboring critical structures. Control of the position of an inserted catheter is achieved by taking CT images with the catheters in situ, and then if necessary correcting the catheter position. This procedure is repeated until all catheters needed to cover the tumor volume have been implanted. After reconstruction of catheters all the graphical information, including body contour, PTV, critical structures and catheters are displayed in a 3D view window. The 3D view is fully scalable and can be rotated. For simplification in an individual patient, the user can select the graphical elements needed to be viewed in 3D, using simple button menus, and exclude all others that may be confusing. The 3D window is extremely useful for real time monitoring of the reconstruction of catheters. It also offers an efficient method of viewing the position of critical organs by reference to the PTV and to the catheters (Kolotas et al., 1999).

3. Gynecological tumors

In gynecological tumors image-guided 3D conformal BT planning postimplant CT images are useful to control and report the dose to treated volume and OARs (e.g. for rectum, sigmoid, and bladder). This allows better assessment of dose distributions in different volumes, such as the gross tumor volume (GTV), clinical target volume (CTV), and OARs. Clinical target volume (CTV), bladder volume, rectum volume, sigmoid colon, and small bowel should be delineated on CT images. Advantages of 3D imaging in gynecologic brachytherapy that may lead to improved patient outcome, irrespective of the dose rate, include avoiding or early detection of a uterine perforation, ensuring target coverage, and avoiding excessive dose to the OAR. Disadvantages include an increased amount of physician and physicist time to coordinate imaging and incorporate this into treatment planning, as well as the need for additional training to gain familiarity with the contouring methodology (Viswanathan & Erickson, 2010). For post-implantation imaging, the advantages of 3D imaging with either CT or MRI include clear target definition as well as better localization and target delineation of the OARs. With MRI, one may contour residual cervical tumor. With CT, one visualizes the cervix and parametrium as one structure, resulting in potential overcontouring of the lateral aspect of the volume (Viswanathan et al., 2007) Nevertheless, CT allows visualization of tumor that may lie beyond Point A, thereby ensuring adequate dosing of the target volume (Viswanathan & Erickson, 2010).

To unify 3D plan evaluation concepts and to provide a common set of terms to be used, Gynecologic (GYN) GEC-ESTRO Working Group (GEC-ESTRO) published guidelines on 3D image-based treatment planning in cervical cancer brachytherapy (Haie-Meder et al., 2005; Pötter et al., 2006).

One of the first reports describing the volumetric dose distributions from BT was published in 1987 (Ling et al., 1987). Since the 1990s, widespread implementation of CT simulation for EBRT treatment planning in radiation oncology departments has enabled physicians to contour and perform dose volume histogram (DVH) analysis of the OARs. Several centers have published results with CT simulation or MRI based gynecologic brachytherapy. To standardize some aspects of nomenclature, the American Brachytherapy Society (ABS) published guidelines for image-guided gynecologic brachytherapy in 2004 (Nag et al., 2004). Viswanathan and Erickson in their recently published (2010) paper determined current practice patterns with regard to three-dimensional (3D) imaging for gynecologic brachytherapy among American Brachytherapy Society (ABS) members. Material was based on a 19-item survey send to physicians from ABS. The results show that after insertion, 70% of physicians routinely obtain a computed tomography (CT) scan. The majority (55%) use

CT rather than X-ray films (43%) or magnetic resonance imaging (MRI; 2%) for dose specification to the cervix. However, 76% prescribe to Point A alone instead of using a 3D-derived tumor volume (14%), both Point A and tumor volume (7%), or mg/h (3%). Those using 3D imaging routinely contour the bladder and rectum (94%), sigmoid (45%), small bowel (38%), and/or urethra (8%) and calculate normal tissue dose–volume histogram (DVH) analysis parameters including the D_{2cc} (49%), D_{1cc} (36%), $D_{0.1cc}$ (19%), and/or D_{5cc} (19%). Authors concluded that more ABS physician members use CT post-implantation imaging than plain films for visualizing the gynecologic brachytherapy applicators. However, the majority prescribes to Point A rather than using 3D image based dosimetry (Viswanathan & Erickson, 2010).

Another authors concluded that calculating dose-volume histograms (DVHs) using 3D-based volumetric planning may provide a more accurate evaluation of the dose to the target volume and OARs (Al-Halabi et al., 2010). In addition, better imaging of the target and OARs allows for a more precise delineation of the target volume and OARs and, consequently, a better assessment of the dose delivered to these structures (Nag et al., 2004). Studies of CT-based 3D brachytherapy planning have shown that the ICRU-defined bladder and rectum doses in fact underestimate the true maximal doses to these organs.

Hellebust et al. recently published recommendations from gynaecological (GYN) GEC-ESTRO Working Group including considerations and pitfalls in commissioning and applicator reconstruction in 3D image-based treatment planning (Hellebust et al., 2010). The aim of these guidelines was to unify 3D plan evaluation concepts and to provide a common set of terms to be used. They concluded that image-guided brachytherapy in cervical cancer is increasingly replacing X-ray based dose planning. In image-guided brachytherapy the geometry of the applicator is extracted from the patient 3D images and introduced into the treatment planning system; a process referred to as applicator reconstruction. Due to the steep brachytherapy dose gradients, reconstruction errors can lead to major dose deviations in target and organs at risk. Appropriate applicator commissioning and reconstruction methods must be implemented in order to minimize uncertainties and to avoid accidental errors. Applicator commissioning verifies the location of source positions in relation to the applicator by using auto-radiography and imaging. Sectional imaging can be utilized in the process, with CT imaging being the optimal modality. The importance of proper commissioning is underlined by the fact that errors in library files result in systematic errors for clinical treatment plans (Hellebust et al., 2010). The next step, reconstruction of the applicator, can be performed by different methods: library plans (LIB), direct reconstruction (DR) or a combination of these two methods. Applicator reconstruction using CT images offers the good visualisation of the lumen of the applicator and this means that a markerstring is not always necessary. Authors indicate some X-ray catheters may produce artifacts in the CT images resulting in larger uncertainties in the reconstruction and contouring process. Slice thickness $\leq$3 mm is recommended to give the best visualization. The lumen of the ring will be visible in several slices, e.g. 3–4 images for 3 mm slice thickness. In order to visualize the ring in one image a multiplanar reconstructed image through the ring can be used. The reconstructed image can be used during direct reconstruction or for positioning of a library applicator (Hellebust et al., 2010). In another paper similar authors analyzed the impact of the applicator orientation and the reconstruction method used on the calculated dose around a reconstructed ring applicator set using CT imaging (Hellebust et al., 2007). Their results showed that it was not possible to identify one applicator orientation that gave lower uncertainties with regard to the calculated dose around the applicator. However, all orientations and all reconstruction methods resulted in limited variation in calculated dose, i.e. both LIB and DR are feasible for applicator reconstruction in CT images. With CT-based reconstruction the visibility of the applicator is usually excellent and it has been shown that the dose variation between different CT reconstruction methods is limited - below 4% (1 standard deviation) in clinically relevant dose points (Hellebust et al., 2010).

Davidson et al. analyzed whether customized 3D plans generated for the first insertion (using CT planning) can be applied to subsequent insertions without significant changes in dose distributions if identical applicators are used (Davidson et al., 2008). They concluded that a duplication of planned dwell times and positions from one insertion to the next does not duplicate dose distributions in HDR cervix applications. A single plan used for an entire course of BT can result in significant increases to OAR doses for tandem and ring (TR) and unpredictable OAR doses for tandem and ovoids (TO) applicators. Treatment plans should be tailored for each insertion to reflect current applicator and anatomical geometry. They emphasized also that ideally, 3D imaging with MRI should be performed after each BT implantation for individual treatment planning of each HDR fraction. This is, unfortunately, not possible for many radiotherapy departments due to limited MRI resources. In cases where MRI is unavailable for BT planning, CT may be a more accessible alternative. Although CT does not provide a clear clinical target volume for BT planning due to poorer soft-tissue contrast than MRI, it can identify surrounding OARs and define dose distributions in 3D. This allows for the determination of problematic volumetric doses to OAR and instances where dose shapes should be altered to reduce the risk of complications (Davidson et al., 2008).

Another authors investigated two-dimensional (2D) radiograph-based plans using 3D dose-volume histogram (DVH) parameters following guidelines from Gynecologic GEC-ESTRO Working Group (Gao et al., 2010). Clinical target volume (CTV), bladder volume, rectum volume, sigmoid colon, and small bowel were delineated on CT images. CTV included the whole cervical mass visualized as aided by implanted marker seeds. DVHs were calculated for these structures. 3D plan evaluation parameters recommended by GYN-GEC-ESTRO guidelines (Pötter et al., 2006) were adopted. CTV coverage was evaluated using D100, D90, and V100 (i.e., dose covering 100% of the volume, dose covering 90% of the volume, and volume covered by 100% of prescription dose). High dose volume in CTV was estimated using V200. For organs at risk (OARs), $D0.1_{cc}$, $D1_{cc}$, and $D2_{cc}$ (i.e., minimum dose received by 0.1-, 1-, and 2-cm^3 tissue volume) were calculated. In conclusions we can read that the DVH analysis of 2D plans revealed a suboptimal coverage of CT-based cervix and a negative correlation between coverage and cervical size. Rectum dose to 2 cc weakly correlated with ICRU point dose. Currently published constraints for bladder in 3D planning were tighter than ABS guidelines in past 2D planning.

Shin et al. compared the conventional point A plan (conventional plan) and computed tomography (CT)-guided clinical target volume-based plan (CTV plan) by analysis of the quantitative dose-volume parameters and irradiated volumes of organs at risk in patients with cervical cancer (Shin et al., 2006). In 30 plans CT images were acquired at the first intracavitary radiotherapy (ICR) session with artifact-free applicators in place. The gross tumor volume, clinical target volume (CTV), point A, and International Commission on Radiation Units and Measurements (ICRU) Report 38 rectal and bladder points were defined on reconstructed CT images. They concluded that the results have shown that CT-guided CTV planning of ICR is superior to conventional point A planning in terms of both conformity of target coverage and avoidance of overdosed normal tissue volumes (Shin et al., 2006).

In another paper Wang et al. evaluated and reported volumetric dose specification of clinical target volume (CTV) and organs at risk with three-dimensional CT-based brachytherapy. They analyzed CTV volumes and correlated the dose specification from CT-based volumes with doses at classical point A and International Commission on Radiation Units and Measurements (ICRU) points (Wang et al., 2009). Their main conclusion was that excellent dose coverage of CTV can be achieved with image-guided CT-based planning with geometric optimization although maximal sparing of rectum was not achieved. Careful dose constraints and standardization of D90 should be considered when optimizing doses to target tissues such that normal tissue constraints can be met (Wang et al., 2009).

These several studies have shown that traditional ICRU reference points underestimate dose to normal organs when compared to CT-based 3-dimensional (3D) imaging. On figure 1 example of typical 3D treatment plan in cervical cancer is presented.

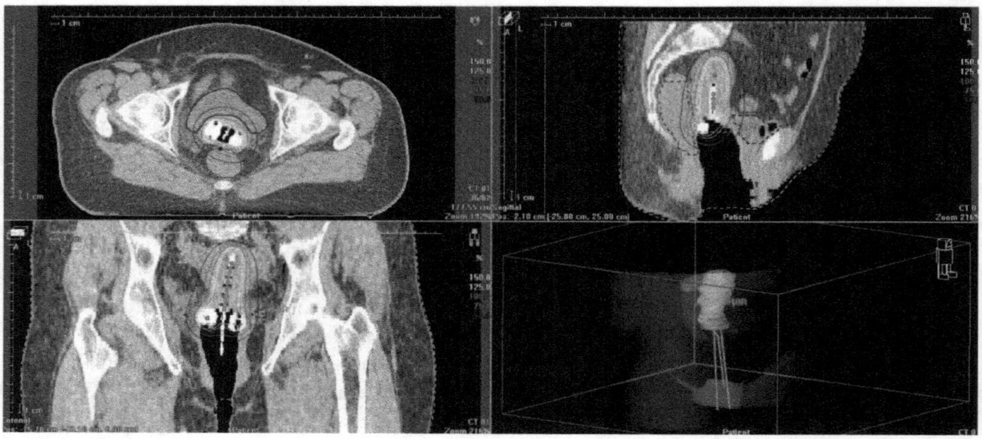

Fig. 1. Cervical cancer - reconstruction of plastic applicator in a 3D CT study. Plastic catheters - intrauterine tube and ovoids are inserted into vaginal vaults and uterus. (a) Para-transverse image at the level of the ovoids, (b) Para-coronal image and (c) Para-sagittal image with a reconstructed tube and ovoids. On (d) 3D-visualisation of application is presented.

4. Prostate cancer

Real-time rectal ultrasonography (US) guidance has been accepted as a standard technique for prostate BT. However, post-implant CT (and MRI) imaging have also been implemented for 3D treatment planning for temporary HDR implants and for the verification of postimplant dose distribution of permanent seed implants. Paper published by Merrick et al. investigated the magnitude of the effect that various methods of treatment volume delineation have on dosimetric quality parameters for a treatment planning philosophy that defines a target volume as the prostate with a periprostatic margin. They noticed that postoperative computed tomography (CT) based dosimetric analysis provides detailed information regarding the coverage and the uniformity of an implant. CT-based postoperative dosimetric analysis provides detailed information regarding the dose distribution to the prostate/periprostatic region, urethra, and rectum (Wallner et al., 1995; Willins & Wallner, 1997; Merrick et al., 1998; Prestidge et al., 1998; Merrick et al., 1999).

Prestidge et al., 1998 found that the majority of institutions performing postimplant assessment employ CT scans, although MRI has also recently been described for this purpose. Typically, scans are taken at 3–5-mm slice intervals from the base to the apex of the gland. The brachytherapist is then asked to outline the prostate on the film of each axial slice on which it is identified. Accurately discerning the prostate from the rectal wall, levator ani musculature, periprostatic venous plexus, preprostatic fat, seminal vesicles, and urethral sphincter requires some experience.

American Brachytherapy Society guidelines for postimplant dosimetric analysis recommend CT-based imaging (Nag et al., 2000). This represents a dramatic improvement over prior postimplant dosimetric methods. The weakness of this method is poor definition of prostate volume by CT imaging relative to MRI or ultrasound imaging (Roach et al., 1996). This is especially true in the postimplant state, when significant anatomical distortion is present due to implanted radioactive sources (seeds) and edema. MRI imaging by pelvic coil or rectal coil provides greater definition of the prostate volume postimplant. Ideally, this clarity of the prostate volume could be combined with the clarity of seed definition by CT to allow improved postimplant dosimetry. Another reason for CT-imaging is assessment of edema associated with ^{125}I or ^{103}Pd prostate brachytherapy and its impact on post-implant dosimetry (Waterman et al., 1998). Pelvic CT scanning is used to determine the necessity of preoperative evaluation of pubic arch interference in patients with small prostate volumes. Bellon et al. concluded that the degree of pubic arch interference is highly variable from one patient to the next and the TRUS volume cannot reliably predict patients who do or do not need a pelvic CT to detect potential arch interference (Bellon et al., 1999).

Another authors compared real-time intraoperative ultrasound-based dosimetry with postoperative computed tomography-based dosimetry for prostate brachytherapy (Nag et al., 2008). Although dosimetry using intraoperative US-based planning provides preliminary real-time information, it does not accurately reflect the postoperative CT-based dosimetry. Until studies have determined whether US-based dosimetry or postoperative CT-based dosimetry can better predict patient outcomes, the American Brachytherapy Society recommendation of CT-based postimplant dosimetry should remain the standard of care (Nag et al., 2008).

An interesting conclusion drew Al-Qaisieh et al. They analyzed computed tomography (CT)-based dosimetry performed to evaluate the variability of different observers' judgements in marking the prostate gland on CT films, and its effect on the parameters that characterize the prostate implantation quality. They observed that the evaluation of prostate gland volume on CT films varies between different observers. This has an effect on the dosimetric indices that characterize the implant quality in particular the D90 (Al-Qaisieh et al., 2002).

CT-imaging is also useful in HDR brachytherapy of prostate cancer. Mullokandov & Gejerman investigated the constancy of catheter position and its impact on dose distribution using serial dosimetric CT scans. During initial CT treatment planning, transverse images of the implant volume were collected, and all structures were digitized into the Planning System. They concluded that interstitial catheters did not slip within the template and were not caudally displaced independently but rather in conjunction with the template (Mullokandov & Gejerman, 2004).

Figure 2 presents example of CT-dosimetry after permanent implants application in Greater Poland Cancer Centre.

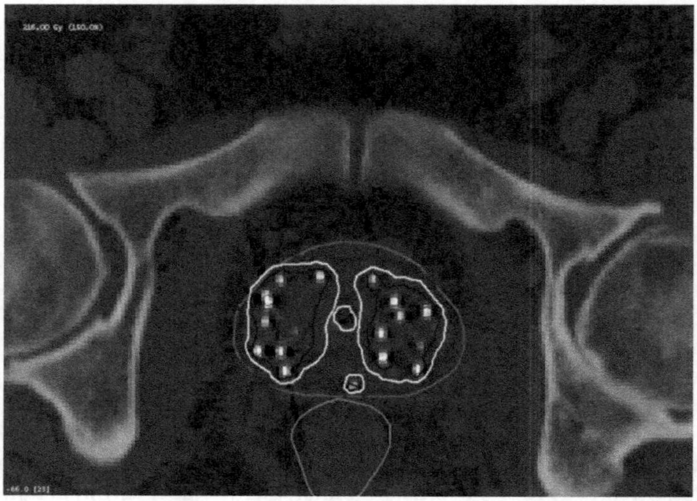

Fig. 2. Prostate cancer - Scan made on next day after permanent seeds implantation. Example of CT-dosimetry after application in Greater Poland Cancer Centre. Prostate is underlined with red line, violet line presents the 100% isodose, yellow line - 150% and blue - 200%, respectively. Urethra (yellow in the middle of prostate) and rectum (brown line) are marked too. Seeds are clearly visible.

5. Breast cancer

Today the availability of modern diagnostic imaging facilities allows to detect early stage of breast cancer, what along with the integration of sophisticated RT techniques, the Breast Conserving Therapy (BCT) makes widely accepted an alternative to mastectomy in the management of early breast cancer (Gerbaulet et al., 2002). The main purpose of radiation in BCT is to prevent any local recurrence without effecting cosmetic outcome (Van Limbergen et al., 1987). Conventionally RT in the BCT includes Whole Breast Radiation Therapy (WBRT) that is usually delivered by tangential beams. A supplementary tumor bed boost dose of 10-20 Gy (either through electrons, photons or an interstitial implants) is added to decrease the rate of local recurrence. The use of BT as additional irradiation to the tumor site with early stage breast cancer has increased significantly over the past several years (Polgar et al., 2002). The big advantage of BT above external beam radiotherapy (EBRT) results in much smaller and more conformal irradiation to the target volume due to the rapid dose fall-off (Frazier et al., 2001; Hammer et al., 2009). Nowadays the indication of the boost after BCT and selection of proper technique in order to deliver extra dose, should be depending on clinical and morphologic criteria as well as patient agreement. At present there are several techniques used in maintaining better coverage of the target volume. However, the irregular 3-D shape of the excision cavity and the normal tissue structures can only be accurately localized by visual information acquired from cross-sectional imaging (Kubaszewska et al., 2008). The use of surgical clips and CT at the same time seems to be the best method to determine the target volume, since both titanium clips and borders of the excision cavity can be visualized exactly from slice to slice (Polgar et al., 2000). CT scan with visible clips is presented in figure 3a, the target volume is then outlined (figure 3b).

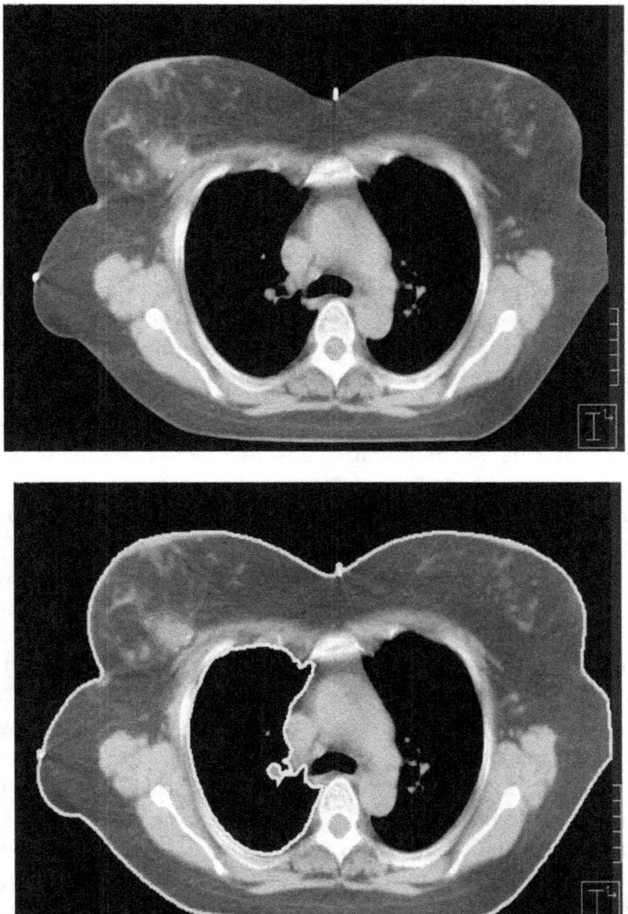

Fig. 3. Breast cancer – (a) CT scan after breast conserving surgery before catheter implantation. Visible three clips, (b) the target (tumor bed) volume (red line), lung and skin (OARs) are outlined.

CT based treatment boost planning - target volume delineation

Every individual case of BT target volume is based on combined information from the pathologic evaluation (factors considered included excision specimen size, tumor location within the resected specimen, characteristic of surgical margins, histological type) mammographic and ultrasound findings, clinical examination (scar position, size and location of any palpable seroma), localization of surgical clips, as well as CT pre-implant cross-sectional imaging (both exact visibility of titanium clips and borders of the slice to slice excision cavity). An intraoperative implantation demands good collaboration and time management between the surgeons and radiation oncologists. The majority of authors suggested the best orientation given by titanium clips marker that are implanted intraoperatively (Hammer et al., 1999; Polgar et al., 2000). Placing of 6 clips into the walls of the excision cavity according to latero - medial, antero - posterior, inferior and superior dimensions seem to be the ideal approach. However, the titanium clips do not alter the dose distribution during RT and the quality of diagnostic MR images after the procedure. The irregular 3 dimensional (3D) shape of the target volume and the normal tissue structures can only be correctly localized on the basis of visual information obtained from cross-sectional CT-imaging. In addition to this, better local control rate with fewer side effects might be achieved with this technique based on CT-imaging (Polgar et al., 2000). The combined use of surgical clips and CT or MRI appear to be the best method to determine the target volume, since both titanium clips and borders of the excision cavity can be visualized exactly from slice to slice. Vicini et al. implemented 3D virtual brachytherapy based on two sets (pre- and postimplant) of CT scans. In their researches, the 3D BT showed excellent agreement in target volume coverage between the preplanned virtual implant geometry and the actual positioning of the final afterloading needles (Vicini et al., 1998).

CT based treatment planning procedure

The advantages of conformal brachytherapy boost treatment planning in the management of breast cancer are as follow: 1. as a useful tool helps to avoid geographical miss, 2. the irregular 3D shape of the target volume and the normal tissue structures can only be localized correctly on the basis of visual information obtained from cross-sectional CT-imaging (better local control rate with less side effects might be achieved with these technique based on CT-imaging), 3. the primary role of the treatment planning and dose optimization for a given implantation is to achieve as best coverage of the target volume as possible (the adequate homogeneity is relatively important) 4. verification of the positioning of the plastic tubes with the use of CT unit (Vicini et al., 1997). With CT-based planning, the distances between implant tubes and overlying skin and underlying ribs are directly visible and measurable. The skin dose should not exceed 60% of prescribed dose (executed only in case of a superficial plane implanted at least 10 mm from the skin).

In the 3D treatment planning based on CT sectional-cross the main aspect is to achieve such dose distribution, where all surgical clips would receive at least 85 % of the prescribed dose (Kubaszewska et al., 2008). Planning concepts are based on the 3D reconstruction of the catheters, tumor bed clips maintaining proper distances (at least 10 mm) from critical structures (skin, ribs). The clinical target volume (CTV) is defined by a margin of 2 cm breast tissue of the primary tumor, since this area contains 80% of the microscopic tumor extensions. The planning target volume (PTV) is comparable to the CTV for the reason that extra margin added in case of organ motion or set-up errors is not required in interstitial BT. The CTV of boost irradiation is not focused on such critical structures like ribs and breast skin with tissues beyond the fascia such as thoracic wall muscle. The minimum distance from the PTV to skin and underling ribs should be 10 mm. This helps to define the dimensions of the boost volume, as well as the choice between electron beam boost and interstitial implants. Some examples of 3-D treatment plans are presented in Figures 4-8. The active source positions, dwell times and reference dose points are defined individually in each catheter as well as dose optimization. To avoid skin and rib injury, the most peripheral active source positions are kept at a minimum of 10 mm distance from the skin and rib surface (Kubaszewska et al., 2008).

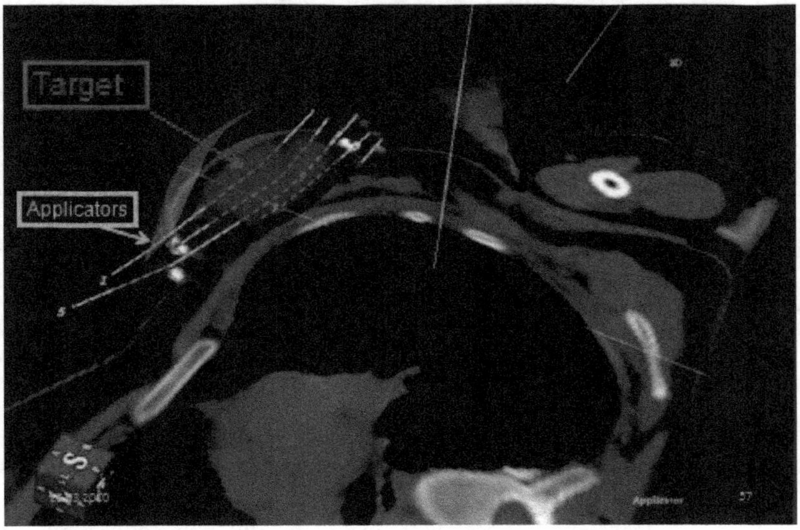

Fig. 4. Breast cancer - CT-based 3D image of Oncentra Planning System® (Nucletron), with target and applicators.

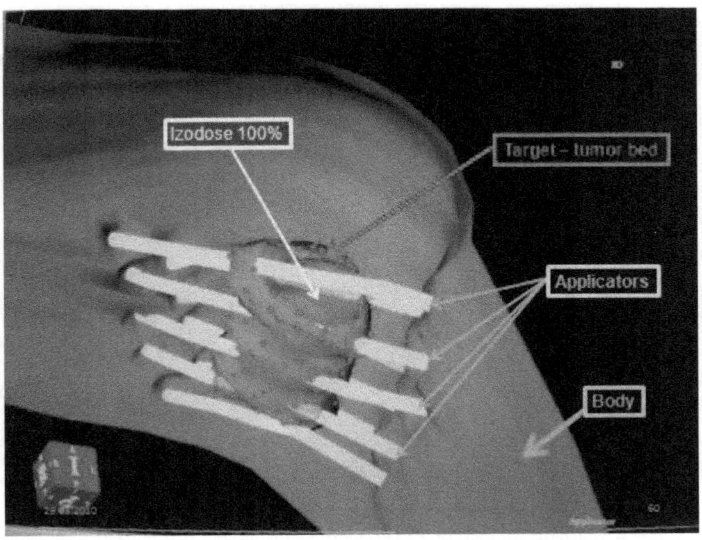

Fig. 5. Breast cancer - CT-based 3D image showing target, applicators and coverage of 100% isodose of target.

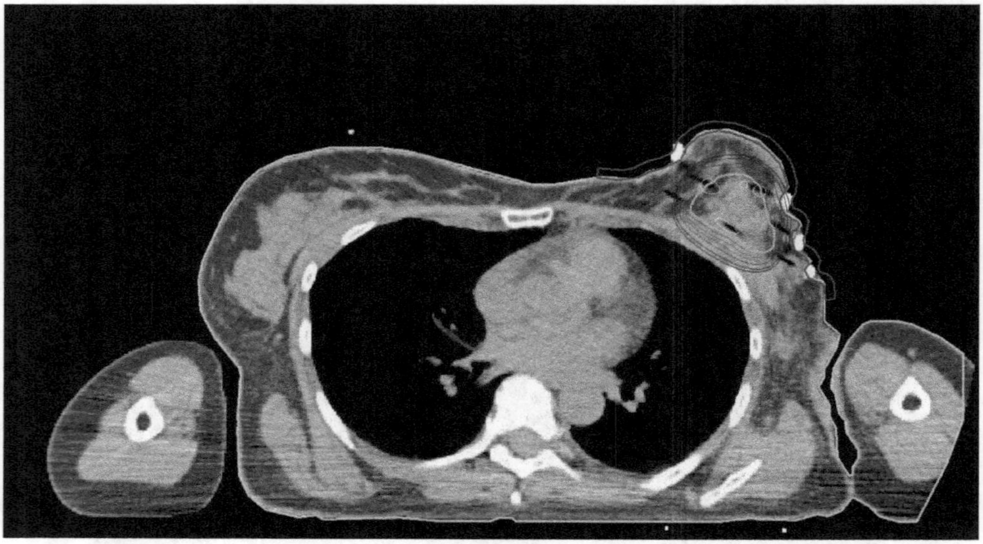

Fig. 6. Breast cancer - Transverse CT scan with final plan - different isodoses allow to assess value of dose in tumor bed (target) lung, skin and other tissues.

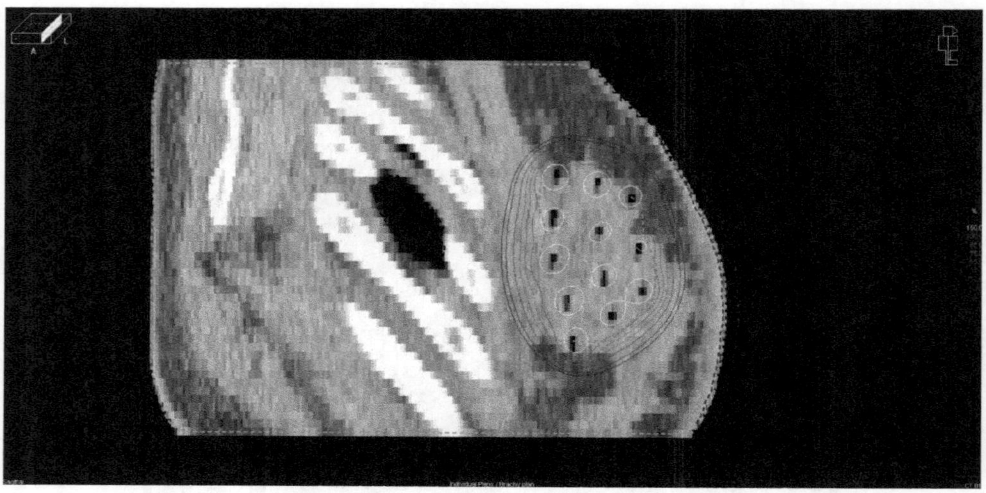

Fig. 7. Breast cancer - Saggital CT scan makes possible assessment of distance from ribs (white structures) and applicators, also from skin to applicators. Values of isodoses are visible.

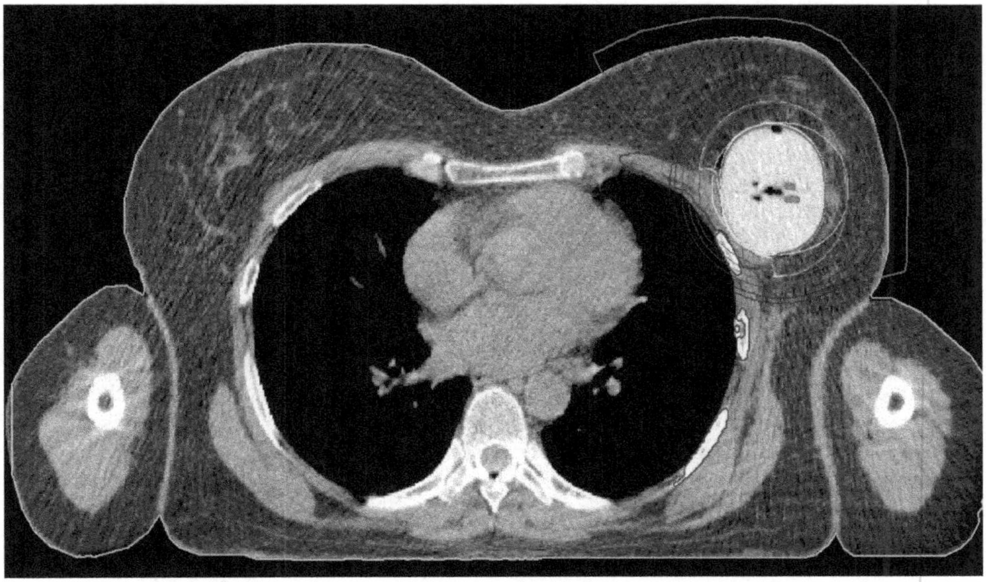

Fig. 8. Breast cancer - Transverse CT scan of Contura® application. Final treatment plan. CT makes possible visualisation of all 5 catheteres within Contura balloon, assessment of isodoses in CTV, lung and skin (OARs).

Polgar et al. compared the conventional 2D, the simulator-guided semi 3D and the recently developed CT-guided 3D brachytherapy treatment planning in the interstitial radiotherapy of breast cancer. With the help of conformal semi 3D and 3D brachytherapy planning they defined reference dose points, active source positions and dwell times individually. This technique decreased the mean skin dose with 22.2% and reduced the possibility of geographical miss. The best conformity between the planning target volume and the treated volume with the CT-image was achieved by 3D treatment planning, however at the cost of worse dose homogeneity. The mean treated volume was reduced by 25.1% with semi 3D planning, however, it was increased by 16.2% with 3D planning, compared to the 2D planning. Authors concluded that the application of clips into the tumor bed and the conformal (semi 3D and 3D) planning help to avoid geographical miss. CT is suitable for 3D brachytherapy planning. Better local control with fewer side effects might be achieved with these new techniques. Conformal 3D brachytherapy calls for new treatment planning concepts, taking the irregular 3D shape of the target volume into account. The routine clinical application of image-based 3D brachytherapy is a real aim in the very close future (Polgar et al., 2000). In conclusion, in breast BT, CT-based PTV definition and implant simulation can be effectively used to obtain improved dose distribution regarding PTV coverage, dose homogeneity and conformality, and dose to OARs (e.g. skin, lung, and heart for left sided tumors). Much better PTV coverage can be achieved with CT image-based implant technique than with conventional one. These dosimetric results reinforce that image-guided BT planning for breast implants can be effectively used to improve dose delivery regarding both target coverage and dose homogeneity, which may turn into improved clinical results.

6. Head and neck cancers

There is limited clinical evidence supporting the routine use of CT image guidance for BT planning of interstitial implants in the H&N region (e.g. oral cavity and base of tongue). Organ (and tumor) motion during implantation limits the possible advantages of preimplant cross-sectional imaging in PTV definition. Thus, clinical examination (palpation) remains the basic element for definition of the target volume for H&N implants. However, CT images are useful to control the dose to OARs for example to avoid radionecrosis of the mandible.

Takácsi-Nagy et al. examined the feasibility and efficacy of interstitial HDR brachytherapy in the treatment of carcinoma of the tongue base (Takácsi-Nagy et al., 2004). Extent of the disease was diagnosed by clinical and computed tomography (CT). Brachytherapy treatment planning was performed by the use of two postimplant isocentric X-ray films or CT images. CT images made possible calculation of the coverage index, which is the fraction of the target volume receiving a dose equal to or greater than the prescribed dose. One of the important conclusions was that successful radiation therapy of base of tongue carcinomas requires total dose above 70 Gy, which, however, increases the risk of osteoradionecrosis and xerostomia. In those locations CT-image based planning reduces this risk.

Another authors analyzed usefulness of CT-imaging in salvage brachytherapy for cervical recurrences of head and neck cancer (Pellizzon et al., 2006). For HDR planning and reconstruction, CT scans were used in order to calculate exactly the dose distribution to the target volume and adjacent healthy tissues. In GEC-ESTRO recommendations we can read, that CT-guided pre-treatment work-up is useful (Mazeron et al., 2009). The CT scan depicts both soft tissue and bone, and is more sensitive than MRI for evaluating lymph nodes. This is the reason for use CT in cases of treatment planning of recurrences in irradiated neck area. Example of CT-image guided brachytherapy is presented in figure 9.

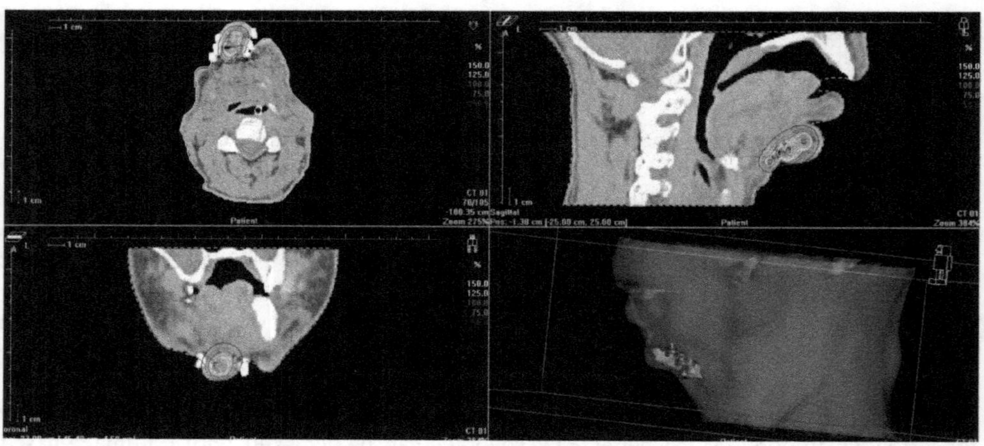

Fig. 9. Head and Neck cancer - CT-image based treatment plan. Tumor (recurrence in lymph node system) is located in chins region. (a) Para-transverse image at the level of the tumor, (b) Para-coronal image and (c) Para-sagittal image. On (d) 3D-visualisation of application is presented.

7. Sarcomas

In 1994 Griffin et al. presented one of the first experiences of using CT-image guided BT. A technique was presented for computer tomography - guided interstitial catheter placement and treatment planning for high-dose-rate brachytherapy. In a 66-year-old woman with adenocarcinoma of unknown origin that had metastasized to the right ilium, interstitial brachytherapy catheters were placed by means of CT guidance. With use of a treatment planning system with dose optimization, an excellent dose distribution was obtained with minimal dose being delivered to the surrounding critical tissues. Authors concluded that for selected patients, this procedure can provide effective and safe local treatment for solid tumors.

Report published by the American Brachytherapy Society (ABS) presents guidelines for the use of brachytherapy for patients with soft tissue sarcoma (Nag et al., 2001). Brachytherapy used alone or in combination with external beam irradiation is an established means of safely providing adjuvant local treatment after resection for soft tissue sarcomas in adults and in children. Brachytherapy options include low dose rate techniques with iridium 192 or iodine 125, fractionated high dose rate brachytherapy, or intraoperative high dose rate therapy. Recommendations are made for patient selection, techniques, dose rates, and dosages. In treatment planning they recommended the cross-section imaging (CT or MRI) which allows for the 3D reconstruction of catheter position and sources within. This approach minimizes errors and furthermore permits 3D treatment planning and dose distribution.

8. Lung cancer and other tumors

There are few reports concerning the use of CT in brachytherapy of lung cancer. Lagerwaard et al. investigated the consequences of using different dose prescription methods for endobronchial brachytherapy (EB), both with and without the use of a centered applicator. A CT scan was performed during EB procedures in 13 patients after insertion of the lung applicator. A dosimetric analysis was subsequently performed in five of these patients using a 3D-brachytherapy treatment planning system (PLATO v13.3®, Nucletron). CT images made possible confirmation of the rapid dose fall-off in EB mucosal dose prescription which should be used with caution in curative treatments where EB, without additional external radiotherapy, was used as the sole treatment modality (Lagerwaard et al., 2000). The CT measurements of the diameter of the different bronchial segments generally correlated well with the calculated values.

In another paper Senan et al. described a CT-based planning method which, by improving target volume definition and volumetric dose information, can improve the therapeutic ratio of EB (Senan et al., 2000). Sixteen CT-assisted EB procedures were performed in patients who were treated with palliative high-dose-rate EB. The CT data were used to analyze applicator position in relation to anatomy. An example of a three-dimensional optimized treatment plan was generated and analyzed using different types of dose-volume histograms. Authors initial experience highlights both the potential benefits and limitations of using "CT-assisted EB", which we have defined as EB characterized by the following: 1. use of CT imaging to supplement the findings of bronchoscopy, particularly in determining the distal extent of the target volume; 2. visualization of the position of the applicator in relation to the target volume; 3. facilitation of dose prescription to the bronchial mucosa by identifying the position of branching of the different subsegments of the bronchial tree and allowing the use of actual measurements of the diameter of each segment; 4. generation of a 3D dosimetric database for correlation with toxicity. Authors concluded that: CT-assisted EB was feasible and underlines the need for using centered applicators for proximally located tumors. By enabling accurate mucosal dose prescription, CT-assisted EB may reduce the toxicity of fractionated EB in the curative setting. However, faster online EB treatment planning is needed for the routine clinical application of this technique (Senan et al., 2000).

In their review article Jansen et al. analyzed usefulness of CT-imaging in treatment planning of brain tumors. They mentioned that delineation of the clinical target volume (CTV) in radiation treatment planning of high-grade glioma is a controversial issue. The use of CT has greatly improved the accuracy of tumor localization in 3D planning. Their review aims at critically analyzing available literature data in which tumor extent of high-grade glioma has been assessed using CT and/or MRI and relating this to postmortem observations. Attention was given to the pattern of tumor spread at initial presentation and to tumor recurrence pattern after external beam irradiation. Special emphasis was given to the site of tumor regrowth after radiation treatment in relation to the boundaries of the CTV. Guidelines for delineating CTV were inferred from this information, taking data on radiation effects on the normal brain into account (Jansen et al., 2000). Hochberg & Pruitt were among the first to demonstrate the value of CT in radiation treatment planning of gliomas. But, they research another subject. They related CT scans in 127 untreated GBM patients with postmortem examination and found that only 3% had multicentric GBM at presentation (Hochberg & Pruitt, 1980). In another study by the same group on 15 patients, CT and postmortem findings were related to the intended radiation treatment plan (Halperin et al., 1989). Studies on CT focused also on reports in which tumor delineation assessed with CT and/or MRI were correlated with documented recurrence patterns after radiation treatment. Accordingly, in a study of 42 patients treated with WBI and followed up with serial CT scanning, 90% of the cases showed tumor recurrence within a 2-cm margin of the primary site (Hochberg & Pruitt, 1980). A similar recurrence pattern was observed after WBI with a cone-down boost field (Gaspar et al., 1992). This results where the basis for limiting the fields in 3D external beam radiation therapy.

In rectal cancer there is an interest in CT-guided needle insertion into tumor or tumor bed. Sakurai et al. described developing of high-dose-rate (HDR) conformal interstitial brachytherapy by means of combined CT-fluoroscopy guidance with CT-based treatment planning for locally recurrent rectal carcinoma. They concluded that CT fluoroscopy guidance ensures safety and increases the accuracy of needles placement in brachytherapy. Conformal high-dose-rate (HDR) interstitial brachytherapy with CT-based treatment planning is a method worth considering for locally recurrent rectal cancer (Sakurai et al., 2004).

9. Conclusions

The target volume is currently generally defined using radiologic imaging (e.g., plane radiography, CT, MRI). The improvements required include increased tissue resolution; improved boundary definition; functional imaging (i.e., PET); and antibody-based imaging. Radiographs are conventionally used for source localization and calculation of the dose distribution around brachytherapy applicators, whether they are placed manually or with a computerized treatment planning system. The doses to normal tissues such as the bladder and the rectum have traditionally been calculated from the implant localization films with contrast in the bladder or catheter bulb and a radiopaque marker or contrast in the rectum. The inability of the orthogonal film pair method to delineate organ boundaries diminishes the reliability of the normal tissue dose point determinations and compromises the understanding of the dose distributions to the non infiltrated soft tissues. An improvement in the spatial resolution may also bring about improved target volume definition of the imaging modality and fusion of various imaging modalities (e.g., transrectal ultrasonography with MRI or CT).

10. Acknowledgements

Author thanks Grzegorz Bielęda, MSc from Greater Poland Cancer Centre, for preparing excellent figures from Oncentra Planning system (Nucletron®, Netherlands).

11. References

Al-Halabi, H., Portelance, P., Duclos, M. et al. (2010). Cone Beam Ct-Based Three-Dimensional Planning In High-Dose-Rate Brachytherapy For Cervical Cancer. *Int J Radiat Oncol Biol Phys;* 77: pp 1092–1097.

Al-Qaisieh, B., Ash, D., Bottomley, D.M. et al. (2002). Impact of prostate volume evaluation by different observers on CT-based post-implant dosimetry. *Radiother Oncol;* 62: pp 267–273.

Barrett, A., Dobbs, J., Morris, S., et al. (2009). *Practical Radiotherapy Planning. 4th Edition.* Hodder Arnold, London. pp 15-19.

Bellon, J., Wallner, K., Ellis, W. et al. (1999). Use of Pelvic CT Scanning to Evaluate Pubic Arch Interference of Transperineal Prostate Brachytherapy. *Int J Radiat Oncol Biol Phys;* 43: pp 579–581.

Davidson, M.T.M., Yuen, J., D'Souza, D.P. et al. (2008). Image-guided cervix high-dose-rate brachytherapy treatment planning: Does custom computed tomography planning for each insertion provide better conformal avoidance of organs at risk? *Brachytherapy;* 7: pp 37-42.

Frazier, R.C., Kestin, L.L., Kini, V., et al. (2001). Impact of boost technique on outcome in early-stage breast cancer patients treated with breast conserving therapy. *Am J Clin Oncol;* 24: pp 26-32.

Gao, M., Albuquerque, K., Chi, A. et al. (2010). 3D CT-based volumetric dose assessment of 2D plans using GEC-ESTRO guidelines for cervical cancer brachytherapy. *Brachytherapy;* 9: pp 55-60.

Gaspar, L.E., Fisher, B.J. & Macdonald, D.R. (1992). Supratentorial malignant glioma: patterns of recurrence and implications for external beam local treatment. *Int J Radiat Oncol Biol Phys;* 24: pp 55-57.

Gerbaulet, A., Pötter, R., Mazeron, J.J. et al. (2002). *The GEC ESTRO Handbook of Brachytherapy.* Brussels. pp 435-454.

Griffin, P.C., Amin, P.A., Hughes, P. et al. (1994). Pelvic Mass: CT-guided Interstitial Catheter Implantation with High-Dose-Rate Remote Afterloader. Radiology; 191: pp 581-583.

Haie-Meder, C., Pötter, R., Van Limbergen, E. et al. (2005). Recommendations from Gynaecological (GYN) GEC-ESTRO Working Group (I): Concepts and terms in 3D image based 3D treatment planning in cervix cancer brachytherapy with emphasis on MRI assessment of GTV and CTV. *Radiother Oncol*; 74: pp 235-245.

Halperin, E.C., Bentel, G., Heinz, E.R. et al. (1989). Radiation therapy treatment planning in supratentorial glioblastoma multiforme: an analysis based on post mortem topographic anatomy with CT correlations. *Int J Radiat Oncol Biol Phys*; 17: pp 1347-1350.

Hammer, J., Mazeron, J.J & van Limbergen, E. (2001). Breast boost - Why, how, when? *Strahlenther Onkol*; 175: pp 478–483.

Hellebust, T.P., Kirisits Ch., Berger D. et al. (2010). Recommendations from Gynaecological (GYN) GEC-ESTRO Working Group: Considerations and pitfalls in commissioning and applicator reconstruction in 3D image-based treatment planning of cervix cancer brachytherapy. *Radioth Oncol*; 96: pp 153–160.

Hellebust, T.P., Tanderup, K., Bergstrand, E.S. et al. (2007). Reconstruction of the ring applicator set using CT imaging; impact of reconstruction method and applicator orientation. *Phys Med Biol*; 52: pp 4893–4904.

Hochberg, F.H. & Pruitt, A. (1980). Assumptions in the radiotherapy of glioblastoma. *Neurology*; 30: pp 907-911.

Jansen, J.P.M., Dewit, L.G.H., van Herk, M. et al. (2000). Target volumes in radiotherapy for high-grade malignant glioma of the brain. *Radiother Oncol*; 56: pp 151-156.

Kolotas, Ch., Baltas, D & Zamboglou N. (1999). CT-Based Interstitial HDR Brachytherapy. *Strahlenther Onkol*; 175: pp 419–427.

Kubaszewska, M., Dymnicka, M., Skowronek, J., et al. (2008). CT-image based conformal High Dose Rate Brachytherapy boost in the conservative treatment of stage I –II breast cancer - introducing the procedure. *Rep Pract Radioth Oncol*; 5: pp 227 - 239.

Lagerwaard, F.J., Murrer, L.H.P., de Pan, C. et al. (2000). Mucosal Dose Prescription in Endobronchial Brachytherapy: A Study Based On CT-Dosimetry. *Int J Radiat Oncol Biol Phys;* 46: pp 1051–1059.

Van Limbergen, E., Van den Bogaert, W., Van der Schueren, E., et al. (1987). Tumor excision and radiotherapy as primary treatment of breast cancer. Analysis of patient and treatment parameters and local control. *Radiother Oncol*; 8: pp 1-9.

Ling, C., Schell, M., Working, K. et al. (1987). CT-assisted assessment of bladder and rectum dose in gynecological implants. *Int J Radiat Oncol Biol Phys*; 13: pp 1577–1582.

Mazeron, J-J., Ardiet, J-M., Haie-Méder, Ch. et al. (2009). GEC-ESTRO recommendations for brachytherapy for head and neck squamous cell carcinomas. *Radiother Oncol*; 91: pp 150–156.

Merrick, G.S., Butler, W.M., Dorsey, A.T. et al. (1998). Influence of timing on the dosimetric analysis of transperineal ultrasound-guided prostatic conformal brachytherapy. *Rad Onc Invest*; 6: pp 182–190.

Merrick, G.S., Butler, W.M., Dorsey, A.T. et al. (1999). The potential role of various dosimetric quality indications in prostate brachytherapy. *Int J Radiat Oncol Biol Phys*; 44: pp 717-724.

Merrick, G.S., Butler, W.M., Dorsey, A.T. et al. (1999). The Dependence Of Prostate Postimplant Dosimetric Quality On Ct Volume Determination. *Int J Radiat Oncol Biol Phys;* 44: pp. 1111–1117.

Mullokandov, E. & Gejerman G. (2004). Analysis of Serial CT Scans to Assess Template and Catheter Movement in Prostate HDR Brachytherapy. *Int J Radiat Oncol Biol Phys;* 58: pp 1063–1071.

Nag, S., Bice, W., de Wyngaert, K. et al. (2000). The American Brachytherapy Society recommendations for permanent prostate brachytherapy postimplant dosimetric analysis. *Int J Radiat Oncol Biol Phys;* 46: pp 221–230.

Nag, S., Cardenes, H., Chang, S. et al. (2004). Proposed guidelines for image-based intracavitary brachytherapy for cervical carcinoma: Report from Image-Guided Brachytherapy Working Group. *Int J Radiat Oncol Biol Phys;* 60: pp 1160–1172.

Nag, S., Shasha, D., Janjan, N. et al. for The American Brachytherapy Society. (2001). The American Brachytherapy Society Recommendations for Brachytherapy of Soft Tissue Sarcomas. *Int J Radiat Oncol Biol Phys;* 49: pp 1033–1043.

Nag, S., Shi, P., Liu, B. et al. (2008). Comparison of Real-Time Intraoperative Ultrasound-Based Dosimetry with Postoperative Computed Tomography-Based Dosimetry for Prostate Brachytherapy. *Int J Radiat Oncol Biol Phys;* 70: pp 311–317.

Pellizzon, A.C.A., Salvajoli, J.V., Kowalski, L.P. et al. (2006). Salvage for cervical recurrences of head and neck cancer with dissection and interstitial high dose rate brachytherapy. *Radiation Oncology;* 1: pp 27-32.

Polgar, C., Fodor, J., Orosz, Z., et al. (2002). Electron and high-dose-rate brachytherapy boost in the conservative treatment of stage I-II breast cancer: First results of the randomized Budapest boost trial. *Strahlenther Onkol;* 178: pp 615–623.

Polgár, C., Major, T., Somogyi, A. et al. (2000). CT-image based conformal brachytherapy of breast cancer: the significance of semi-3D and 3-D treatment planning. *Strahlenther Onkol;* 176: pp 118-124.

Pötter, R., Haie-Meder, C., Van Limbergen, E. et al. (2006). Recommendations from gynaecological (GYN) GEC ESTRO working group (II): Concepts and terms in 3D image-based treatment planning in cervix cancer brachytherapy-3D dose volume parameters and aspects of 3D image-based anatomy, radiation physics, radiobiology. *Radiother Oncol;* 78: pp 67-77.

Prestidge, B.R., Bice, W.S., Kiefer, E.T. et al. (1998). Timing of computed tomography based post-implant assessment following permanent transperineal prostate brachytherapy. *Int J Radiat Oncol Biol Phys;* 40: pp 1111–1115.

Roach, M., Faillace-Akazawa, P., Malfatti, C. et al. (1996). Prostate volumes defined by magnetic resonance imaging and computerized tomographic scans for three-dimensional conformal radiotherapy. *Int J Radiat Oncol Biol Phys;* 35: pp 1011–1018.

Sakurai, H., Mitsuhashi, N., Harashima, K. et al. (2004). CT-fluoroscopy guided interstitial brachytherapy with image-based treatment planning for unresectable locally recurrent rectal carcinoma. *Brachytherapy;* 3: pp 222–230.

Senan, S., Lagerwaard, F.J., de Pan, C. on behalf of the Rotterdam Oncological Thoracic Study Group. (2000). A CT-assisted method of dosimetry in brachytherapy of lung cancer. *Radiother Oncol;* 55: pp 75-80.

Shin, K.H., Kim, T.H., Cho, J.K. et al. (2006). CT-guided intracavitary radiotherapy for cervical cancer: Comparison of conventional Point A plan with clinical target volume-based three-dimensional plan using dose-volume parameters. *Int J Radiat Oncol Biol Phys;* 64: pp 197–204.

Takácsi-Nagy, Z., Polgár, C., Oberna, F. et al. (2004). Interstitial High-Dose-Rate Brachytherapy in the Treatment of Base of Tongue Carcinoma. *Strahlenther Onkol*; 180: pp 768–775.

Vicini, F.A., Horwitz, E.M., Lacerna, M.D. et al. (1997). Long term outcome with interstitial brachytherapy in the management of patient with early breast cancer treated with breast conserving therapy. *Int J Radiat Oncol Biol Phys*; 37: pp 845-852.

Vicini, F.A., Jaffray, D.A., Horwitz, E.M. et al. (1998). Implementation of 3D-virtual brachytherapy in the management of breast cancer: a description of a new method of interstitial brachytherapy. *Int J Radiat Oncol Biol Phys*; 40: pp 629-635.

Viswanathan, A.N. & Erickson, B. (2010). Three-Dimensional Imaging in Gynecologic Brachytherapy: A Survey of the American Brachytherapy Society. *Int J Radiat Oncol Biol Phys*; 76: pp 104–109.

Viswanathan, A.N., Dimopoulos, J., Kirisits, C. et al. (2007). Computed tomography versus magnetic resonance imaging-based contouring in cervical cancer brachytherapy: Results of a prospective trial and preliminary guidelines for standardized contours. *Int J Radiat Oncol Biol Phys*; 68: pp 491–498.

Wang, B., Kwon, A., Zhu, Y. et al. (2009). Image-guided intracavitary high-dose-rate brachytherapy for cervix cancer: A single institutional experience with three-dimensional CT-based planning. *Brachytherapy*; 8: pp 240-247.

Wallner, K., Roy, J. & Harrison, L. (1995). Dosimetry guidelines to minimize urethral and rectal morbidity following transperineal I-125 prostate brachytherapy. *Int J Radiat Oncol Biol Phys*; 32: pp 465–471.

Willins, J. & Wallner, K. (1997). CT based dosimetry for transperineal I-125 prostate brachytherapy. *Int J Radiat Oncol Biol Phys*; 39: pp 347–353.

Waterman, F., Yue, N., Cord, B.W. et al. (1998). Edema associated with ^{125}I or ^{103}Pd prostate brachytherapy and its impact on post-implant dosimetry: An analysis based on serial CT acquisition. *Int J Radiat Oncol Biol Phys;* 41: pp 1069–1077.

Part 4

Advanced CT Imaging and Analysis

10

An Approach to Lumbar Vertebra Biomechanical Analysis Using the Finite Element Modeling Based on CT Images

Haiyun Li
Capital Medical University School of Biomedical Engineering, Beijing, 100069 China

1. Introduction

Lumber disc herniation is one of the most common causes of low back pain. Relevant research indicates that it is generally induced by the degenerated deformation of a disc due to too much labor or spine abnormality. The number and variety of clinical interventions for lumbar disc herniation continue to grow. The lumbar intervertebral disc is a viscoelastic tissue located in the middle of the two intervertebral bodies, which is the largest cartilaginous structure in human body that contributes to flexibility and load support in the spine. They can transfer labor loads, balance body, stabilize spine and absorb vibration[1]. All the functions depend on the intact disc. In pathological cases such as disc herniation caused by excessive load on the spine. The spine will undergo a series of changes in its biomechanical properties.

The interbertebral disc consists of endplate, annulus fiber, and nucleus pulposus. The penetration between endplate and the concellous bone will change feebly if the disc bears an abnormal force and thus can affect the nutrient supply of annulus fiber, which results in the degeneration of the disc. Annulus fiber with poor nutrient supply is likely to rupture if there exists a stress concentration on this region. The nucleus pulposus will dissociate from the disc along the ruptured region. At last, the disc extrudes out[2,3].

In order to biomechanically evaluate the treatment options for spine related diseases and gain a better understanding of spinal biomechanical behaviour, there are three types of methodologies available. *In vitro* biomechanical experimental measurements on spinal components or segments tested in the laboratory have been used extensively to compare different treatment scenarios, but there are inherent limitations in using the specimens[2,4,5]. The limitations include the availability, the range of samples and the representativity of specimens. *In vivo* measurements can provide true subject-specific information on the spine in its physiological state but are confined by the requirement for limited invasiveness. More recently, in silico testing method has become more prevalent in the biomechanics assessment of the spine. In particular, there has been a rapid rise in the use of finite element analysis for this purpose over the last decade. The finite element analysis is a standard engineering technique generally used in the design of airplanes, machines and bridges. Using a special software, it allows the modeling of complex structures by splitting the structure into numerous simple finite elements, each of which is easy to characterize and model mathematically. It is a numerical method for solving problems of engineering and mathematical physics[6]. Finite element modelling and calculating can be applied to show detailed biomechanical characteristics of lumbar and provide intrinsic parameters (stress, strain, strain energy, etc). Finite element models of the spine have been developed to evaluate surgical interventions, and also to investigate the risk of fracture in the vertebrae and the progression of degeneration in the intervertebral discs.

Our study is to analyze the biomechnical characteristics of lumbar in the compression using the finite element method based on medical image. We are sure that better understanding on the biomechnical characteristics of surgical procedures will ultimately get to better diagnosis and treatment on intervertebral disk herniation.

2. Methodology

In this chapter, a CT image based computational method has been presented which is applied to perform biomechanical analysis for lumbar vertebrae *in vivo*. The method involves establishing a subject-specific geometric model and a finite element model for vertebra. The geometric model derived from CT images represents three-dimensional anatomy characteristics of the vertebra. the finite element model based on geometric model provides a useful tool to perform biomechanical calculation for the vertebra. These numerical models are created from CT image data, in a process, which draws from an array of segmentation and mesh generation tool to define the geometry model. The geometry model is then augmented into finite element model with material properties, boundary conditions and interactions between multi-element models. We can get the stain and stress distribution of the whole structure by studying the relation between the displacement of particle and force for every element[6,7]. It is a feasible method for resolving biomechanical characteristic problem of complex structure.

2.1 Geometric model

The subject-specific geometric model is established by segmenting vertebrae in CT slice images and performing three-dimensional reconstruction slice-by-slice using extracted vertebrae morphology information.

A reliable segmentation of vertebrae is essential for subject-specific geometric model. Although bony structures show high contrast in CT images, a precise segmentation of vertebrae still remains challenging. Many factors could influence the accuracy and robustness of the vertebrae segmentation, e.g., complex anatomical structure, degenerative deformations, unclear object boundaries and similar structures in close vicinity, and these factors also could complicate the application of fully automated segmentation. Several approaches to precise segmentation of lumbar vertebrae in CT images were proposed so far. Admittedly, exact vertebrae segmentation has not been addressed. It has to be noted that these methods were developed for specific vertebrae regions. Several methods have been presented aiming at automated segmentation and labelling of the vertebrae, combining respective characterics of MRI and CT image. In MRI images, bony tissue structures show as dark regions with sparse details and low contrast whereas the intervertebral disks often appear brighter. In comparison with MRI, CT offers higher contrast for bony tissue structures while it is somewhat difficult to distinguish the intervertebral disks from surrounding soft tissue in CT images.

We developed a method to establish three-dimensional subject-specific geometric model of vertebrae based on the CT and MRI data-based anatomical structure of spine by using reconstruction software VTK. A GE Lightspeed 16 CT scanner (General Electric, Fairfield, CT) was used to scan the human subject. A young man with no history of present and past disc disease was selected as normal subject. Initially L1-L2 motion segment data were taken in the axial direction, from which we could get 30 contiguous slices images from the CT scans. The CT slice images had a slice thickness of 0.8mm, and each pixel size is 0.33×0.33mm. The 3D modeling procedure was in the VTK software. We obtained three groups of 3D data from CT scans, the disc, L1, and L2 vertebral bones. The original 2D image slices from CT scans has 512×512 resolution. Considering the cost of the calculation time, in order to get the balance between the accuracy and time cost, we reconstructed the 3D image by using the 2D subsampled image slices which had 64×64 resolution substituted of the original 2D image slices with a 512×512 resolution. The subsample ratio is 8:1. Then, we have these slice images segmented. In order to precisely extract the morphology of vertebrae in CT images, we apply both automated and manual segmentation methods for slice images. First we adopted gray threshold segmentation algorithms for 2D image slices. As we know, the gray value of bone is greater than those of other tissues. We can separate the bone tissue from other tissue by setting a proper gray value. However, the automated gray threshold segmentation may result in artificial isolated section or discontinuous boundary as the gray value of cancellous bone is lower than that of cortical bone and similar to those of other tissues such as soft tissue. That's why we employ the manual segmentation to modify the contour and boundary of the 2D slice images of the vertebrae. The manual segmentation is a live-wire-based semi-automatic segmentation method.
MRI image is used as a reference priori knowledge for radiologist to identify the corresponding anatomical structure in CT image. The radiologist could interactively modify the segmented result using the manual method after the automated gray threshold segmentation.
The 3D L1-L2 segmentation modeling was fundamentally performed based on a set of segmented image data of axial slices in VTK software using Maching cubes algorithm, a surface reconstruction method. The segmentation result shows in Fig. 1, and the reconstructed 3D model of the segment shows in Fig. 2.
All reconstruction models were saved in a VTK file format. Its content included space coordinates of keypoints as well as topologic structure on the surface of the model. We

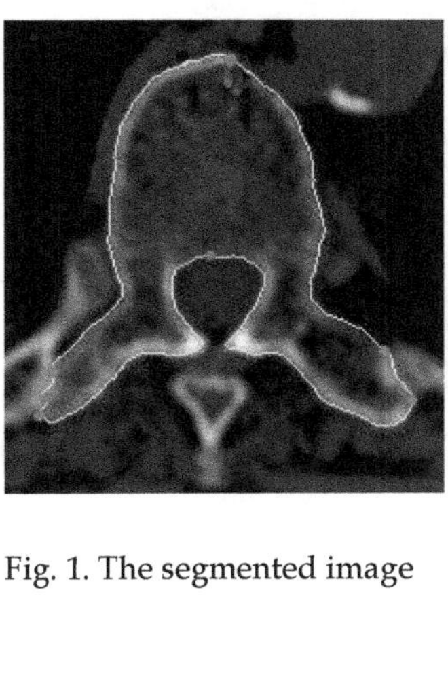

Fig. 1. The segmented image

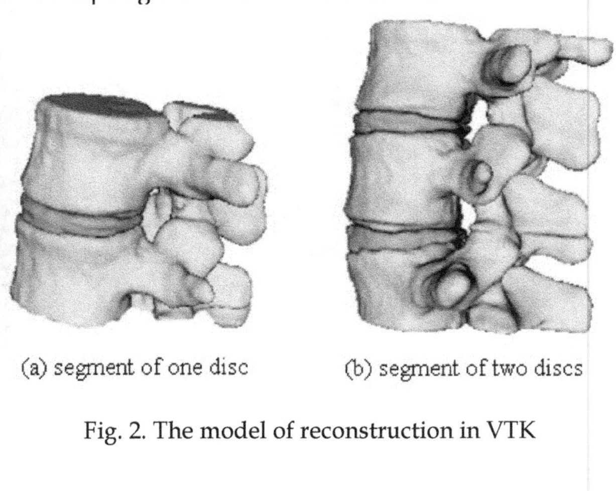

(a) segment of one disc (b) segment of two discs

Fig. 2. The model of reconstruction in VTK

translate the data from the VTK file format to the macro file format in order to import the data to the finite element method software Ansys6.0. We finally create the geometric model of the L1-L2 segment in Ansys6.0. The space coordinates of the keypoints in the VTK software correspond to the keypoints in Ansys6.0. It is convenient to transfer data between the geometric model in VTK and the finite element model in Ansys6.0. The geometric model which was imported into Ansys6.0 is an entity model. We divided it into a grid of elements by applying the finite element meshing on it to form the finite element model.

2.2 The finite element model

The generation of a subject-specific finite element model consists of the determination of the geometrical parameters, the creation of a finite element mesh and the definition of the material properties, and all the procedures should be associated to the given subject. The common method for creating a subject-specific mesh of the vertebrae is the direct conversion from image voxel to hexahedral mesh elements. In this method, the segmented region of the image is extracted and each image voxel is directly converted to a brick element in the mesh. Materials properties are defined on an element-by-element basis using densities derived from the image data. The density value is generally derived for each element based on the image intensity in that region, then the density is applied to calculate the Young's modulus value for that element. Several formulae used for this calculation conversion have been published, as yet there is no consensus as to which of these formulae is most appropriate. How to get more accurate material properties of vertebrae tissue is still challenging for most image-based models.

We applied the Ansys to create an isotropic, 3D, nonlinear finite element model of an intact human L1-L2 motion segment. Details of the model developing have been given and are briefly summarized here: the shape of the lumbar segment is reconstructed from data obtained from CT scans of a human L1-L2 segment. The finite model created is shown in Fig. 3.

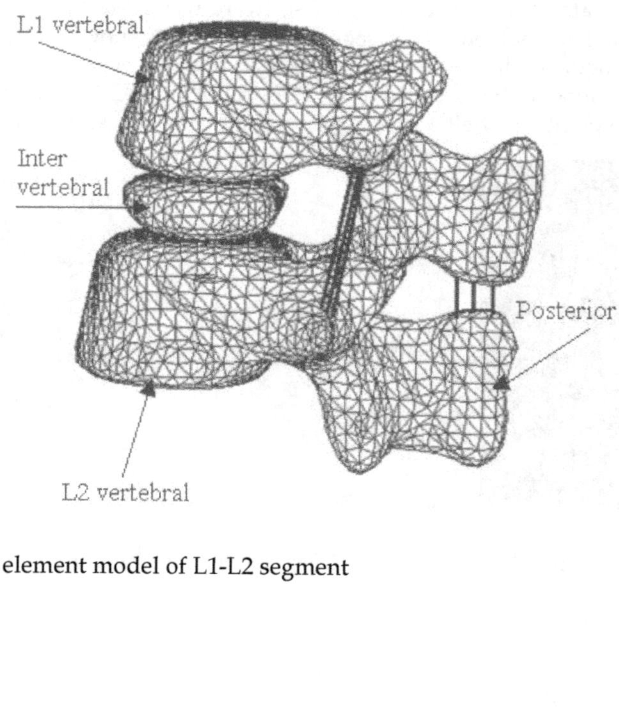

Fig. 3. The finite element model of L1-L2 segment

Each vertebral bone was modeled as 20-node isoparametric material elements using homogeneous and isotropic material properties[8]. The intervertebral disc was modeled using solid elements to simulate an incompressible behavior with a low Young modulus and a Poisson ratio close to 0.4999[8]. In order to appropriately model the changes of contacting areas of facet articulating surface which were applied upon with the load, facet articulations were modeled using contact elements. The ligaments were modeled as two-node axial cable elements that sustained tension only, oriented along the respective ligament fiber alignment. Their attachment points to the bony prominence were determined by referring to anatomy books in order to mimic anatomic observations as close as possible. The cross-sectional areas used were averages of the values reported previously. The material properties used in the study were derived from the literature[8-10]. The behavior of material properties in the model response better reflected those of published experimental lumbar response. Here, we hypothesize that the strain of spine is small. Table 1 lists the type, number and material properties of element used to model the various components of the L1-L2 motion segment and the complete model consists of 37449 elements.

Material	Element type	Element number	Young's modulus(MPa) /Possion rate
Cortical bone of L1	20-node brick (solid 95)	16596	200/0.3
Cortical bone of L2	20-node brick (solid 95)	18663	200/0.3
Disc bone	20-node brick (solid 95)	2082	4/0.4999
Facet joint Ligaments	Contact(CONTA 174) 3D-cable(tension only)	42	

Table 1. Element type and material properties

2.3 Boundary conditions

With regard to the validation and accurateness of model analysis, we applied the boundary conditions on the finite element model. The boundary conditions on the model use pressure and restraints assigned to surface areas of the model. The inferior surface of L2 vertebral body and its spinous process were fixed in all directions. The restraints were used to limit the models movement with six possible values at the node on the surface, three translations and three rotations. The value of freedom was zero. Then couple the inferior surface of vertebral L1 body and the upper surface of the intervertebral disc body, as well as the bottom intervertebral disc body and the upper surface of the L2 vertebral body in all directions of translation. The facet articulation was modeled as a 3D contact unit using interface elements [8].

2.4 Load cases

In this study we will analyze the stress and strain distribution of the spine. The evaluation was performed by following methods: (1) load-displacement behavior. We can observe the displacement change of the vertebral and the strain distribution of L1-L2 segment under different loads. (2) A load of 1600N axial compression was applied to the superior surface of the model in the form of a uniformly concentrated load over all L1 superior surface nodes. We can observe the stress distribution of L1-L2 segment by applying the load and clue on the high stress concentration region as the most likely fracture areas. (3) Disc bulge: disc herniation is an important part in our study for the L1-L2 segment. It is of clinical significance to analyze the disc bulge degree under different directions at 400N axial compression, and such analysis can instruct the surgical treatment for disc herniation. (4) Nucleus populous resection: appling 500N loads on the L1-L2 segment with denucleated disc to observe stress and strain distribution on lumbar and the difference between normal disc and denucleated disc. From the load cases, we know that the finite element model can be used to predict the change of biomechanical behavior of the human lumbar spine under pressure.

3. Results

The stress and strain distributions of the vertebral column were obtained from biomechanical analysis by applying different axial compression loads using our proposed CT image based numerical modelling method. The results are presented in the following sections.

3.1 Load displacement

The loads we applied on the L1 superior surface were: 500, 1000, 1500, 2000, and 2500 N. The L1 superior surface bears a 500N load when a healthy person weighted 70 kg stands straight in a relaxation state. However, the number goes up to 2000N when he lifted 100N with two arms stretching straight. The heavier he lifts the more L1 superior surface bears. The results of load-displacement behavior in axial compression are shown in Table 2. From the table we can see an increase tendency of displacement of L1 superior surface with the increase of load. The tendency is approximately linear which also illustrates that the vertebral bone has flexible biomechanical characteristics.

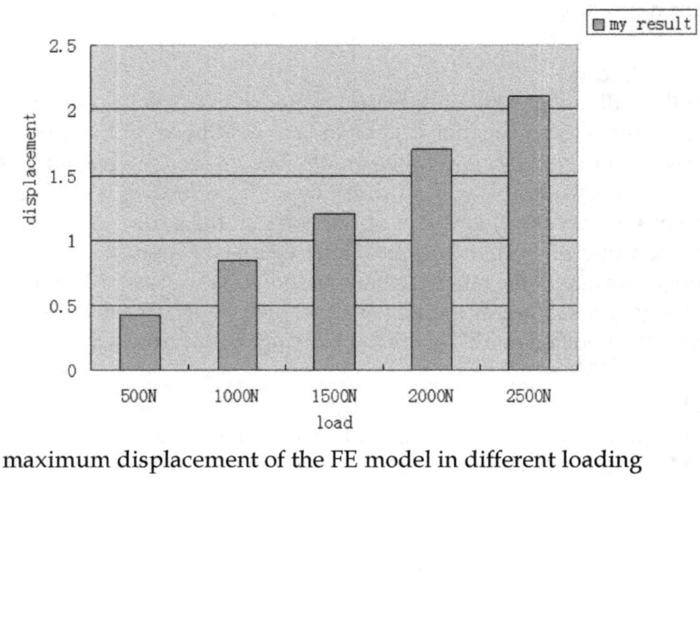

Table 2. The maximum displacement of the FE model in different loading

3.2 Stress distribution of model

Fig. 4 shows the stress distribution of the spine when an 1500N load is applied. It shows that the high stress concentrations are around the vertebral body and pedicle region due to the way the load applied. That is, they are mainly focusing on the upper body of vertebral. These areas show Von Mises stress that ranges gradually from blue, 1.7E−01mN/mm^2 to the Maximum Von Mises stress of 1.57E−02mN/mm^2 indicated in red. The stress on the vertebral body (the value ranges from 35 to 87) is higher than that on the pedicle (about 17), which makes it a common place for injuries due to loading. The stress concentration may be higher in pedicle region if the pedicle area is loaded with a greater proportion.

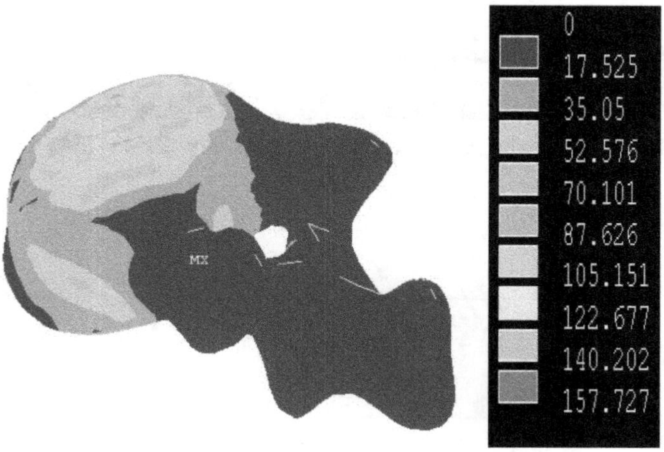

Fig. 4. The Vos Mises distribution of L1-L2 segment

As to the L1 vertebral displacement, the vertebral body and the superior articular processes are compressed downward. Consequently, the movement of vertebral due to the applied load and restraints placed on the model induces the high areas of stress in the pedicle.

3.3 Disc bulge

3.3.1 Disc stress distribution

The disc consists of annulus fiber and nucleus pulposus. In a normal healthy disc, the hydrated nucleus pulposus exerts a hydrostatic pressure (intradiscal pressure, IDP) on the annulus fibrosus (annulus) fibers [11]. The fiber bears a higher IDP than the nucleus pulposus [12,13]. Applying 1000N axial compressive loads on the normal disc, we can see that the value of stress on fiber shows in green, and the range of the stress is from 1.77E−01 to 2.67E−01mN/mm^2. From the annulus fiber to the nucleus pulposus, the intensity of stress grows weaker and weaker (Fig. 5). It indicates that the nucleus pulposus can absorb some compressive loads. That's why the fiber shows higher stress than the nucleus pulposus. From the figure, we can also see that the stress and strain distribution of lumbar is mainly concentrated on the posterior and bilateral posterior of annulus fibers in the normal disc.
We can also observe that the stress becomes higher correspondingly as the loads applied to the disc increases. The relationship between IDP and the external load is approximately linear as is shown in Table 3, indicating that intervertebral disc has flexible properties in a certain extent.

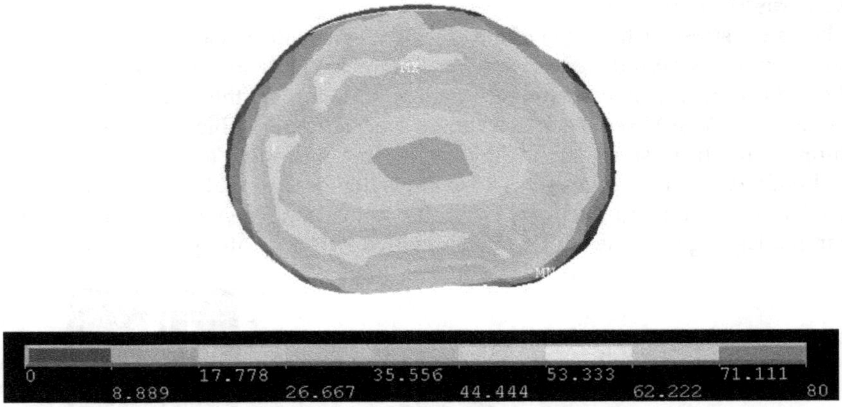

Fig. 5. Vos Mises distribution of disc at 1000N axial compressed load

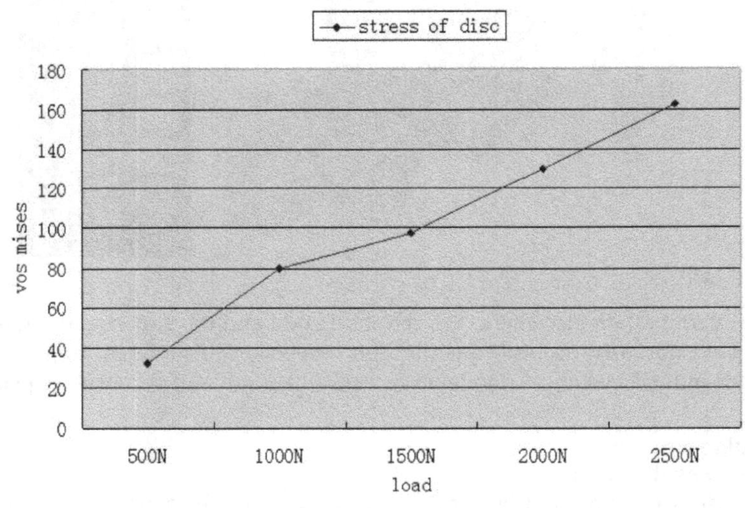

Table 3. The maximum stress of disc in different loading

3.3.2 Bulge direction and magnitude

Four nodal points on the intervertebral disc were taken to represent the directions of bulge, left lateral, and right lateral, left posterior and right posterior. They were marked to determine the bulge displacement of the disc at the 500N axial compression (Fig. 6) [9]. We observed the degree of the bulge at four directions. The result indicates that the displacement of posterior disc extrusion is more obvious than that of bilateral.

Table 4 displays the disc bulge magnitude at different directions on the 500N load. Table 5 lists the disc displacement magnitude at different axial compressive loads from 500 to 2500 N. The values of displacement at all directions increase with the increase of loads. The posterior direction has a more obvious tendency to extrude than others; at the same time, the bilateral direction has a greater tendency to extrude out than the anterior. This agrees

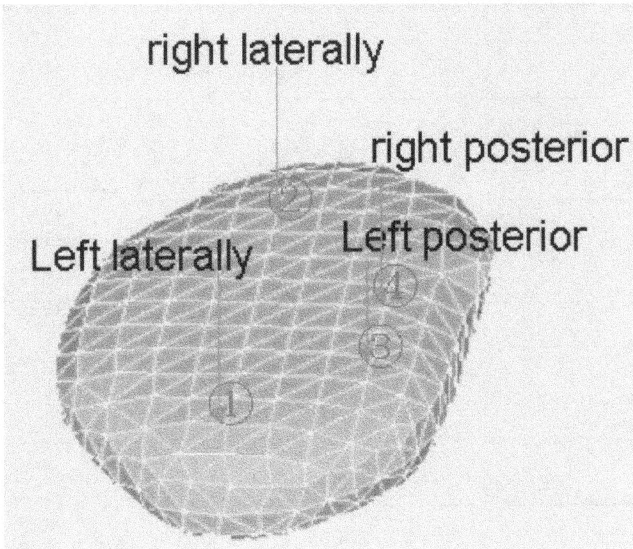

Fig. 6. The selection of four directional node

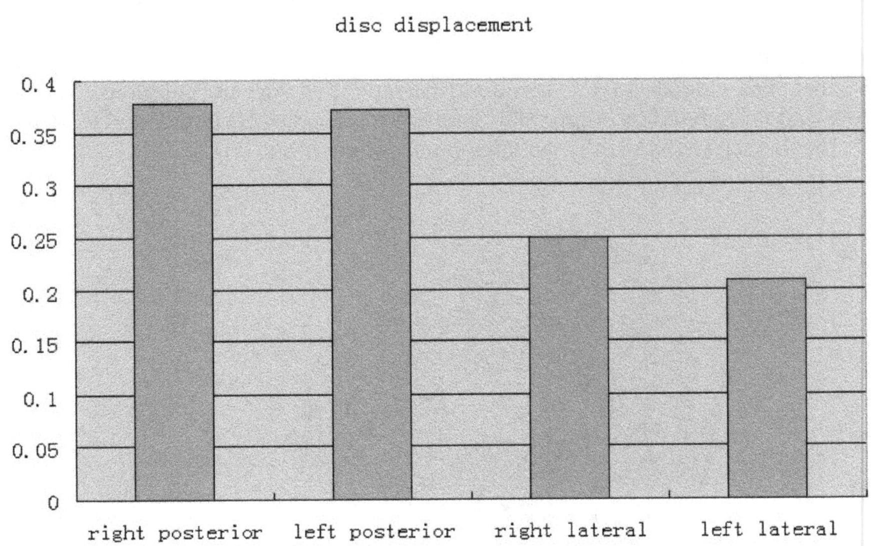

Table 4. Disc bulge displacement at axial load of 500N

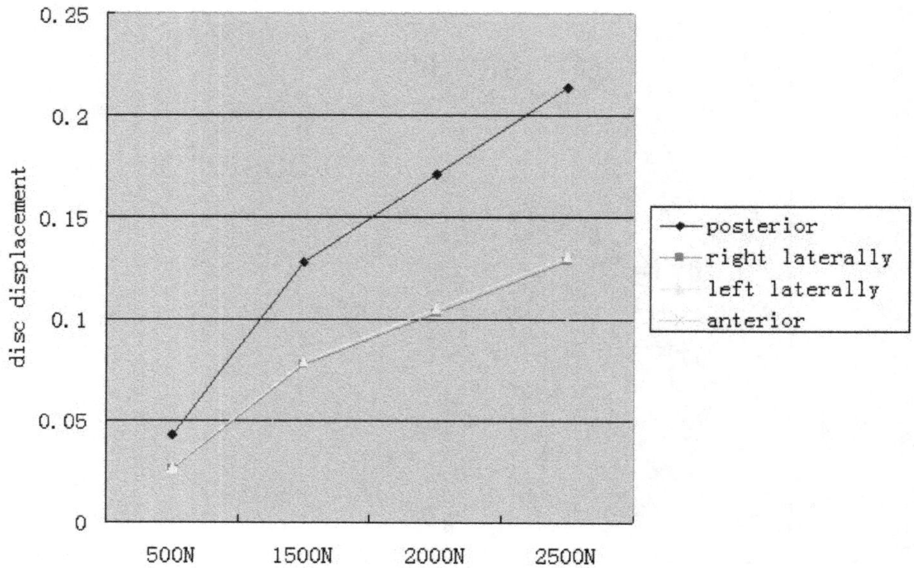

Table 5. Disc displacement at different axial loads

with what we observed on the patients. Our clinical experience tells us that posterior-lateral of the disc is the region where annulus fiber ruptures and nucleus populous extrusion occurs easily. As we reviewed above, this is also the region with higher stress. It indicates stress focusing on the region defined has certain relation with disc herniation.

3.4 Removal of the nucleus

The normal disc consists of the annulus fiber and the nucleus populous. The nucleus populous was considered incompressible and was modeled as 3D tetrahedral solid elements [11,14]. The denucleated disc only includes annulus fiber tissue (Fig. 7).

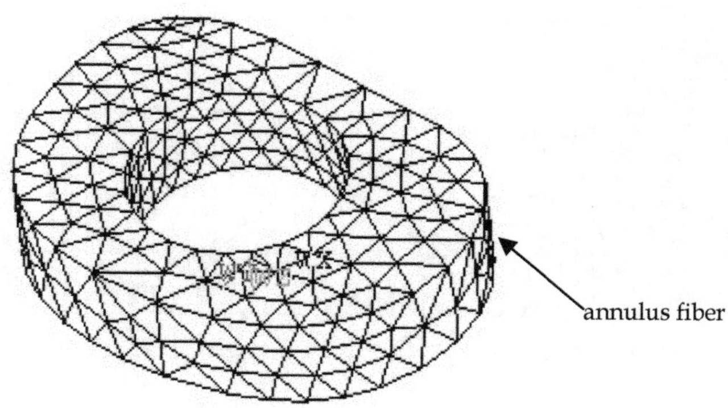

Fig. 7. The finite element model of an intact denucleated disc

Consequently, the process of modeling is similar to that of a normal disc except setting IDP of nucleus to zero. The whole model of the L1–L2 segment with a denucleated disc was developed as shown in Fig. 8.
The disc plays an important role in the stabilization of lumbar. The nucleus populous is the fulcrum during lumbar activity [15,16]. It maintains the height of the lumbar, and distributes the stress evenly around the annulus fiber, as shown in Fig. 9.

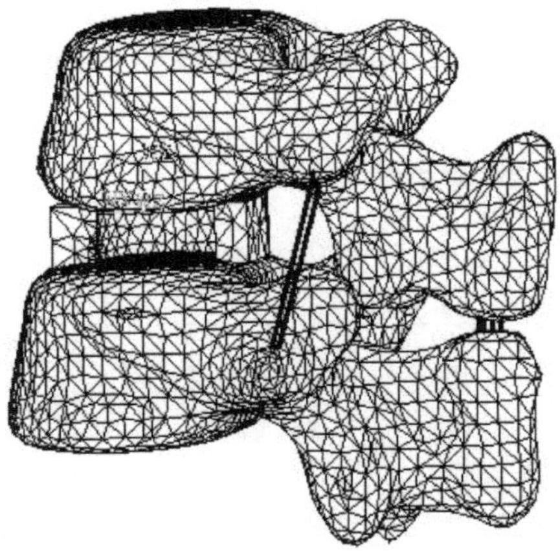

Fig. 8. The L1-L2 segment model with denucleated disc

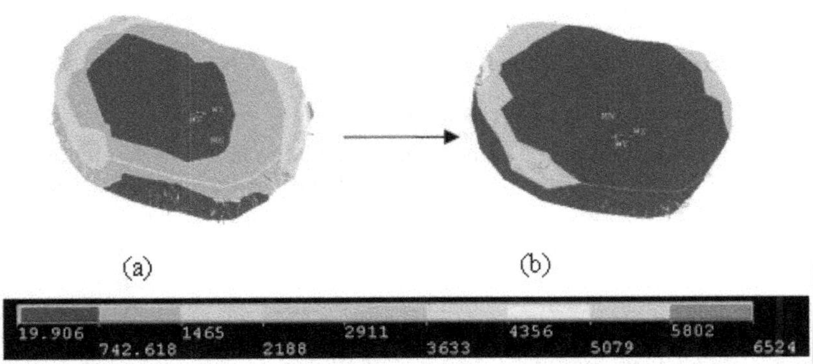

Fig. 9. Von Mises of the intervertebral disc: (a) Intact Disc,(b) Intact denucleated Disc.

We applied 500N load on the L1 upper surface body of the normal disc and observed changes in the stress. As is shown in Fig.9a, the central area of the disc shows low stress indicated in blue. The area outside the disc bears higher stress indicated in green. Fig. 9b shows the results of the Von Mises stress on the denucleated disc, we can see almost the whole disc bears low stress indicated in blue, illustrating that the IDP on the denucleated disc falls without the nucleus populous' function of sustaining surface tension of annulus fibers near the nucleus. The results from the analysis show that resection operations can relax the IDP of the disc, relieve the pain in the patients, and attain the goal to cure disc herniation through operation.

Table 6 lists the axial displacement of normal disc and denucleated disc. Three nodes in different locations representing three directions (anterior, posterior, lateral) are selected to determine the displacement of disc. The histogram in blue in the table represents the axial displacement of normal disc, and the red represents that of denucleated disc.

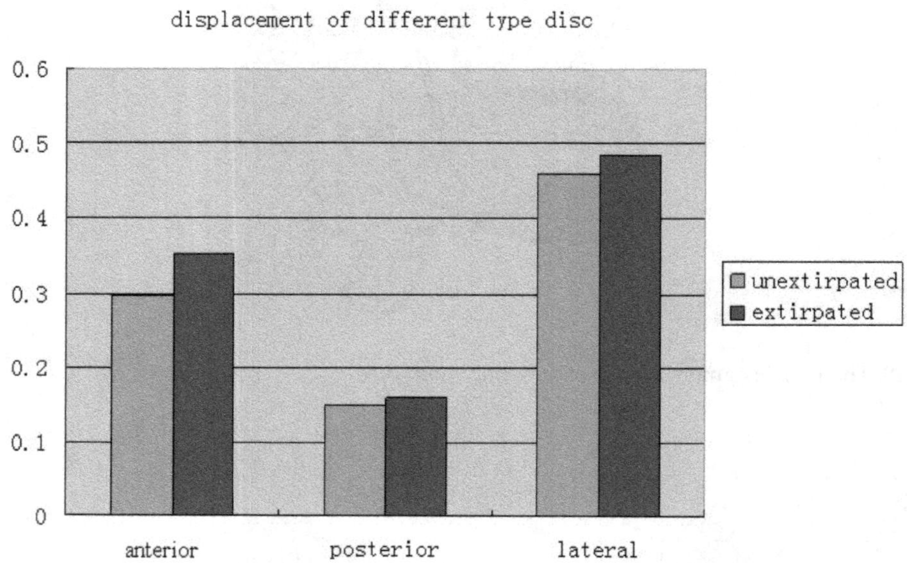

Table 6. Axial displacement of two types of discs

From the table, we can see that the value of axial displacement of of the denucleated disc is larger than that of the normal, illustrating that the height of intervertebral disc will become smaller when the nucleus pulposus is resected. The disease or the operation on the disc will make the cubage of the disc and the height it maintains disappear. They also destroy the compact structure between upper and lower intervertebral bodies. Then, the stress on small joints on both sides may change. Finally, the cartilage on it degenerates, leading to deformation of the disc.

As we know, the nucleous populous serves as the fulcrum of the spine and maintains the stability of the lumbar [17]. Once resected, the function of fulcrum disappears, and the disc will tend to extrude frontal, resulting in instability of the spine.

4. Discussion

The CT image based finite element modelling can provide a thorough understanding of the biomechanical influence on the lumbar and may offer reasonable explanations to biomechanically linked pathologies. It allows us to implement simulation calculation of biomechanical parameters of lumbar tissues, thus to analyze the influence of a single component within the construct investigated. It is useful in analyzing stress and strain distribution patterns of lumbar, leading to an optimal design of the surgeon[3]. It does, however, not mean that biomechanical *in vitro* approaches should be replaced by such a model. The current finite element model also has limitations, even if its modeling is based on the characteristics of physiological material and the geometric shape of lumbar. The anatomic structure of spine is complicated, and such properties of the small articulation as friction coefficient are not very clear. So all the material parameters adopted for the model have been simplified or based on hypothesis on some degree. It is a simplified model. In the future study, more nonlinear materials will be modeled. Any finite element model does only represent a mathematical model and thus is only an approximation to the specimen and even further from real life conditions[18-20]. It cannot reflect the variability of shape and material properties of the bone within an individual or among individuals. The interface between two bones only simulates appropriately the condition *in vitro* or *in vivo*. The model is just one segment of the whole spine. The results may vary if done with the whole spine. There are lots of differences and uncertain factors induced by the individual diversity during modeling. Based on the above reason, even though a finite element model has some limitations, it simulates the biomechanical characteristics of the lumbar preferably[19-21].

5. Conclusions

The lumbar is an important organ for bearing the weight. Wherein, the intervertebral disc can keep the height of the spine, linking the adjoining vertebral body. Experiment tests show that the nucleus pulposus bears a load of 45–60 kg when one lies down with muscles relaxed. A normal disc can bear a load of 30 kg while it goes up to several times when exercising violently or lifting heavy things. The nucleus pulposus is more likely to be injured and extrude out while the loading threshold is exceeded. We apply the load from 500 to 2500 N, which are in the range that the human being can bear. The result accords with the biomechnical characteristics in the normal disc[22–24]. In our research, we applied small distortion parameters to simulate the stress and strain distribution of the lumbar. The height of L1 is about 23 mm. When a load is applied on the L1, small distortion appears, reflecting the flexion properties, which indicates that the cancellous bone and cortical bone bear the force together, and the high stress is concentrated on the pedicle. The high stress is on the lateral and posterior region of the normal disc. From the tables, we learn that the extrusive magnitude for the posterior and the lateral is larger than in other directions. The tendency is more distinct with the increase of the load. A 3D nonlinear finite element model of lumbar motion segment was established to simulate the loading state of the spine. The study indicates the biomechanical characteristics as follows:

1. The strain of L1–L2 segment under axial compressive load increases with the performed load.
2. Large stress concentrations are found in the pedicle region, a common place for injuries. Under the axial compressive load, the body of vertebrate and articular process was compressed downward. The magnitude of stress in the pedicle region depends on the proportion of load applied on the superior articular processes. The stress on the pedical region is higher with greater proportion.

3. Excessive loads could cause the disc bulge. The bulge extent depends on the magnitude of the applied load. Under the same load, the disc tends to bulge laterally than posteriorly.
4. The denucleated disc shows a lower IDP than the normal disc. The resection surgery relieves the stress of the disc and alleviates the low back pain in the patients. However, after the nucleus populous is resected, the denucleated disc is liable to extrude outward frontal, and the height of the disc is lower than that of the normal. All of these will result in changes of biomechanics in the spine, such as lumbar instability and the inhomogeneous stress distribution on the annulous fiber, as well as the loss of the function of nucleus on the disc. This study has enriched some understandings of the biomechanical characteristics under loadings and can help surgeons make better decisions for the treatment of low back pain. In the study, an initial model of vertebral is developed, which includes solid cortical bone, disc, facet joints and several ligaments. In the further study, the models will include cortical bone, cancellous bone, and ligaments, which can also improve the accuracy of results and evaluation validity. Our next step is to study more on stress and strain distribution under torsion and shear conditions and to simulate the biomechanical characteristics of lumber during an operation. We aim at the operation simulation and surgery navigation by developing and analyzing the finite element model. The finite element model of L1–L2 segments based on medical images can analyze biomechanical characteristics of lumbar effectively and facilitate the optimization of individualized therapy in the future.

6. Acknowledgement

This study was supported by Scientific Research Key Program of Beijing Municipal Commission of Education(Grant No. kz200810025011) and National Natural Science Foundation of China(Grant No.30670576).

7. References

[1] Lee KK, Teo EC. Effects of laminectomy and facetectomy on the stability of the lumbar motion. Med Eng Phys 2004;26:183-192.

[2] Riches PE, Dhillon N, Lotz J, Woods AW, McNally DS. The internal mechanics of the intervertebral disc under cyclic loading. J Biomech 2002;35(9):1263-1271.

[3] Liyang Dai. Some basic biomechanical questions of human being lmbar. Mech Evol 1990;20:352.

[4] Frei, Hanspeter, Oxland, Thomas R, Nolte Lutz-P. Thoracolumbar spine mechanics contrasted under compression and shear loading. J Orthop Res 2002;20(6):1333-1338.

[5] Iatridis JC, James C, MacLean JJ, Jeffrey J, Ryan DD, David A. Mechanical damage to the intervertebral disc annulus fibrosus subjected to tensile loading. J Biomech 2005;38(3):557-565.

[6] Nabhani F,Wake M. Computer modeling and stress analysis of the lumbar spine. J Mater Process Technol 2002;127:40-47.

[7] Francisco Ezquerro, Antonio Simo'n. Combination of finite element modeling and optimization for the study of lumbar spine biomechanics considering the 3D thorax pelvis orientation. Med Eng Phys 2004;26(32):11-22.

[8] QinY-XS. Proceeding of the First Joint BMES/EMBS Conference Serving Humanity. 1999. p. 13-16.

[9] Christian Wong P, Martin Gehrchen, Tron Darvann. Nonlinear finiteelement analysis and biomechnical evaluation of the lumbar. IEEE Trans Med Imag 2003;6(22).

[10] Tanaka E, del Pozo R, Tanaka M, Asai D, Hirose M, Iwabe T, et al. Threedimensional finite element analysis of human temporomandibular joint with and without disc displacement during jaw opening. Med Eng Phys 2004;26(6):503-511.

[11] Wagner, Diane R, Lotz, Jeffrey C. Theoretical model and experimental results for the nonlinear elastic behavior of human annulus fibrosis. J Orthop Res 2004;22(4):901-909.

[12] Dolan, Patricia, Adams Michael A. Recent advances in lumbar spinal mechanics and their significance for modeling. Clin Biomech 2001;16:8-16.

[13] Joshi, Abhijeet, Fussell, Garland, Thomas, Jonathan, et al. Functional compressive mechanics of a PVA/PVP nucleus pulposus replacement. Biomaterials 2006;27(2):176-184.

[14] Meakin, Judith R, Reid, Janet E, Hukins, David WL. Replacing the nucleus pulposus of the intervertebral disc. Clin Biomech 2001;16(7):560-565.

[15] Abjiject Joshi. The effect of nucleus implant modulus on the mechanical behavior of lumbar functional spinal. IEEE 2003.

[16] Meakin, Judith R, Redpath, Thomas W, Hukins, David WL. The effect of partial removal of the nucleus pulposus from the intervertebral disc on the response of the human annulus fiber to compression. Clin Biomech 2001;16(2):121-128.

[17] Kumaresan, Srirangam,Yoganandan, Narayan, Pintar, Frank A, et al. Finite element modeling of the cervical spine: role of intervertebral disc under axial and eccentric loads. Med Eng Phys 1999;21(10):689-700.

[18] Martinez JB, Oloyede VOA, Broom ND. Biomechanics of load-bearing of the intervertebral disc: an experimental and finite element model. Med Eng Phys 1997;19(2):145-156.

[19] Jerome Noailly, Hans-Joachim Wilk, Jose A. Planell, Damien Lacroix, How does the geometry affect the internal biomechanics of a lumbar spine bi-segment finite element model? Consequences on the validation process. J Biomech 2007;40(12):2414-2425.

[20] Alison C. Jones, Ruth K. Wilcox, Finite element analysis of the spine: Towards a framework of verification, validation and sensitivity analysis. Med Eng Phys 2008;30(9):1287-1304.

[21] Ian A. Sigal, Michael R. Hardisty, Cari M. Whyne, Mesh-morphing algorithms for specimen-specific finite element modeling. J Biomech 2008;41(2):1381-1389.

[22] Wang J-L, Parnianpour M, Shirazi-Adl A, Engin A-E. The dynamic response of L 2/L 3motion segment in cyclic axial compressive loading. Clin Biomech 1998;13(1):16-25.

[23] Cheung, Jason Tak-Man, Zhang, Ming, Chow, Daniel Hung-Kay. Biomechanical responses of the intervertebral joints to static and vibrational loading: a finite element study. Clin Biomech 2003;18(9):790-799.

[24] Iatridis, James C, Setton, Lori A, Foster, Robert J, et al. Degeneration affects the anisotropic and nonlinear behaviors of human anulus fibrosus in compression. J Biomech 1998; 31(6):535-544.

11

Novel Computational Approaches for Understanding Computed Tomography (CT) Images and Their Applications

Oyeon Kum
School of Electronics Engineering, Kyungbook National University, Daegu
Korea

1. Introduction

We discuss three closely relevant computational approaches for understanding computed tomography (CT) images: X-ray imaging, medical image analysis, and the application of radiotherapy planning. The computational approaches have been widely used in X-ray research for more than three decades (Colijn, 2004; Feldkamp et al., 1984; Ju et al., 2010; Kak, 1999; Kum, 2010; KumPark, 2010; Kum, 2007; 2005; Kim, 2006; Kum et al., 2009; Peterzol et al., 2008). To understand CT images is to understand photon and/or electron scattering in matter, which can easily be done by the Monte Carlo method. Our research is mostly based on our in-house Monte Carlo code, PMCEPT code, which was developed recently (Ju et al., 2010; Kum, 2007; 2005; Kim, 2006; Kum et al., 2009; Peterzol et al., 2008).

Image processing to delineate tumor and to extract body contours and organ boundaries for dosimetric modeling in radiotherapy planning has become a routine process since CT scanners became available in the late 1970s (Gu et al., 2006; Haris et al., 1998; Kum et al., 2007; Kim et al., 2007; Kum, 2007; Kum et al., 2008). Moreover, pixel by pixel dose computation for planning is performed on the bulk inhomogeneous human body via the CT image. Recently, almost all major treatment machine manufacturers have been influenced by these technically advanced attributes to mount a cone beam CT(CBCT) 3D-imaging system on their linear accelerators for radiotherapy (Moore et al., 2006). They are using flat panel transducers to acquire a rotation fluoroscopy image sequence for input to 3D filtered back-projection algorithms. However, the development of cone beam tomography for radiotherapy is far from complete, with X-ray source, image transducer, reconstruction algorithms, and techniques for image profile collection still being researched (Feldkamp et al., 1984; Kak, 1999; Lagravere et al., 2008; Miceli et al., 2007; Wang et al., 1993; Zhao et al., 2009).

Simulation is a helpful tool to develop and optimize a new CBCT imaging system and to understand the influence of the various adjustable parameters. It acts as a virtual experimental workbench to offer powerful means for choosing the most suitable components and for predicting the future imaging system performance. It may enable the behavior of the whole imaging system to be investigated in complex situations by using simulated images which can be obtained in little time and at low cost (Colijn, 2004; Duvauchelle et al., 2000; Freud et al., 2006; 2004; Li et al., 2008; Miceli et al., 2007).

Although Monte-Carlo simulation is a powerful method for the investigation of the production of scattered particles in a medium in detail, deterministic calculations based on ray tracing algorithms are known as a powerful alternative to the Monte Carlo approaches to simulate X-ray imaging system whenever computation time is a critical issue (Freud et al., 2006; 2004). We focus on a simpler ray tracing approach in this chapter to describe our X-ray imaging system.

One of the important issues in medical imaging is to precisely segment structures of interest from a huge dataset, accurately represent them, efficiently visualize them, and perform measurements appropriate for diagnosis and therapy guidance, or other applications (Gu et al., 2006; Haris et al., 1998; Jos, 2001; Lagravere et al., 2008; Moga et al., 1998; Vincent, 1991). Advances in the area of computer science have a tremendous impact on the interpretation of medical images. Computer Aided Diagnosis systems aim to provide computer output as a second opinion in order to assist physicians in the detection of abnormalities, quantification of disease progress, and differential diagnosis of lesions, which enhances the physicians' capabilities and reduces the time required for accurate diagnosis.

Image segmentation is the process of dividing images into regions according to its characteristics involved in the images. The segmented objects are in the form of images that are more meaningful, easier to understand, and easier to analyze. In order to locate objects and boundaries in images, either data-based methods or pixel classification methods are used. Data-based approaches involve mathematical morphology, model-fitting, level-set methods, thresholding, edge-detection, and knowledge-based classification. Pixel classification techniques have used neural networks, Markov random field modeling, and active contours. The simplest idea for segmenting CT images is to classify the Hounsfield units (CT numbers) of the DICOM file into clusters. Intuitively, the Hounsfield unit of a pixel is interpreted as its altitude in the relief of each cluster, which leads to the watershed image segmentation algorithm. We discuss this algorithm in this chapter to provide semi-automatic segmentation of CT image, including the pre- and post-processing procedures for alleviating the drawbacks of a pure watershed algorithm.

Images are digitally processed to maximize the perception of medically important features. Physically meaningful Hounsfield values (CT numbers) in the computer memory are adjusted to suit grey values on a display monitor for the special application requirements. The customized radiation therapy applications are easily available with the information of the clustered Hounsfield values segmented by the watershed algorithms. The physico-chemical information from each patient's CT image such as the mass density and the chemical elements' weights of atomic compositions in each voxel corresponding to each pixel of the CT image is extracted via segmentation process because the Hounsfield unit includes quantitative information about the radiological properties of the different tissues (Lagravere et al., 2008; Scheneider et al., 2000). Tissue inhomogeneities are expressed in terms of different Hounsfield values, which makes the corrected dose calculations available for inhomogeneous target materials such as human body.

Exact estimate of clinical dose distribution in a patient body is the ultimate goal for the radiotherapy treatment planning (Moore et al., 2006). The exact dose calculation can be done by direct simulation of the interactions between the radiation and the patient tissue, the mass density and the chemical composition of the tissues, with Monte Carlo code such as PMCEPT code (Kum, 2007; 2005). With the advances of the computing power, applications of the Monte Carlo method for patient dose calculations have recently become more and more common by using the patient's CT images. Since this idea is closely correlated to the Hounsfield values, radiotherapy treatment planning is closely relevant to the CT imaging techniques, reconstruction algorithms, and segmentation algorithms in the computer simulations.

In this context, our laboratory initiated a comprehensive simulation research program of "from CT imaging to radiotherapy treatment planning with the state of the art information technologies." The major subject of this research program is to use our in-house Monte Carlo code, PMCEPT code to simulate directly the interactions between the radiation and the patient body. However, for better understanding of the complex physical phenomena involved in the radiation interactions with matter, this program involves closely relevant augmented novel computational approaches for each phase which are introduced in this chapter in order better to understand the CT images.

2. Cone beam computer tomography simulator

2.1 Virtual cone beam imaging technique

The major advantages of cone-beam acquisition are the reduction of data collection time and lower patient absorbed dose per scan. This is particularly important for real-time imaging of moving structures such as the beating heart, or the use of image guided radiotherapy treatment (IGRT) (Moore et al., 2006). With the advances in planar detector technology, it is expected that next generation scanners will adopt the cone beam geometry. This is the reason we developed a CBCT simulator in our laboratory.

CT image is acquired by the physical principle that the X-ray interacts with the body's tissues while it is passing through the body. If it does not experience some type of interaction, such as absorption, attenuation, and scattering with the body, the detected signal would not contain any useful information regarding the internal anatomy, and thus it would not be possible to construct an image of the anatomy with the detected information (Kum, 2010).

Although a medical image has an aesthetic appearance, the acquisition of an image is closely related to both the technical quality of the image and the adjustment of the input parameters. Thus, image quality in medical imaging involves very little artistic evaluation but a great deal of technical appraisal. For example, better CT images can be obtained when the radiation dose to the patient is high. However, patient safety and comfort must be considered first while acquiring medical images. Consequently, excessive patient dose in the pursuit of a perfect image is not acceptable, rather, a power balance is required to satisfy both the patient safety and image quality.

The procedure involved in obtaining CT image is that the patient remains stationary on the examination table while the X-ray tube rotates in a circular orbit around the patient in a plane perpendicular to the length-axis of the patient. The data acquired from the detectors are fed in to a computer which, after numerous calculations, produces a tomogram of the patient, i.e., a map of linear attenuation coefficients whose value is assigned a grey scale value on the display-monitor and is presented in a square picture element (pixel) of the image. In the 2D tomography, after a complete rotation of X-ray tube, the table with the patient is moved a small distance and the next slice can be measured. Thus, it takes a comparatively long time and gives high dose to the patient. Moreover, it is not possible to obtain, in particular, real-time imaging of moving structures, such as the beating heart, or contrast agent flow through the body in 2D fan beam CT imaging.

CBCT is a three-dimensional extension of two dimensional fan beam tomography. X-rays diverging as a cone from the source irradiates on the body, and data corresponding to passing X-rays is recorded on a planar detector surface (receptors) (Freud et al., 2006; 2004). Such cone beam projections are collected for a multitude of source positions along a source orbit which

may be a complete circle or not. The main advantages of cone beam acquisition system are the reduction of data collection time, reduced dose to the patient, and real-time imaging of moving structures. High quality CBCT images may be generated with high patient exposures and a large number of X-ray image profiles for reconstruction. However, this is not practical in view of the general regulations that embodies the principle of doses being "as low as reasonably practical" in the context of risks and benefits to the patient. Thus, there still remain many important research problems in CBCT imaging technology (Moore et al., 2006).
The apparent drawback of the CBCT image is the significant degradation of image quality due to the contamination of X-ray projection data with scattered photons and/or secondary electrons, resulting in a decrease of low-contrast detectability, cupping artifacts and streak artifacts between different objects (Peterzol et al., 2008). The amount of scatter contamination depends strongly on the type of imaging and detector geometry used as well as the object under study. Monte Carlo methods are known to be the best to accurately simulate scatter in X-ray imaging. Our in-house Monte Carlo code, PMCEPT code, has a capability to simulate the photon energy as low as 1 KeV and as high as 1 GeV against the targets of about hundred chemical elements, their compositions, and mixtures (KumPark, 2010; Kum, 2005). However, when low noise scatter projections have to be simulated, these Monte Carlo simulations tend to be very time consuming even though we use high performance parallel computing (Kim, 2006). Thus, it is worthwhile to add the most simplified approach to simulate CBCT X-ray projection by using ray tracing algorithms which is discussed in detail in the following.

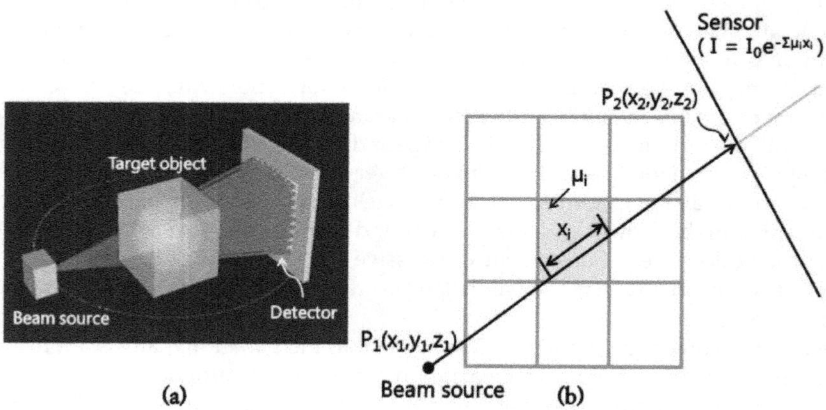

Fig. 1. Cone beam simulator model. (a) A set of ray beams is emitted towards every pixel center of the detector. (b) Radiological path is determined by summing up the length times the corresponding attenuation value.

Cone beam X-ray projector can be modeled with a bunch of rays that are emitted by a source point towards irradiated objects. This is the simplest and fastest in algorithm speed but the scattering effects and quantum noise are not taken into account. A plane panel detector is described by the grid of pixels with perfect quantum efficiency in a 3D scene. The right-handed Cartesian coordinate system is appropriate to describe the position and orientation of the source, object, and detector in the three dimensions. As shown in Fig. 1 (a), from the X-ray source, a set of ray beams is emitted towards every pixel center of the detector. The exact radiological path through the phantom volume is calculated on the basis of the calculation of ray-box intersection (see Fig. 1 (b)) because the phantom volume makes up the grid of cuboid cells (meshes or voxels). Determining the total path length with a cuboid grid is simpler than it is with a triangulated surface model. Radiological path is determined by summing up the length times the corresponding attenuation coefficient of the ray segments that cut each cell together along the ray path (see Fig. 1 (b)). There are many algorithms to calculate the exact radiological path through the phantom volume. Among them, our system adopted the well-known Siddon's fast or improved algorithms (Siddon, 1985). Our code was purposefully developed from scratch (no recourse to existing 'black-box' code libraries), including specifically designed and optimized ray casting algorithms.

The X-ray attenuation law, together with ray tracing techniques forms the basis of our code. The detector measures the attenuation in the phantom volume along the path of a particular ray. The attenuation of X-rays with a typical mean energy of 50–150 keV is determined by three different physical processes; Compton scattering (σ^{com}), photoelectric absorption (σ^{pho}), and Rayleigh scattering (σ^{ray}). The particle fluence of the transmitted X-rays entering the detector behind the phantom (Kum, 2010) is

$$\Phi(E) = \Phi_o(E)exp(-\int_0^l \mu(E,s)ds), \tag{1}$$

where $\Phi_o(E)$ is the initial particle fluence of the X-rays and $\mu(E,s)$ is the linear attenuation coefficient of the phantom material at position s and energy E. The attenuation coefficient depends on the atomic compositions at point s,

$$\mu(E) = \rho N_A \sum_{i=1}^{n} (\frac{w_i}{A_i}\sigma_i(E)), \tag{2}$$

where ρ is overall mass density (g/cm^3) at point s, N_A the Avogadro constant, i the element index, w_i the element weight, A_i the atomic mass (g/mol), and σ_i the total cross section, $\sigma_i^{com} + \sigma_i^{pho} + \sigma_i^{ray}$. The corresponding attenuation coefficients, associated with any elementary or compound substance, can be obtained from available databases, such as EPDL97 (Cullen et al., 1997).

The measured detector signal is either proportional to the particle fluence (i.e. energy fluence) or, to the energy deposition per mass if the detector is an ionization chamber. In general, projection value r which is calculated as the logarithmic ratio of the signal measured without a phantom (Φ_o) in the CT scanner and the signal of the X-rays attenuated by the phantom (Φ_E), i.e. $r = ln(\Phi_o/\Phi_E)$. In the case of monochromatic X-rays, we have:

$$r = ln(\frac{\Phi_o}{\Phi_E}) = \int_0^l \mu(E,s)ds \equiv \sum \mu(E,s_i)\Delta s, \tag{3}$$

where the sum runs from 0 to l. Reconstructing these line integrals would give the values $\mu(E)$ of the different material, i.e. a well defined physical quantity.

Although most commercial CT scanners produce more or less polychromatic X-rays, even though the bandwidth is not so broad, we only use the monochromatic X-rays in this simpler ray casting model, which is different from the full Monte Carlo model. Thus, we neglect the unavoidable beam hardening effect with polychromatic X-rays in this model. However, we consider the different CT scanner effect of having wide range of measured attenuation values. We obtain comparable attenuation values for different CT scanners by rescaling them with respect to that of water because most soft tissues have linear attenuation coefficients very similar to that of water over a large photon energy interval. The CT number or Hounsfield value (H) is defined as follows:

$$H = 1000(\frac{\mu}{\mu_{H_2O}} - 1) \tag{4}$$

where μ_{H_2O} is the mean attenuation coefficient of water. Thus, water has always the value 0 and air the value -1000. Note that the ratio of (μ/μ_{H_2O}) depends slightly on the spectral function $\hat{f}(E)$ of the commercial CT scanner, and therefore the CT number is a scanner-dependent quantity with fixed values for water and air (Scheneider et al., 2000).
These investigations show that we can also define uniquely patient body's mass density and chemical composition according to the Hounsfield values of the patient's CT data. Thus, we emphasize that the process of clustering pixels in a medical image dataset according to Hounsfield values classifies anatomical structures with corresponding physiological properties. This classification has a wide variety of applications in medical research and visualization, i.e. computer-aided diagnosis and radiotherapy treatment planning. Therefore, these three areas are closely relevant (KumPark, 2010).
A straightforward ray tracing technique would require computing time that scales with the array size N^3. Siddon (Siddon, 1985) proposed a fast method to trace the rays whose computing time scales with 3N. In this study, a refinement to Siddon's algorithm is investigated. Our new algorithm uses an incremental or decrement operation for computing the voxel indeces which improves computing time a little bit. Moreover, like the PMCEPT Monte Carlo code, ray tracing algorithm uses MPI based parallel computing algorithm for the projection angle on a Linux PC cluster. It is very efficient parallel algorithm because there is no intercommunication between nodes while computing. The final project data in the form of 'RAW' file is used for reconstruction, which is discussed in the following.
The two kinds of algorithm, ray tracing and Monte Carlo are not exclusive, but complementary. The Monte Carlo approach is slow but correct. Several hours or even days may be needed to get an image with an acceptable noise level (e.g. 1%), but it incorporates all the photon-material interactions into account, such as scattering, fluorescence, and electron processes. The ray tracing approach is fast and does not produce any noise. To simulate realistic images, a few statistical noise models in each photon energy channel can be added. A full sinogram can be simulated from computer-aided design (CAD) models in a few minutes using a current computer for the directly transmitted photons. This ray tracing with CAD model is also closely related to the optimization simulation used for the optimized radiotherapy planning.

2.2 Reconstruction technique

A reconstruction algorithm is a mathematical method to find the attenuation coefficients, μ-values, in each voxel based on all the measured data in the projection profiles. The procedure to reconstruct the image, based on the many projections at different angles, is performed with a reconstruction algorithm. Several types of reconstruction algorithms are available: filtered backprojection, direct Fourier, and algebraic reconstruction techniques. For the acquisition geometry of circular rotation of a cone about a fixed iso-center, Feldkamp, Davis, and Kress (FDK) algorithm (Feldkamp et al., 1984; Kak, 1999) which uses weighted filtered back-projection is used most often in practice, although it is an approximate method. Specifically, this algorithm is appropriate for the incomplete data set which is prone to inherent artifacts, in particular, away from the source plane.

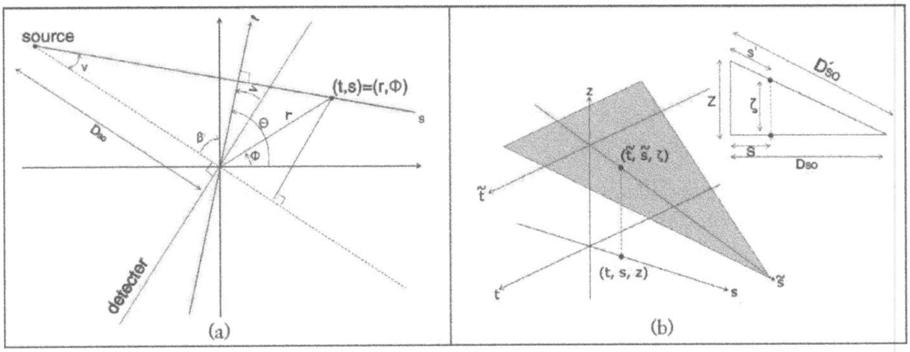

Fig. 2. Geometry of cone beam reconstruction. (a) Fan beam reconstruction geometry corresponding to the mid-plane of cone beam. (b) Tilted fan geometry of FDK algorithm.

Figure 2(a) shows mid-plane geometry of cone beam tomography (equivalent to fan beam reconstruction geometry or 2D parallel projection), and (b) shows tilted fan geometry of FDK algorithm. Three dimensional Radon transformation delivers integration values over planes formed by the detector plane, rather than along lines (formed by the receptors). The cone beam reconstruction algorithm is driven from the fan beam reconstruction algorithm (mid-plane geometry of cone beam) for the point (t, s) which represents the 2D parallel projection.

$$g(t,s) = \frac{1}{2}\int_0^{2\pi} \frac{D_{SO}^2}{(D_{SO}-s)^2} \int_{-\infty}^{\infty} R_\beta(p) f\left(\frac{D_{SO}t}{D_{SO}-s} - p\right) \frac{D_{SO}}{\sqrt{D_{SO}^2+p^2}} dp d\beta. \tag{5}$$

where,

$$t = x\cos\beta + y\sin\beta, \tag{6}$$
$$s = -x\sin\beta + y\cos\beta, \tag{7}$$
$$x = r\cos\phi, \tag{8}$$
$$y = r\sin\phi. \tag{9}$$

$R_\beta(p)$ represents the 2D projection data, p describes a linear detector array intersecting the origin of the reconstruction coordinate system, D_{SO} denotes the (source) distance between the X-ray source and the origin of the reconstruction coordinate system, and $f(\cdot)$ is the reconstruction filter defined as Kak and Slaney (Kak, 1999),

$$f(p) = \int_{-W}^{W} |\,\omega\,| \exp(j\omega p) d\omega. \tag{10}$$

In a cone beam reconstruction, all the fans except the mid plane are tilted out of the plane of rotation so that the size of the fan and the coordinate system of the reconstructed point change. Thus, a new coordinate system $(\tilde{t}, \tilde{s})$ is defined that represents the location of the reconstructed point with respect to the tilted fan shown in Fig. 2(b). Because the geometry of the fan size changes, both the source-to-origin distance, D_{SO}, and the angular differential, β, are changed. The new source-to-origin distance is given by

$$D_{SO}'^2 = D_{SO}^2 + \zeta^2, \tag{11}$$

where ζ is the height of the fan above the center of the plane of rotation. In addition, for the tilted fan the increment of angular rotation $d\beta'$ must be,

$$D_{SO}d\beta = D'_{SO}d\beta' \Rightarrow d\beta' = \frac{D_{SO}d\beta}{\sqrt{D_{SO}^2 + \zeta^2}}. \tag{12}$$

If we replace the 2D reconstruction variables, D_{SO} and β, by the 3D reconstruction variables, D'_{SO} and β', respectively, Eq. 5 becomes

$$g(\tilde{t}, \tilde{s}) = \frac{1}{2}\int_0^{2\pi} \frac{D'^2_{SO}}{(D'_{SO} - \tilde{s})^2} \int_{-\infty}^{\infty} R_{\beta'}(p, \zeta) f\left(\frac{D'_{SO}\tilde{t}}{D'_{SO} - \tilde{s}} - p\right) \frac{D'_{SO}}{\sqrt{D'^2_{SO} + p^2}} dp d\beta'. \tag{13}$$

To return the reconstruction to the original orthogonal (t, s, z) coordinate system we replace the 3D reconstruction variables D'_{SO} and β', by the 2D rotating plane variables, D_{SO} and β, respectively, in Eq. 13 by using a coordinate transformation,

$$g(t, s, z) = \frac{1}{2}\int_0^{2\pi} \frac{D^2_{SO}}{(D_{SO} - s)^2} \int_{-\infty}^{\infty} R_{\beta}\left(p, \frac{D_{SO}z}{D_{SO} - s}\right) f\left(\frac{D_{SO}t}{D_{SO} - s} - p\right) \frac{D_{SO}}{\sqrt{D^2_{SO} + p^2 + \zeta^2}} dp d\beta, \tag{14}$$

where a coordinate transform is,

$$\tilde{t} = t, \quad \frac{\tilde{s}}{D'_{SO}} = \frac{s}{D_{SO}}, \quad \frac{\zeta}{D_{SO}} = \frac{z}{D_{SO} - s}. \tag{15}$$

In the numerical algorithm the final formula $g(t, s, z)$ in Eq. 14 is usually converted again into $g(x, y, z)$ in the usual 3D Cartesian coordinate system by using the inverse coordinate transformations of Eqs. 6-9. The Eq. 14 is called the generalized Feldkamp's cone beam reconstruction formula. The important problem in the reconstruction algorithm is to choose the reconstruction filter $f(\cdot)$. We assume that the projection data are sampled with a sampling interval of τ cm. If there is no aliasing, this means that in the Fourier domain the projections don't contain any energy outside the frequency interval $(-W, W)$ where

$$W = \frac{1}{2\tau}\text{cycles/cm}. \tag{16}$$

Since the highest frequency of the projections is finite, we have

$$\int_{-\infty}^{\infty} R'_{\beta}(w, \zeta) \mid w \mid \exp(j2\pi wt) dw = \int_{-\infty}^{\infty} R'_{\beta}(w, \zeta) F(w) \exp(j2\pi wt) dw, \tag{17}$$

where $R'_{\beta}(w, \zeta)$ is the one-dimensional Fourier transform of $R_{\beta}(p, \zeta)$ with respect to p,

$$F(w) = \mid w \mid b_W(w). \tag{18}$$

and

$$b_w(w) = \begin{cases} 1, & \mid w \mid < W \\ 0, & \text{otherwise.} \end{cases} \tag{19}$$

$F(w)$ represents the transfer function of a filter with which the projections must be processed. Thus, the impulse function, $f(t)$, of this filter is given by the inverse Fourier transform of $F(w)$ and is

$$f(t) = \int_{-\infty}^{\infty} F(w)\exp(+j2\pi wt)dw \tag{20}$$

$$= \frac{1}{2\tau^2}\frac{\sin(2\pi t)/2\tau}{2\pi t/2\tau} - \frac{1}{4\tau^2}\left(\frac{sin(\pi t)/2\tau}{\pi t/2\tau}\right)^2, \tag{21}$$

where Eq.16 is used. Since the sampling interval of the projection data is τ, the impulse response, $f(t)$, needs only to be known with the same sampling interval for the digital processing. The samples are given by

$$f(n\tau) = \begin{cases} 0 & n: \text{ even} \\ \frac{1}{4\tau^2} & n = 0 \\ -\frac{1}{n^2\pi^2\tau^2} & n: \text{ odd.} \end{cases} \tag{22}$$

The cone beam reconstruction algorithm can be formulated as three steps:
Step 1: Calculate the pre-weighted projection data,

$$R'_\beta(p,\zeta) = \frac{D_{SO}}{\sqrt{D_{SO}^2 + p^2 + \zeta^2}} R_\beta(p,\zeta). \tag{23}$$

Step 2: Convolve the weighted projection $R'_\beta(p,\zeta)$ with $f(p)/2$ by multiplying their Fourier transforms with respect to p,

$$Q_\beta(p,\zeta) \equiv R'_\beta(p,\zeta) * \frac{1}{2}f(p). \tag{24}$$

Note that this convolution is done independently for each elevation, ζ.
Step 3: Back-project over the three-dimensional reconstruction grid,

$$g(t,s,z) = \int_0^{2\pi} \frac{D_{SO}^2}{(D_{SO}-s)^2} Q_\beta\left(\frac{D_{SO}t}{D_{SO}-s}, \frac{D_{SO}z}{D_{SO}-s}\right) d\beta. \tag{25}$$

The two arguments of the convolved projection, Q_β, represent the transformation of a point in the object into the coordinate system of the tilted fan shown in Fig. 2(b). Note that the cone beam system can not correctly reconstruct the whole object because the beam projection region is a sphere of radius $D_{SO}\sin(\Gamma_m)$, where Γ_m is half the beamwidth angle of the cone and some points outside this region may not be included in any of the projections (Lagravere et al., 2008; Wang et al., 1993).
For the fast ray-tracing, a target object is, in general, included in the smallest cuboid which includes the object, and the cuboid is divided into the same size of small voxels as shown in cylindrical object in Fig. 3(a). Radiological path is calculated by multiplying the attenuation coefficients of the target materials. The void voxels have zero attenuation values (vacuum) and automatically subtracted from the radiological path as shown in Fig.3(b), top-view of the cylindrical object. Thus, there may exist negligible error for the curved objects. In this example, the height of the target cylinder is 160 mm and is divided into 64 slices, so that each slice is 2.5 mm in thickness. The number of pixels in each slice is 512 $\times$ 512 and the width between the pixels is 0.5 mm. 720 projections were simulated for the evenly divided

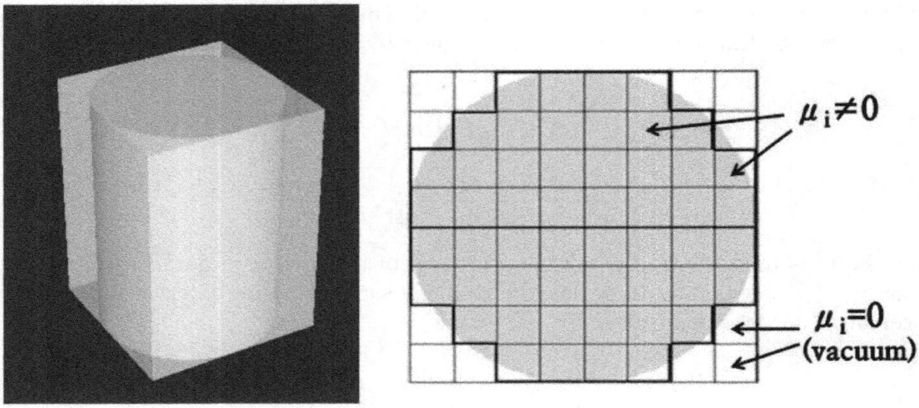

(a) (b)

Fig. 3. CAD description of target object. (a) Cylinder object included in cuboid. (b) Top-view of the cylindrical object.

angles. On the plane of rotation (z = 0) the cone beam algorithm is identical to a equi-spatial fan beam algorithm, as discussed above, and the quality of the reconstruction varies with the elevation of the plane because farther from the central plane each point in the reconstruction is irradiated from all directions but now at an oblique angle. Figure. 4 shows reconstruction at z=15 mm, the sixth slice above from the plane of rotation. However, as shown in Fig. 4, there is no noticeable degradation in the reconstruction in our algorithm.

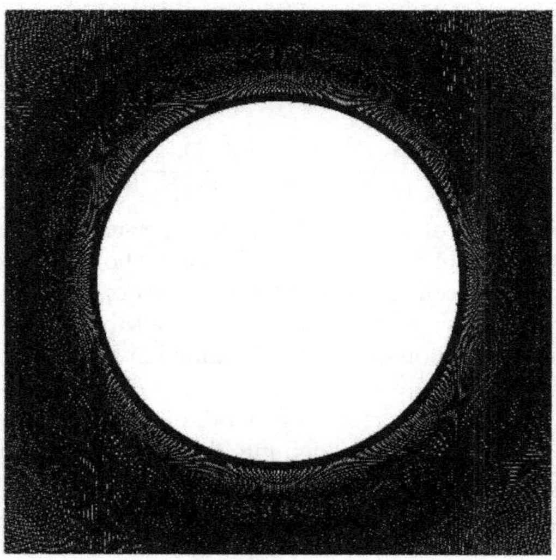

Fig. 4. Reconstructed image (512 $\times$ 512) of the slice at z=15 mm above the rotational plane.

3. Image segmentation

3.1 Watershed segmentation algorithm

Image segmentation is one of the most important issues in computer aided medical imaging. It is now frequently used in the analysis and diagnosis of numerous applications, such as the study of anatomical structure, localization of pathology, treatment planning, and computer-assisted surgery. Computers are indispensable for the analysis of large amounts of data, for tasks that require complex computation, or for the extraction of quantitative information. There are two important reasons for the use of computer aided segmentation: one is to improve upon the conventional expert (human)-based segmentation, and the other is to acquire segmentation prior to visualization or quantification for the analysis of medical images (Gu et al., 2006; Haris et al., 1998; Moga et al., 1998).

The watershed transform is the method of choice and widely used for medical image segmentation. It is classified as a region-based segmentation method and an important field in mathematical morphology. It can provide a hierarchical image segmentation from which a single region or set of regions can be extracted *a priori* by using a threshold or interactively with the help of a graphical user interface (Kim et al., 2007). To study the physical or physiological properties for each group of pixels in a medical image, a hierarchical image segmentation is important because it can provide a set of several segmentations at different levels of segmentation detail. The segmentations at coarser levels of detail can be produced by simple merges of regions from segmentations at finer levels of detail. A unique feature of hierarchical image segmentation is that the segmented region boundaries are maintained at the full image spatial resolution at all levels of the segmentation hierarchy.

The intuitive idea underlying the watershed transform is that of a landscape or topographic relief flooded by water. In flooding a landscape or topographic relief with water, watersheds are the dividing lines of the domains of attraction of rain falling over the region. An alternative approach is to imagine the landscape being gradually immersed in a lake, with holes pierced at the local minima. Basins (called 'catchment basins') will fill up with water starting at these local minima, and, at points where water coming from different basins would meet, dams are built. When the water level has reached the highest peak in the landscape, the process is stopped. As a result, the landscape is partitioned into regions or basins separated by dams, called watershed lines or simply watersheds. One of the difficulties with this intuitive concept is that it leaves room for various formalizations. Different watershed definitions for continuous functions can be given (Jos, 2001). Our main interest in this study is in digital images, for which there is even more freedom to define watersheds because in the discrete case, there is no unique definition of the path that a drop of water follows. This produces various algorithmic specifications and implementations. In this study, we followed Insight Image Segmentation and Registration Toolkit (ITK) (ITK, 2010) and Vincent-Soille transforms (Vincent, 1991) in digital spaces, which are now used as a fundamental step in many powerful segmentation procedures.

ITK is a cross-platform application development framework widely used for the development of image segmentation and image registration programs. ITK was developed with funding from the National Library of Medicine in the USA as an open resource of algorithms for analyzing the images of the Visible Human Project. The toolkit provides a top-down watershed algorithm that first computes a complete partition of the image into basins and subsequently finds watersheds by boundary detection. This assumes a multi-scale differentiable operator and, consequently, floating point operations in two, three, and more dimensions. The software is implemented in C++, and it is wrapped for Tcl, Python, and

Java. On the other hand, Vincent-Soille transforms, developed in early 90's, are faster and flexible with adaptations to any kind of underlying grid (different connectivities) and easily extendable to n-dimensional images and to graphs. They are appropriate to the CT images because they used an integer-sorting algorithm of the pixels in increasing order of Hounsfield values and fast breadth first scanning of the plateaus enabled by a first-in-first out type data structure. The algorithm first finds basins; then, the watersheds are the voxels not included in any basin.
Mathematically rigorous algorithmic definition of the digital watershed is presented based on the Vincent and Soille's idea. In fact, other watershed algorithms could be defined in a similar manner.

Definition: Image function Let $\mathbb{Z}$ be a set of integer and $\mathbb{D} \subseteq \mathbb{Z} \times \mathbb{Z} \equiv \mathbb{Z}^2$. Define a digital image map I: $\mathbb{D} \rightarrow \mathbb{Z}$, where $\mathbb{D}$ is the domain of the image and $I(p)$ denotes the Hounsfield value of the pixel $p \in \mathbb{D}$.

Definition: Path Let $\mathbb{G} \subseteq \mathbb{Z}^2 \times \mathbb{Z}^2$ denote the pixel grid. Define a path P of length l between two pixels p and q be an $l+1$-tuple $(p_0, p_1, \cdots, p_{l-1}, p_l)$ such that $p_0 = p$, $p_l = q$ and $\forall$ $i \in [0, l) : (p_i, p_{i+1}) \in \mathbb{G}$.

Definition: Connected A set of pixels $\mathbb{M}$ is called *connected* if and only if for every pair of pixels p, $q \in \mathbb{M}$ there exists a path between p and q which only passes through pixels of $\mathbb{M}$.

Definition: Connected component A *connected component* is defined as a nonempty connected set of pixels of maximal size.

Definition: Minimum A *regional minimum* (or *minimum* for short) of I at altitude h is a connected component of pixels p with $I(p) = h$ from which it is impossible to reach a point of lower altitude without having to climb.

Definition: Geodesic distance Let $\mathbb{A} \subseteq \mathbb{Z}^2$, and a, b two points in $\mathbb{A}$. The *geodesic distance* $d_{\mathbb{A}}(a,b)$ within $\mathbb{A}$ is the minimum of the lengths of all paths from a to b in $\mathbb{A}$:
$d_{\mathbb{A}}(a,b) = \min\{l(P) : P \text{ path between a and b which is totally included in } \mathbb{A}\}$.

Definition: Geodesic influence zone Let $\mathbb{A} \subseteq \mathbb{Z}^2$ and contain a set $\mathbb{B}$ made of several connected components, $\mathbb{B}_1, \mathbb{B}_2, \cdots, \mathbb{B}_k$. The *geodesic influence zone* of the set $\mathbb{B}_i$ within $\mathbb{A}$ is defined as:
$iz_{\mathbb{A}}(B_i) = \{p \in \mathbb{A} \mid \forall j \in [1, \cdots, k] \setminus \{i\} : d_{\mathbb{A}}(p, B_i) < d_{\mathbb{A}}(p, B_j)\}$.

Definition: Skeleton by influence zones (SKIZ) Let $\mathbb{A} \subseteq \mathbb{Z}^2$. The *skeleton by influence zones* (SKIZ) of the set $\mathbb{B}_i$ within $\mathbb{A}$ is defined as a complement of the union of the geodesic influence zones of the connected components of $\mathbb{B}$:
$\text{SKIZ}_{\mathbb{A}}(B) = \mathbb{A} \setminus IZ_{\mathbb{A}}(B)$ with $IZ_{\mathbb{A}}(B) = \bigcup_{i \in [1;k]} iz_{\mathbb{A}}(B_i)$.

Note that SKIZ consists of all points which are equally distant from at least two connected components. However, SKIZ does not necessarily separate the different geodesic influence zones and is often made of disconnected and thick one, meaning that a set of pixels equally distant from two connected components may be thicker than one pixel.
The key feature of the Vincent-Soille algorithm is a recursive computing from the lowest pixel value (h_{min}) to the highest one (h_{max}). To explain the recursive algorithm, we define the threshold set of I at level h as follows:

Definition: Threshold set of I at level h $\mathbb{T}_h(I) = \{p \in \mathbb{D} \mid I(p) \leq h\}$.

Let $\min_h$ denote the union of all regional minima at level h. Then, the *catchment basins and watersheds by immersion* can be defined as follows.

Definition: Catchment basins and watersheds by immersion The set of the catchment basins of the image I is equal to the set $X_{h_{max}}$ obtained after the following recursion:
(1) $X_{h_{min}} = T_{h_{min}}(I)$,
(2) $X_{h+1} = \min_{h+1} \cup IZ_{T_{h+1}(I)}(X_h), \forall h \in [h_{min}, h_{max} - 1]$.

Finally, the watersheds ($\mathbb{W}_I$) of the image I correspond to the set of the pixels of $\mathbb{D}_I$ which do not belong to any catchment basin, i.e., $\mathbb{W}_I = \mathbb{D}_I \cap (X_{h_{max}})^c$. The fact that computing X_{h+1} needs X_h expresses the sequential recursive nature of this algorithm. An example of the watershed transform on the square grid according to the immersion process is shown in Fig. 5.

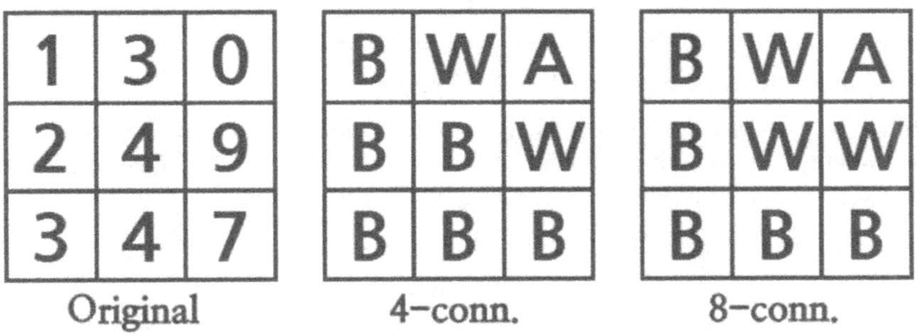

Fig. 5. Example of watershed transform. Original image is in the left-hand side, watershed with 4-connectivities in the middle, and 8-connectivities in the right-hand side.

The drawback of watershed segmentation is that it produces a region for each local minimum, resulting in oversegmentation. To alleviate this problem, a graph merging algorithm which is generally complicated, is used with a threshold value of the watershed depth, which sometimes impedes the efficient implementation of the graphical user interface. In this study, we propose an effective watershed method without a post merging process. Moreover, a steppedup graphical user interface provides a function of interactive and semi-automatic medical image segmentation.
The initial oversegmentation depends on the gradient image intensity variations because of the high sensitivity of the watershed algorithm. Thus, as a pre-processor, the noise reduction algorithm can reduce the oversegmentation appreciably. However, the image edges should be preserved to represent the boundaries of the image objects which have different physiological properties. We implemented a well-known statistical edge-preserving noise reduction algorithm. To preserve the edges, small bi-modal window filters were used. Also, the noise reduction process depends on the value of parameter of the filter size which may be user defined or can be evaluated based on the estimated noise variance. The output of the noise reduction procedure is the starting point of the gradient-based boundary sharpening process. This process is closely combined with a watershed technique, resulting in an effective watershed method without a post merging process. The gradient-based boundary sharpening technique reduces the oversegemntation by thresholding the gradient magnitude priori to

detect the watersheds of the image. To detect the boundary, a first order derivative is used in two-dimensional image:

$$\nabla I = \begin{bmatrix} G_x \\ G_y \end{bmatrix} \tag{26}$$

i_1	i_2	i_3
i_4	i_5	i_6
i_7	i_8	i_9

Fig. 6. An example of local image mask in 3 × 3 region.

Many different gradient operators can be used in the boundary sharpening step. Combination of the two operators also makes the edge sharper and thinner. For the mask shown in Fig. 6, the standard and cross gradient operators are given, respectively:

$$G_x = i_6 - i_5, \; G_y = i_8 - i_5, \tag{27}$$

$$G_x = i_8 - i_6, \; G_y = i_9 - i_5. \tag{28}$$

The mean value of the two gradient magnitudes results in the value of the gradient. Thresholding the gradient magnitude is performed interactively by using the graphical user interface (moving bar).

3.2 Application: Defining anatomical structures

Defining anatomical structures and the extraction of the objects in CT images are essential parts of medical imaging applications, such as diagnostic imaging, 3D treatment planning, and image-guided surgery. The volume definition process may provide for delineating the specific shape of an organ on a digital image as accurately as possible, especially for 3D rendering, radiation therapy, and surgery planning. Specifically, in the radiation treatment planning the accuracy and reproducibility of this process affects targeting, optimization based on dose-volume histograms or other volume-based measures, and the development of biological models for tumor control and complication probabilities (Kum et al., 2007).

This can be done either through manual user interactions or by applying imaging processing techniques for the automatic detection of specific structures in the image using segmentation techniques. The automatic segmentation process might involve complicated structures, and in this case usually only an expert can perform the task of identification manually on a slice-by-slice basis. Humans can perform this task using complex analyses of shape, intensity, position, texture, and proximity to surrounding structures. Thus, despite the advances in automatic segmentation methodology, many medical image research labs continue to rely on manual delineation. This reluctance to accept automation may be due to insufficient reliability and high specificity of fully automatic methods and the lack of inexpensive user-friendly tools implementing semi-automatic methods. To address this difficulty, we developed the semi-automatic hierarchical watershed segmentation algorithms. A semiautomatic approach combines high efficiency, accuracy, and repeatability of automatic methods with expertise and quality control that can only come from human supervision.

The hierarchical watershed segmentation algorithms divide the whole medical image into many groups of pixels according to the corresponding Hounsfield values. The number of divided groups depends on the threshold value given by the user. In our current experience, a single fixed threshold has not produced adequate results, so semi-automatic human-aided adjustment is necessary. For this purpose, we have supplied a user interface with which regions can be added, replaced, or subtracted semi-automatically via the command input window in 3D and a mouse click in 2D. With a user-friendly interface tools, the watershed method is an especially elegant segmentation technique that requires the expert to provide an initialization, set control parameters, and terminate the segmentation. Moreover, it was designed to make segmentation and parameter selection as easy as possible for users without a mathematical background. The detailed pixel information for each group is included in the ASCII format output file, from which we may extract any region of interest. We found that the semiautomatic method was useful to avoid errors incurred by both human and machine sources and, in addition, provided clear and visible information for pedagogical purposes.

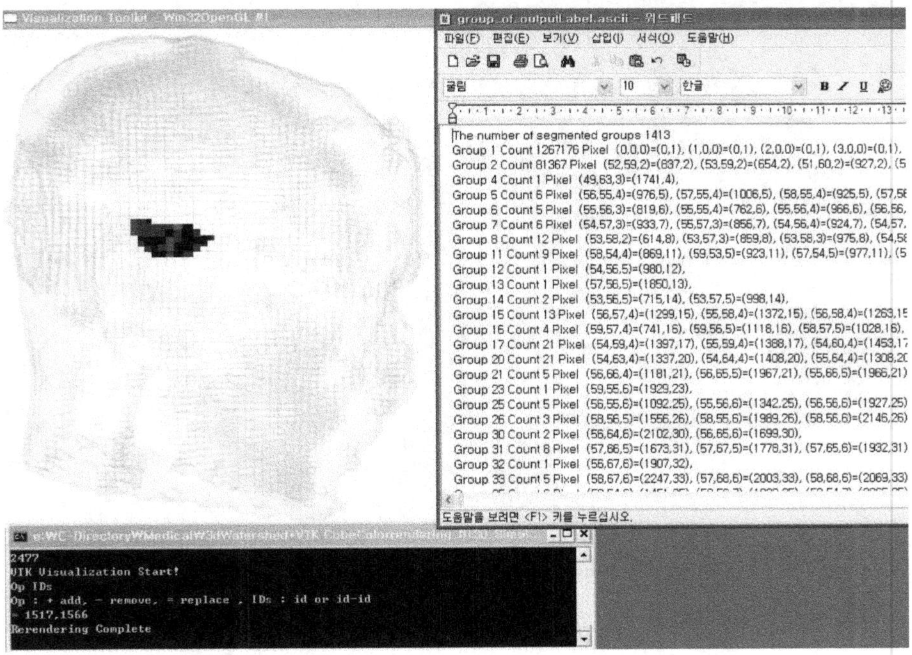

Fig. 7. Three-dimensional semi-automatic region extraction and registration procedures from the head phantom CT data.

Figure 7 shows three-dimensional semi-automatic region extraction and registration procedures from the head phantom CT data. The figure shows three windows, the three-dimensional transparent image output window with a selected volume, the ASCII file output window including group information and Hounsfield value for each pixel, and the command input window (Kim et al., 2007). The number of segmented groups is automatically contingent on the given threshold value. It is more than just an implementation of a given computational method, which contains innovative tools for manual outlining and quality control in addition to the automatic segmentation work flow.

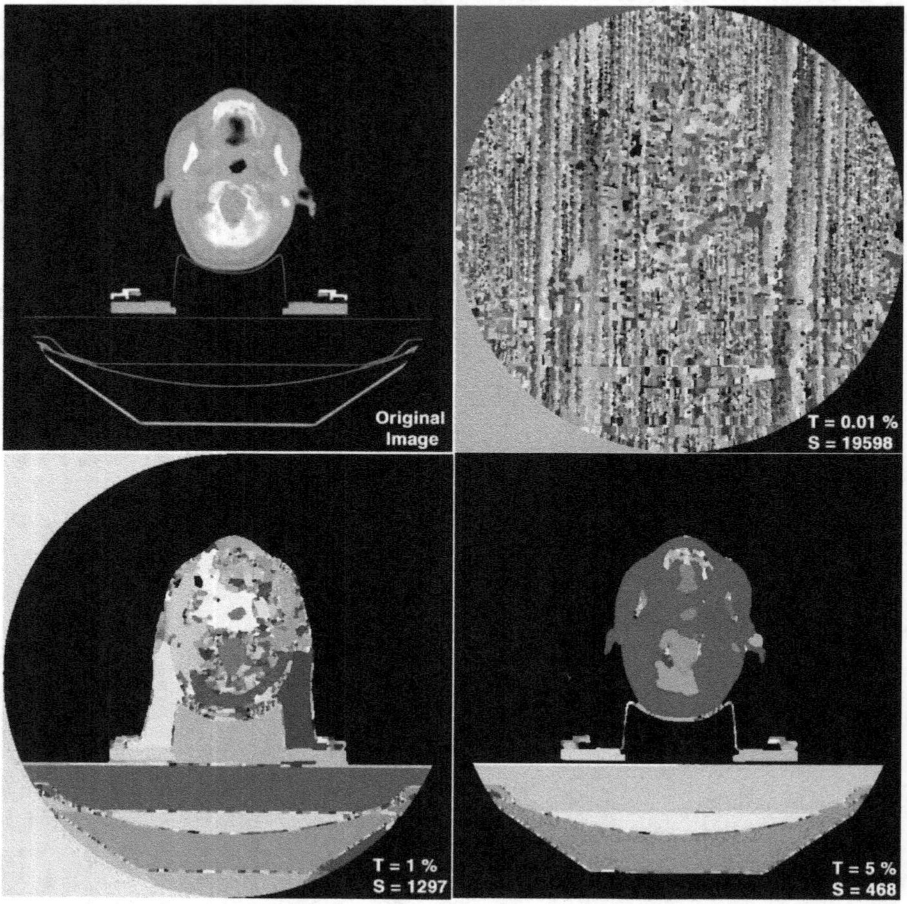

Fig. 8. Two-dimensional segmentation of the head phantom CT data.

Figure 8 shows two-dimensional segmentation of the head phantom CT data. The original CT slice is on the upper left-hand side. The threshold value is given as a percentage of maximum depth. As the threshold value (T) increases, the number of segmentations (S) decreases. This property is very useful to select a focused anatomical region automatically. A graph merging algorithm is used to adjust the number of regions. The computing time for two-dimensional problem is only a few seconds using a desktop PC. During radiation therapy, irradiating beams pass through a patient, killing both carcinoma and normal tissues. Thus, the radiation treatment must be carefully planned to deliver a clinically prescribed dose to the target volumes containing carcinoma cells, while nearby organs at risk and normal cells are spared. To optimize the beams, we need to extract pixel numbers for each group of organs. The ASCII format output file (including group numbers and pixel addresses) is very useful to find the exact pixel numbers for the focused region.

Defining anatomical structures is an especially useful procedure for the treatment planning. The state of the art of modern treatment planning requires very tight margin and dose escalation. To meet these requirements, we obtain exact pixel addresses of the interesting anatomical regions for the calculation of an optimization matrix, whose rows represent pixel numbers and columns gantry angles, for example, in conformal 3D treatment planning. Prior to optimization, each pixel's (or voxel's) dose in the target volume and neighboring organs is calculated with respect to the gantry angle as a matrix ($d_{i,j}$), where i is the pixel address and j is the gantry angle. In general, the matrix size is too big to include all elements for the optimization. We choose a small number of pixels in the simulation, but the choice of insufficient number of pixels can cause a dose inhomogeneity problem. Frequently, we may observe hot spots that may have critical effects on the organs at risk. Thus, the pixel address information is essential for the best treatment planning. Our algorithm was developed specifically for segmenting anatomical structures and is considerably easier to master than the other packages due to its tightly focused and simple functionality.

3.3 Application: Hepatic tumor analysis

The primary goals of a CT examination of the liver are the detection and the characterization of focal hepatic lesions. The choice between surgical or palliative treatment depends on the size, number, and location of metastases as determined by the image. The detection of hepatic tumors with CT theoretically improves as lesion conspicuousness increases. Because most hepatic tumors are hypo-vascular, increased conspicuousness may be accomplished by increasing the degree of enhancement of normal surrounding liver. CT contrast agents, sometimes referred to as "dyes," are used to highlight specific areas so that the organs, blood vessels, or tissues are more visible. In this study, we show a sample patient's CT image whose liver has a comparatively large-area tumor. The results show that the use of our segmentation algorithms for studying various radiological problems, such as liver CT enhancement with contrast material, is indeed feasible. However, this is not an exhaustive radiological study for the effects of contrast materials or CT protocols (Kim et al., 2007).

Two different methods based on watershed segmentation are applied to the analysis of the hepatic tumor (see Fig. 9). The segmented images and corresponding frequency distributions of the Hounsfield values are shown in the left-hand and the right-hand columns, respectively. In each column, the four images from top to bottom represent the progressive levels of contrast materials, pre-contrast (PRE), arterial phase (ART), portal venous phase (POR), and delayed phase (DEL), respectively. Once the contrast is injected into the bloodstream, it circulates throughout the body. Advanced CT scanners with rapid acquisition times and short delay between acquisition of groups of scans permit scanning of the liver in an exclusively and separately a pre-contrast phase, an arterial phase ($\sim$ 30 sec), and a separate portal venous phase ($\sim$ 70 sec) consecutively. A couple of minutes after the portal venous phase, a delayed phase ($\sim$ 3 min in general) can be obtained. Watershed segmentation produces hierarchical region segmentations contingent on the threshold value. For the first automatic segmentation step, we adjusted the threshold values to get better segmentations, though the results were not complete. The pictures shown here were automatically segmented with the best adjusted threshold value in each phase. After this procedure, we adjusted the segmented regions semi-automatically via the command input window or mouse click.

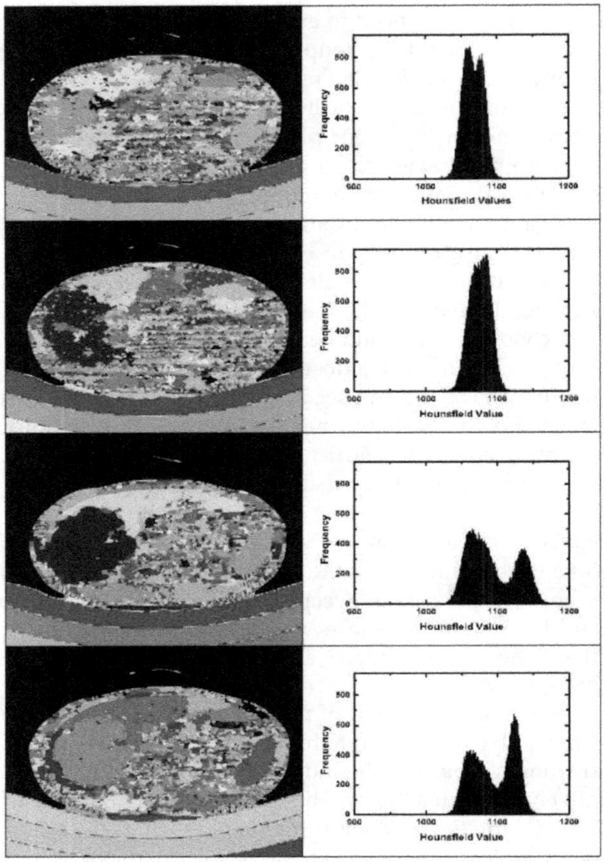

Fig. 9. Segmented images and corresponding frequency distributions of the Hounsfield values in the left-hand and the right-hand columns, respectively. In each column, the four images from top to bottom represent the progressive levels of contrast materials, pre-contrast (PRE), arterial phase (ART), portal venous phase (POR), and delayed phase (DEL), respectively.

For the appropriate region of interest chosen semi-automatically, we analyze radiological properties using regional average and median Hounsfield values, which represent X-ray transport properties.

The pre-enhanced segmented image on the top left-hand side shows many clustered regions, which are different basins in the Hounsfield values. Although there are many different basins, their average Hounsfield values are not significantly different as shown in the corresponding right-hand side histogram. Separation between tumor and normal liver is negligible, so that it is not easy to identify the hepatic tumor area from this picture. For better identification of the lesion area, it is necessary to develop augmented tools or analysis techniques. They are included in one of our on-going research activities. The segmented image of the artery phase on the left-hand side shows the focal hepatic region, although it is still not quite satisfactory.

Hepatic metastases are supplied almost exclusively by hepatic arteries, but most of these lesions are hypo-vascular and are not well visualized on images obtained during the hepatic arterial phase. On the other hand, a strongly enhanced liver lesion is readily perceived before the minimally enhanced surrounding normal liver parenchyma during the arterial phase. This result is shown clearly in the right-hand side corresponding histogram. Frequencies in tumor area are increased, compared to those of normal area. The CT's X-ray beam is weakened as it passes through the blood vessels and organs that have "taken up" the contrast. These structures are enhanced by this process and show up as white areas on the CT images. The segmented image in the third row from the top shows clearly the focal tumor region in a portal venous phase. The frequency distribution shown in the right-hand side also shows the two different groups of Hounsfield values. During the portal venous phase, the liver lesion is normally seen as a filling defect in the strongly enhanced normal liver parenchyma because approximately 70% − 75% of the hepatic parenchymal blood flow arrives from the portal vein and the remaining 25% −30% arrives from the hepatic artery (Greenway, 1971). The liver lesion, however, can be more conspicuous in either phase, depending on the vascularity of the tumor. The metastases are most conspicuous when imaging is performed with techniques that optimize portal venous enhancement, during which phase they appear as regions of low attenuation against a background of the brightly enhanced liver parenchyma. Therefore, the biggest difference in attenuation value between a liver lesion and the normal liver tissue will be visible shortly after maximum portal venous enhancement, with the lesions appearing as hypo-attenuating within a highly enhanced liver parenchyma. The length of this phase is, however, limited in time and depends on multiple parameters, among which are the volume and the rate of injection of the contrast material. Thus, the results shown in two phases (ART and POR) suggest that this patient has a hepatic metastases. The delayed phase segmented image in the bottom of the left-hand column shows clearly the focal regions. The frequency distribution in the right-hand side shows more clearly the 'V'-shape focal regions. It looks similar to the portal venous phase, which is explained by the staying time of the contrast material in the liver area. The results suggest that segmented images cannot exceed or overpower the effects of the contrast material for the liver CT scan to find the tumor area, and the histogram estimations can be used as a good measure to find tumor areas as shown in Fig. 9. However, the segmentation algorithm is useful for studying quantitative variations of the Hounsfield values in the tumor. In the histogram calculations, we used unsigned integers by adding 1000 to Eq. 4 for computational purposes so that the Hounsfield value of water is not 0 but 1000.

Segmentation is absolutely necessary to cluster Hounsfield values for each region of interest. Specifically, the semi-automatic algorithm was helpful in reducing errors incurred by both human and machine sources. The whole liver image included approximately 35000 pixels in total. Two separated peaks explain the existence of the different groups of Hounsfield values. This phenomenon explains explicitly the existence of the hepatic tumor. Frequency analysis using the segmentation algorithm shows more clearly the existence of the tumor (quantitatively) than the segmented image (qualitatively). The evidence is very clear in this sample because its tumor size is almost half of the whole liver area. It may, however, not be easy to detect a tumor from frequency analysis if the tumor size is comparatively small, but a watershed segmentation algorithm is still very helpful even for a small tumor.

Figure 10 shows the changes in the average Hounsfield values with one standard deviation as a function of the phase (PRE, ART, POR, and DEL) for both the lesion area and the normal area. In the lesion area, the mean enhancement values differed by 12, 15, 11 at the ART, the POR, and

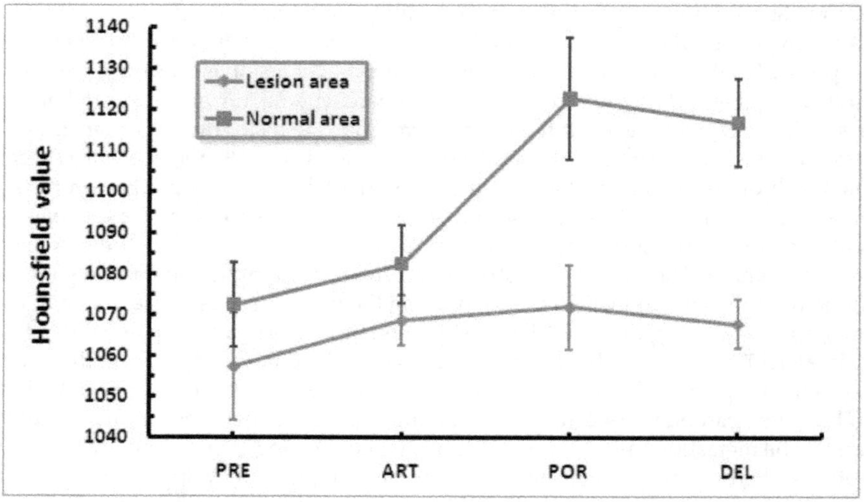

Fig. 10. Changes in the average Hounsfield values with one standard deviation as a function of the phase (PRE, ART, POR, and DEL) for both the lesion area and the normal area.

the DEL phases, respectively. On the other hand, in the normal liver region, the differences were 10, 50, 44 at the ART, the POR, and the DEL phases, respectively. Thus, in both areas, the maximum difference occurred at the POR phase. The results suggest that the liver is mostly surrounded by portal veins, and discrimination between the normal parenchyma and liver lesions is considered to be most effective in the early portal venous phase. These results also suggest that the tumor may be hepatic metastases.

Statistical analysis between different phases were performed by using t and one-way ANOVA tests for means and variances. We used the SPSS software program for the statistical analysis. The means were considered significantly different if P was less than 0.01. For each test parameter, the confidence interval was obtained by using the standard normal distributions. The statistical analysis showed that for the normal liver region, the mean Hounsfield value was 1072.4, and its standard deviation and standard error were 20.6 and 0.2, respectively. Thus, in the 95 % confidence interval, the minimum value is 1072.1, and the maximum is 1072.7. For the lesion area, the mean Hounsfield value was 1057.3 and its standard deviation and standard error were 26.1 and 0.2, respectively. This results in a minimum of 1057 and a maximum of 1058 in the 95 % confidence interval. Thus, both areas are included in the same group by Schneider et al.'s classification table (see the Table 1 in the reference) (Scheneider et al., 2000). Their densities, however, are slightly different because the density is linearly proportional to the CT number (see Fig. 7 in the same reference).

4. Analysis of radiological properties

Both the exact anatomical structures of the patient's body and quantitative information about radiological properties of the different tissues can be extracted from the CT scans as described by Eq. 2. Although the Monte Carlo simulations are the most accurate methods for radiation treatment planning, without accurate input data, they can only produce incorrect results. For the customized cancer treatment planning, each patient's physico-chemical data of the body, such as mass density and the elemental mass fractions of the patient's tissues, is required. The Monte Carlo method for high-energy photon and charged particle transport is the most accurate for dose calculations, specifically for tissue inhomogeneities. Thus, the radiological properties relative to the beam quality used in radiotherapy planning must be obtained by conversion of the CT numbers because most CT scans are taken at X-ray energies of approximately 120 keV (fixed value).

The general approach in this direction was to divide the scale of CT numbers into different groups to correlate the CT numbers with the elemental mass fractions of the tissues, but there was no rule about how to determine the threshold values correctly. Thus, the results might, in general, depend on the therapeutic beam quality. In this direction, we used Schneider et al.'s results (Scheneider et al., 2000) to evaluate the physico-chemical properties for the normal liver and lesion areas in the first trial because they extracted the information about the tissue parameters from the CT number irrespective of the therapeutic beam quality.

However, by using the segmentation tools, we can extract different organ areas and estimate the average Hounsfields values and standard deviation from the pixels consisting of the area. Although the distribution of the CT numbers may be different for the same material (except water) due to both beam hardening effects and small machine dependent band widths, we can adjust the differences with the graphical user interface as shown in Fig. 7. For a better study, many experiments are required with the CT scanner being used for generating this CT data set. It remains as one of our on-going projects to study exhaustively the radiological properties of the patient's CT data sets. CT imaging simulations are the most efficient methods for the exhaustive study. In addition, statistical analysis for differentiating the tissues is performed as shown in hepatic tumor analysis.

Ray-tracing algorithm (used in virtual CT imaging) with Monte Carlo method may be used in the next step to optimize the treatment planning. Although the Monte Carlo method is the most accurate for dose calculations, specifically, for tissue inhomogeneities, it costly in terms of computation time in general. Therefore, deterministic calculations based on ray-tracing techniques are used as a powerful alternative to the Monte Carlo approach to optimize the treatment planning, especially with the results based on the Monte Carlo calculations, whenever computation time is a critical issue. The most popular method for the optimization is a simplex method, which is closely relevant to the optimization of the segmentation problems. Thus, a few novel computational approaches such as ray-tracing, segmentation, Monte Carlo, and optimization cover the simulations of almost all subjects ranging from CT imaging to treatment planning and quality assurance in radiotherapy. Moreover, they turned out to be all closely relevant and affect to each other in the simulations of CT imaging and its applications.

5. Conclusions

As a part of the larger numerical simulation project, "from CT imaging to customized cancer radiation treatment planning," which includes virtual X-ray imaging, image reconstruction, medical image segmentation and structure definition, radiological property analysis of the CT data, irradiating beam optimization, and scientific data visualization, we have been developing a few novel numerical approaches such as ray tracing algorithm for virtual cone beam imaging, cone beam image reconstruction algorithm, in-house general purpose Monte Carlo code (PMCEPT), semi-automatic watershed segmentation schemes to analyze CT data based on radiological and/or physical principles. In this feasibility study, we found that the Monte Carlo method was a powerful simulation approach which covered from CT imaging to customized cancer radiation treatment planning whenever computation time is not a critical issue. However, we also found that a simpler augmented deterministic algorithm such as ray tracing was a useful alternative to the Monte Carlo approach to simulate X-ray imaging systems. The same ray tracing algorithm is also used for the fast radiotherapy treatment optimization. Moreover, a simplex optimization algorithm can be applied to optimize the image segmentation. Thus, we found that a few closely relevant numerical algorithms could be used for almost all simulations ranging from CT imaging to treatment optimization.

In this chapter, we presented some results such as the virtual X-ray imaging and reconstruction algorithms for cone beam CT, semi-automatic medical image segmentation algorithm and its applications to define anatomical structures of a head phantom CT and to analyze hepatic lesion areas with contrast material, and to calculate radiological and chemico-physical properties of the patient's liver CT data. The algorithms show outstanding performance and several characteristic features, which make it possible to apply the proposed algorithms to build a larger numerical simulation project, from CT imaging to treatment optimization. In combination with our in-house Monte Carlo code (PMCEPT code), these augmented algorithms were very useful to study CT image and its various applications. According to our experiences on this study, the algorithms are not separated but closely relevant to each other, so that the experience of an algorithm accelerates the study of other algorithms. Eventually, they can be combined into one system for studying almost all areas of CT imaging, which is one of our on-going research activities.

6. Acknowledgments

We first thank Prof. William G. Hoover for his careful proofreading and thoughtful comments. This research was supported by Basic Science Research Program through the National Research Foundation of Korea(NRF) funded by the Ministry of Education, Science and Technology(grant number: 2010-0003983).

7. References

Colijn, A., & Beekman, F. (2004). Accelerated simulation of cone beam X-ray scatter projections. *IEEE Transections on Medical Imaging*, Vol.23, No. 5, pp 584-590. May, 2004.

Cullen, D., Hubbell, J., & Kissel, L. (1997). EPDL97: The evaluated photon data library '97 Version. *UCRL-LR-50400*, Vol.6, Rev 5., Sept. 1997.

Duvauchelle, P., Freud, N., Valérie, K., & Babot, D. (2000). A computer code to simulate X-ray imaging techniques. *Nuclear Instruments and Methods in Physics Research B*, Vol.170, pp 245-258. 2000.

Freud, N., Duvauchelle, P., Létang, J., & Babot, D. (2006). Fast and robust ray casting algorithms for virtual X-ray imaging. *Nuclear Instruments and Methods in Physics Research B*, Vol.248, pp 175-180. 2006.

Freud, N., Duvauchelle, P., Pistrui-Maximean, S., Létang, J., & Babot, D. (2004). Deterministic simulation of first-order scattering in virtual X-ray imaging. *Nuclear Instruments and Methods in Physics Research B*, Vol.222, pp 285-300. Jan, 2004.

Feldkamp, L., Davis, L., & Kress, J. (1984). Practical cone-beam algorithm. *J. Opt. Soc. Am. A*, Vol.1, No. 6, pp 612-619. June 1984.

Greenway, C., & Stark, R. (1971). Hepatic vascular bed. *Physiol. Rev.*, Vol.51, No. 1, PP 23-65. Jan. 1971.

Gu, L., Xu, J., & Peters, M. (2006). Novel multistage three-dimensional medical image segmentation: Methodology and validation. *IEEE Transactions on Information Technology in Biomedicine*, Vol. 10, No. 4, PP 740-748. Oct. 2006.

Haris, K., Efstratiadis, S., Maglaveras, N., & Katsaggelos, A. (1998). Hybrid image segmentation using watersheds and fast region merging. *IEEE Transactions on Image Processing*, Vol. 7, No. 12, PP 1684-1699. 1998.

ITK-homepage, www.itk.org.

Roerdink, J., & Meijster, A. (2001). The watershed transform: Definitions, algorithms and parallelization strategies. *Fundamenta Informaticae*, Vol. 41, PP 187-228. 2001.

Ju, S., Han, Y., Kum, O., Cheong, K., Shin, E., Shin, J., Kim, J. & Ahn, Y. (2010). Comparison of film dosimetry techniques used for quality assurance of intensity modulated radiation therapy. *Med. Phys.*, Vol.37, No.6, pp 2925-2933. June, 2010.

Kak A., & Slaney, M. (1999). *Principles of Computerized Tomographic Imaging*. IEEE Press, The Institute of Electrical and Electronics Engineers, Inc., New York. ISBN 0-87942-198-3.

Kum, O. (2010). *Medical Statistics with Monte Carlo Methods*. Jinhan M&B Press, Seoul, Korea. ISBN 978-89-8432-471-8.

Kum, O. & Park, K. (2010). *Biomedical Engineering*. Jinhan M&B Press, Seoul, Korea. ISBN 978-89-8432-446-6.

Kum, O., Kim, H., & Max, N. (2007). Semi-automatic watershed medical image segmentation methods for customized cancer radiation treatment planning simulation. *Int. J. CARS*, Vol.2, (Suppl) No.1, pp S44-S45. June, 2007.

Kim, H., Kum, O., & Max, N. (2007). Computer-aided CT image analysis aased on clustered Hounsfield values. *J. Korean Phys. Soc.*, Vol.51, No.1, pp 235-244. July, 2007.

Kum, O., & Kim H. (2007). Semi-automatic segmentation of CT image using watershed algorithm and graphical user interface (abstract). *Med. Phys.*, Vol.34, No.6, pp 2394-2394. June, 2007.

Kum, O. (2007). Telematics-based online client.server/client collaborative environment for radiotherapy planning simulations. *Med. Bio. ENg. Comput.*, Vol.45, No.11, pp 1053-1063. November, 2007.

Kum, O., Lee H., Kim, J., Song T., Park K., & Han, Y. (2007). Simpler and faster watershed medical image segmentation algorithm (abstract). *Med. Phys.*, Vol.35, No.6, pp 2663-2663. June, 2008.

Kum, O.,& Lee, S. (2005). Development of a parallel electron and photon transport code (PMCEPT) I: Method and absorbed dose computation in water. *J. Korean Phys. Soc.*, Vol.47, No.4, pp 716-725. October, 2005.

Kim, H.,& Kum, O. (2006). Development of a parallel electron and photon transport (PMCEPT) code II: Absorbed dose computation in homogeneous and heterogeneous media. *J. Korean Phys. Soc.*, Vol.49, No.4, pp 1640-1651. October, 2006.

Kum, O., Park, K., & Han, Y. (2009). Semantic web-based PMCEPT Monte Carlo code simulations in medical physics. *J. Korean Phys. Soc.*, Vol.55, No.5, pp 2242-2247. November, 2009.

Lagravére, M., Carey, J., Ben-Zvi, M., Packota, G., & Major, P. (2008). Effect of object location on the density measurement and Hounsfield conversion in a NewTom 3G cone beam computed tomography unit. *Dentomaxillofacial Radiology*, Vol.37, pp 305-308., 2008.

Li, N., Zhao, H., Cho, S., Choi, J., & Kim, M. (2008). A fast algorithm for voxel-based deterministic simulation of X-ray imaging. *Computer Physics Communications*, Vol.178, pp 518-523. Jan. 2008.

Miceli, A., Thierry, R., Flisch, A., Sennhauser, U., Casali, F., & Simon, M. (2007). Monte Carlo simulations of a high-resolution X-ray CT system for industrial applications. *Nuclear Instruments and Methods in Physics Research A*, Vol.583, pp 313-323. Sept., 2007.

Moga, A., Cramariuc, B., & Gabbouj, M. (1998). Parallel watershed transformation algorithms for image segmentation. *Parallel Computing*, Vol. 24, PP 1981-2001. 1998.

Moore, C., Amer, A., Marchant, T., Sykes, J., Davies, J., Stratford, J., McCarthy, C., MacBain, C., Henry, A., Price, P., & Williams, P. (2006). Developments in and experience of kilovoltage X-ray cone beam image-guided radiotherapy. *The British Journal of Radiology*, Vol.79, pp S66-S78. Jan., 2006.

Peterzol, A., Létang, J., & Babot, D. (2008). A beam stop based correction procedure for high spatial frequency scatter in industrial cone-beam X-ray CT. *Nuclear Instruments and Methods in Physics Research B*, Vol.266, pp 4042-4054. July, 2008.

Scheneider, W., Bortfeld, T., & Schlegel, W. (2000). Correlation between CT numbers and tissue parameters needed for Monte Carlo simulations of clinical dose distributions. *Phys. Med. Biol.*, Vol. 45, PP 459-478. 2000.

Siddon, R. (2010). Fast calculation of the exact radiological path for a three-dimensional CT array. *Med. Phys.* Vol.12, No.2, pp. 252-255, Mar/Apr 1985.

Vincent, L., & Soille, P. (1991). Watersheds in digital spaces: An efficient algorithm based on immersion simulations. *IEEE Transactions on Pattern Analysis and Machine Intelligence*, Vol. 13, NO. 6, PP 583-598. 1991.

Wang, G., Lin, T., Cheng, P., & Shinozaki, D. (1993). A general cone-beam reconstruction algorithm. *IEEE Transactions on Medical Imaging*, Vol.12, No. 3, pp 486-496. Sept. 1993.

Zhao, X., Hu, J., & Zhang, P. (2009). GPU-based 3D cone-beam CT image reconstruction for large data volume. *International Journal of Biomedical Imaging*, Vol.2009, Article ID 149079, pp 1-8. June 2009.

12

Use of Pseudocolor for Detecting Otologic Structures in CT

Moon Suh Park, MD, Jae Yong Byun, MD,
Seung Geun Yeo, MD and Ho Yun Lee, MD
Kyunghee University
Republic of Korea

1. Introduction

Visualization of the fine structures of the ear is not easy because they may not be well contrasted and their shapes in ear may be variable in CT; for instance the incudostapedial joint often cannot be visualized separately and the stapes foot plate is barely visible in CT. Black-and-white images may not reflect actual anatomy in CT because the human eye is capable of detecting only 30 different shades of gray and intensity variations of less than 200 Hounsfield units (HU) are invisible to the naked eye(Tringali et al., 2007). However, the human eye can discriminate between hundreds of colors and human beings have a superior memory for colors, which means that color has wider dynamic range than gray scale(Addrews et al., 1972). There were some reports to support the effectiveness of the pseudocolor for the interpretation and detection of small periodontal defects (Brägger U et al., 1989; Reddy et aL., 1991). An endoscopic pseudocolor imaging system has been used for color processing of ulcer images observed using an electronic endoscope (Tamada et al., 1996) and images of paranasal sinuses for endoscopic sinus surgery (Christmas et al., 1999). Besides there was an experiment showing that contrasting-color scales was the most efficient to detect small changes in radionuclide images (Crowe et al., 1988).

Recently color transformation of radiologic images has come into wide use because of the popularization of picture archiving and communication systems (PACS) for digital radiology. This has made it easier to manipulate image enhancement systems such as pseudocolor transformation. Converting a gray scale intensity level to a specific pseudocolor would be helpful for detecting small and difficult-to-find lesions in temporal bone CT(Park et al., 2009).

Pseudocolor could be used with various combinations. The rainbow scale is a standard and popular process that has been applied to density data to improve visual clarity, which is the result of traversing the color solid along a path through all the hues of the rainbow. Even the single pseudocolor could be applied for easy concentration on a specific area, for example otosclerotic foci in CT if needed.

Otosclerosis is a primary focal disease of the otic capsule. This disease involves principally the stapes footplate and the bone around the base of the stapes, which reduces normal sound transmission resulting in a conductive hearing loss. In temporal bone CT, the appearance of otosclerotic foci differs depending on the stage of the disease. In the active stage, they appear to be radiolucent areas due to active bone resorption and remodeling of the otic capsule. But, in the inactive stage, they look like the normal adjacent bone of the cochlear capsule. In the active stage of otosclerosis, otosclerotic foci tend to occur in the area just in front of the oval window (fissula ante fenestram, FAF), round window, and pericochlear area. If the size of the lesions or the difference of radio-opacity is too small to detect, it will be not easy for otolaryngologists without much experience to find out them in CT images and to explain them to patients.

It has been known that the normal otic capsule has about 1800 to 2000 HU; however the optic capsule with otospongiotic change has about 1000 to 1400 HU (Huizing et al., 1987). So, the difference which numerical value of normal otic capsule and otospongiotic change occurred ranges from 400 to 1000 HU, which is correspondent to only several shades when the values is converted to gray color scale. But, if we convert the difference of HU to various colors or specific color then there will be lots of color shades. The pseudocolor transformation of the original image can widen capability of dynamic range. So, we supposed that converting gray scale intensity level to specific pseudocolor would be helpful to detect small lesions as well as fine structures of the ear in temporal bone CT.

2. Methods

2.1 Pseudocolor transformation of normal ossicles

Thirty-six CT studies of healthy ears were studied. Healthy ears were defined as having normal hearing ability with hearing loss of less than 20dBHL and showed a typical type A tympanogram. There was no past history of ear infection or inner ear diseases.

Both axial and coronal CT images were used. One mm thick contiguous non-overlapping sections were acquired. The scanner used was a Lightspeed 16(GE, Milwaukee, USA). The window width and level were adjusted to 3200 and +400 respectively.

The entire middle ear of the temporal bone was scanned; *i.e.* 24-32 planes were taken. The software used was Image- Pro Plus 4.0. (Media Cybernetics, MD, USA).

Pseudocolor transformation of the middle ear was performed using the following procedures: 2 planes of the axial CT image immediately below the plane showing the incudomalleolar joint were selected. After the CT images were scanned, they were converted to gray-scale images, because the pseudocolor command is only relevant to monochrome images. In Process menu, the intensity range was specified using the upper limit and lower limit buttons. The specified range was divided into the numbers of intervals and a default color was assigned to each interval, i.e. 255 colors were selected using the Divisions tool that showed entire and colorized part of the intensity range. Because red to blue and blue to red patterns of color spread (rainbow scale) were chosen in the pseudocolor scale's predefined assignments the process of the color assignments changing and refining of the intensity division widths were omitted. Blue to red arrays the colors in a spectrum with blue assigned to a lower value than red. Red to blue arrays the colors in a spectrum with red assigned to a lower value than blue. Two planes of the coronal CT image showing the bony lip of the oval window were selected and pseudocolor transformation was performed in the same manner. However typical variables such as the continuous zone of soft tissue or higher attenuation between the incus and stapes were excluded in this study.

Two otolaryngologists examined each image twice: plain, blue to red and red to blue transformed. They knew nothing about the history and audiometric findings for the subjects. They were informed that the images were given from randomly selected temporal bone CTs. They compared the detectability of the stapes and IS joint using pseudocolor-transformed images with that of plain images.

Using Lemmerling's rating; scale the examination of CT images was done. For each image one of 5 scores concerning the visibility of the stapes (head of stapes, anterior & posterior crura, footplate, oval window) and IS joint (lenticular process, IS joint, crus of stapes) was given: 1-not seen, 2-probably not seen, 3-not sure, 4-probably seen, 5-definitely seen. The stapes footplate was defined as the structure that had higher attenuation than the fluid in the vestibule at the interface. The oval window was defined as the structure at the interface between the air in the tympanum and the fluid in the vestibule and the IS joint was defined as the small gap of hypoattenuation between the most medial part of the lenticular process of the incus and the most lateral part of the stapes head(Lammering et al., 1997). The determination of visualization sensitivity was done through statistical analysis using a paired t-test.

2.2 Pseudocolor transformation of otosclerotic foci

Temporal bone CT images of sixty patients were reviewed. Of them, thirty-two ears were normal and twenty-eight ears were diagnosed as otosclerosis by radiologists experienced in evaluating otosclerosis in CT images.

Two otolarynogologists with experience of 3 years independently evaluated the sixty temporal bone CT images, randomly selected in a conventional manner (gray scale). They knew nothing about the history and audiometric findings for the subjects. 1 month later, they were educated about the technique of real time pseudocolor transformation (RTPT) and reevaluated the images randomly selected using it. The sensitivity, specificity, and inter-observer agreement rate were evaluated.

The method of RTPT is as follows: The axial CT images were used. 0.6mm thickness contiguous non-overlapping sections were acquired. The CT was a BRILLIANCE TM CT 64 Slice (PHILIPS, Yerusalem, Israel). The entire middle ear was scanned. The whole scanned images were transported to Picture Archiving and Communication System (PACS). The PACS was a STARPACS 5.0.8.1 (INFINITT, Seoul, Korea)

After opening the images of a selected patient in PACS, one or two planes of the axial CT image showing the anterior portion of oval window or stapes crura were selected and the observers amplified the image twice using zoom button menu, built-in PACS. And the observers chose "T" button menu located upper tool bar and selected the "Pseudo" sub-menu, then pseudocolor mapping working window appeared. There were variable predefined pseudocolor scales in the palette menu. But, we selected the same gray-scale for the reference. Using the color mask function, we chose specific color (red color in this case) to be applied to the specific intensity range of scanned image. Moving the control bar of the "color mask" up and down between soft tissue density and bone density range, red color was dressed on the selected gray-scale intensity area (figure 1).

If observers find out the presence of focal thickenings of red color in the otic capsule, especially in FAF, oval window, and pericochlear area, then it can be diagnosed as otosclerosis. It is excluded that focal thickening at the boundary where soft tissue and bone are contiguous, because it shows false radiolucent area where soft tissue and bone are abut by the interference during scanning the image.

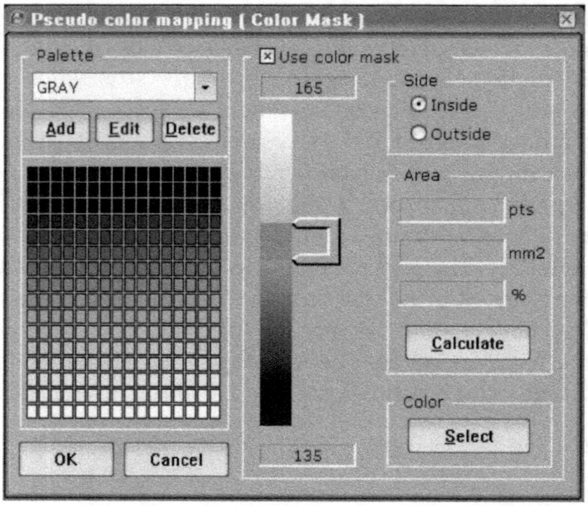

Fig. 1. Pseudocolor mapping task window showing the range of intensity to be applied by red color.

3. Results

3.1 Pseudocolor transformation of normal ossicles

The result indicated increased visibility of the stapes and IS joint in CT images after pseudocolor transformation. But, pseudo-colored images often showed slightly distorted bony structures.

Figure 2 shows an example of plain and pseudocolor-transformed images of the stapes. The footplate and oval window were more easily identifiable in the pseudocolor image compared with the plain image. In the red to blue image (b), the green-colored crura showed sharp contrast. The air in the tympanum appeared as blue, the fluid in the vestibule appeared as green to sky blue. The radiolucent area between the otic bones in the plain image was a light green color after the transformation, which was considered the area of the

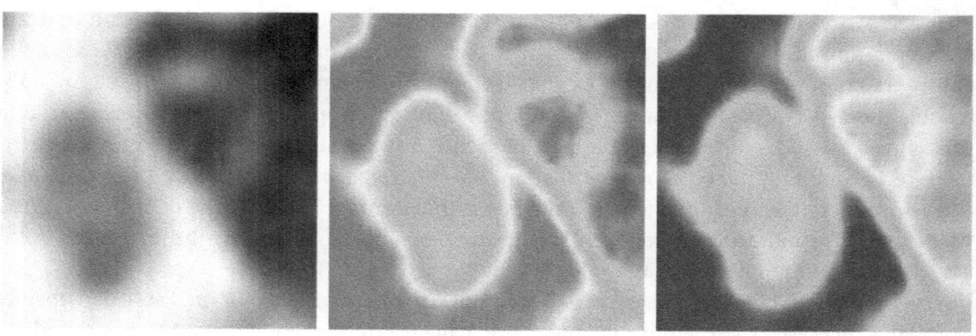

(a) (b) (c)

Fig. 2. Axial image of CT showing pseudocolor transformation of stapes. a) plain image b) pseudocolor transformed image(red to blue) c) pseudocolor transformed image (blue to red)

foot plate. In the blue-to-red image(c), the otic bone appeared blue. The crura of the stapes appeared thicker compared with the plain image.
Figure 3 shows an example of plain and pseudocolor-transformed images of the IS joint. The gap of hypoattenuation in the IS joint appeared to be more prominent in the pseudocolor-transformed image.

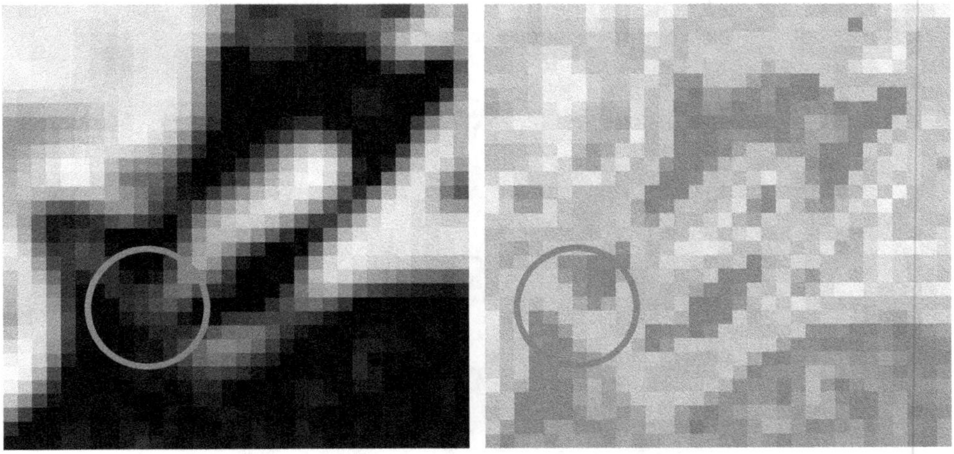

(a) (b)

Fig. 3. Coronal image of CT showing pseudocolor transformation of incudostapedial joint. a) plain image. b) pseudocolor transformed image(red to blue). Red circles indicate incudostapedial joint.

The visibility of the stapes was increased after pseudocolor transformation. The oval window and footplate in particular were more easily distinguishable in both pseudocolor-transformed images compared with the plain images ($p<0.05$) (Figure 4). The visualization sensitivity of the IS joint including surrounding structures was increased after pseudocolor transformation. In particular the IS joint was more easily identifiable in both pseudocolor-transformed images as compared with plain images ($p<0.05$).

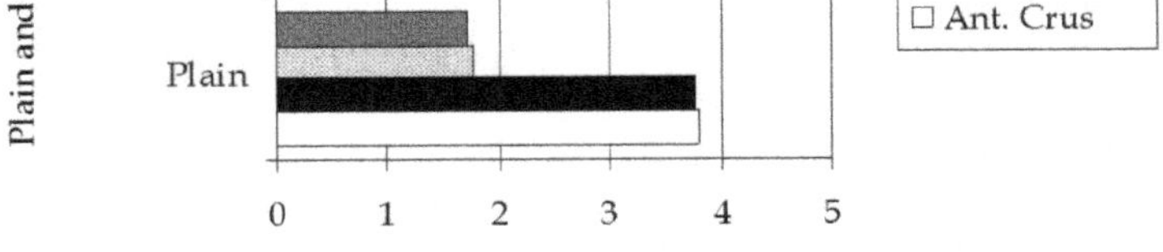

Fig. 4. Changed visibility of the stapes structures after pseudocolor transformation

3.2 Pseudocolor transformation of otosclerotic foci

The study cases consisted of 30 patients (60 ears), including 16(53.3%) women and 14(46.7%) men. Age ranged from 26 to 65 years, with a mean of 46.8 years. 15 patients were healthy and 15 patients (28 ears) were otosclerosis. Among otosclerotic patients, 13 patients had bilateral otosclerotic foci and 2 patients had unilateral foci. Distribution of otosclerotic foci consisted of fenestral(71.43%), cochlear(7.14%), and mixed type(21.43%). Figure 5 showed one CT image of otosclerosis after pseudocolor transformation.

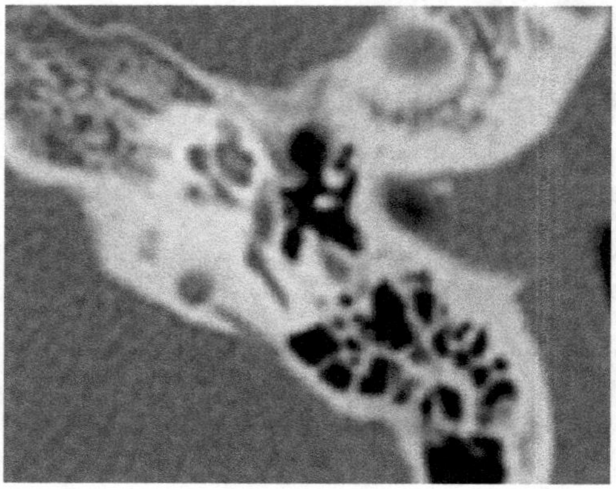

(a)

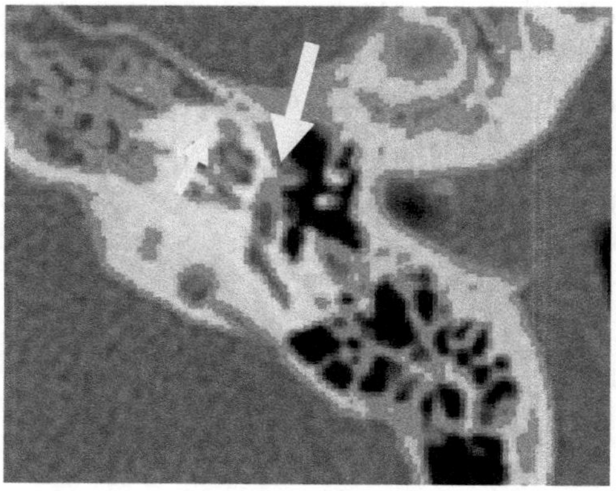

(b)

Fig. 5. Axial image of CT showing foci of radiolucent area anterior to the oval window (yellow arrow) and the apex of cochlear (small yellow arrow). a) plain image, b) pseudocolor transformed image.

When they were classified according to the distribution of otosclerotic foci, the sensitivity was increased in fenestral and mixed type and was equal in cochlear type (Fig.6).
Inter-observer agreement rate of conventional technique and RTPT technique was similar each other. The kappa value was 0.528($p<0.05$) in conventional technique and 0.539($p<0.05$) in RTPT.

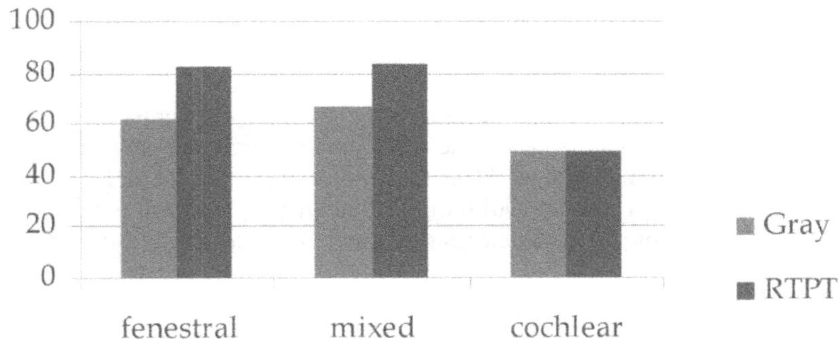

Fig. 6. Comparison of the sensitivity according to the distribution of otosclerotic foci. Increased sensitivity of fenestral and mixed type was seen when using the RTPT than conventional technique and same sensitivity of cochlear type was seen in each techniques

4. Conclusion

Nowadays, digital technology has been commonly used to transform an original image into various forms without damaging it. And the creative combinations of pseudocolor could make it possible to producing various impressive images. In our studies, a new visualization method using pseudocolor transformation was described to increase detection rate of ossicles in many CT images. And also we showed that pseudocolor transformation could be helpful for detecting ear pathology such as otosclerosis. These procedures may be performed by use of the image analyzer or PACS with real time processing.
Variable color transformation can be examined for increasing detectability of CT image in the future.

5. References

Addrews HC, Tescher AG, Kruger RP. (1972) Image processing by digital computer. *IEEE Spectrum* 9(7): 20-33.

Brägger U, Pasquali L (1989). Color conversion of alveolar bone density changes in digital subtraction images. *J Clin Periodontol.* 16:209-14.

Christmas DA, Mirante JP, Yanagisawa E.(1999) Rainbow scale in computer-aided sinus surgery. *Ear, Nose & Throat Journal* 78:670-2.

Crowe EJ, Sharp PF, Undrill PE, Ross PG.(1988) Effectiveness of colour in displaying radionuclide images. *Med Biol Eng Comput.* 26:57-61.

Huizing EH, de Groot JA.(1987) Densitometry of the cochlear capsule and correlation between bone density loss and bone conduction hearng loss in otosclerosis. *Acta Otolaryngol.* 103:464-8.

Lemmerling MM, Stambuk HE, Mancuso AA, Antonelli PJ, Kubilis PS. (1997)Normal and opacified middle ears: CT appearance of the stapes and incudostapedial joint. *Radiology* 203:251-6.

Park MS, Byun JY, Cha CI. (2009)Pseudocolor transformation for visualization of ossicles in CT images. *Acta Otolaryngol.* 129:515-20.

Reddy MS, Bruch JM, Jeffcoat MK, Williams RC.(1991) Contrast enhancement as an aid to interpretation in digital subtraction radiography. *Oral Surg Oral Med Oral Pathol.* 71:763-9.

Tamada F, Hirohata S, Honsako Y, Kumada H, Kashio Y, Konishi M, et al. (1995) Quantitative analysis of the gastric ulcer healing process using video endoscopic pseudocolor imaging systems. J Clin Gastroenterol; 20 (Suppl 2): 52-5.

Tringali S, Pouget JF, Bertholon P, Dubreuil C, Martin C. (2007)Value of temporal bone density measurements in otosclerosis patients. *Ann Otol Rhinol Laryngol.* 116:195-8.

13

Advanced Neuroimaging with Computed Tomography Scanning

Béatrice Claise[1], Jean Gabrillargues[1,4], Emmanuel Chabert[1,4], Laurent Sakka[3,4], Toufik Khalil[3,4], Vivien Mendes-Martins[3,4], Viorel Achim[3], Jérôme Costes [3,4], Thierry Gillart[2,4] and Jean-Jacques Lemaire[3,4]

[1]*Neuroimaging Unit, Department of Radiology, University Hospital of Clermont-Ferrand, Hôpital Gabriel Montpied, B.P. 69, 63003 Clermont-Ferrand cedex 1*

[2]*Intensive Care Unit, Department of Anaesthesiolgy, University Hospital of Clermont-Ferrand, Hôpital Gabriel Montpied, B.P. 69, 63003 Clermont-Ferrand cedex 1*

[3]*Department of Neurosurgery, University Hospital of Clermont-Ferrand, Hôpital Gabriel Montpied, B.P. 69, 63003 Clermont-Ferrand cedex 1*

[4]*Univ Clermont 1, UFR Médecine, Image-guided clinical neuroscience and connectomics (ICCNC), Auvergne University, Clermont-Ferrand, F-63001 France*

1. Introduction

For the first 20 years of clinical use, CT scan explored morphology of the body with axial slices. Within the head, CT-scan allowed to analyze broadly the brain like any organ of the body, whereas the skull like others bones was finely detailed.

The appearance of helical and multi-slice CT scans in the 1990's, with high speed processes, led to volumetric and dynamic data, such as angio CT and CT perfusion.

Since 2005, there has been a constant development in new techniques.

1. The improved travelling table systems allow thicker dynamic studies, especially useful for cerebral perfusion.
2. Dual energy allows reduction of metallic and bony artefacts, making possible to obtain material decomposition images (quantitative evaluation of density).

However, these improvements often lead to increased patient irradiation. Techniques aiming to limit this important drawback are currently being developed, allowing reducing irradiation dose.

We review the basic principles of advanced techniques, including irradiation dose reduction, and then describe their neuroradiological applications in daily practice.

2. Material

In our institution, we use a 40-mm CT scanner (General Electric Discovery CT 750 HD, with Gemstone Spectral Imaging and Volume Helical Shuttle Perfusion), with Adaptative Statistical Iterative Reconstruction (ASIR).

3. Dual-energy CT

First experiments in Dual Energy CT (DECT), performed initially in the 1970s, demonstrated that DECT improved tissue characterization (Rutherford, Pullan, et Isherwood 1976). Until recently, this technology was impractical because of limiting factors such as insufficient spatial resolution, length of scan duration and important noise in the low-energy (low-kilovolts, low-kv) images. Two datasets must be acquired separately, at different times, increasing the risk of patient movements during the two phases that can reduce image quality (Thorsten R C Johnson et al. 2007).
Recent avdances in CT technology allow simultaneous acquisition of datasets at different energy levels (Coursey et al. 2010); such acquisitions have become possible either with two tubes mounted orthogonally, or with a generator able to switch between 80 and 140 kv targets in a very short time, less than 0.5 msec.

3.1 Principles

In Computed Tomography, differenciation of materials or tissues depends on X-ray attenuation, which is a function of X-ray energy, determined by photoelectric effect and Compton scattering (fig.1)

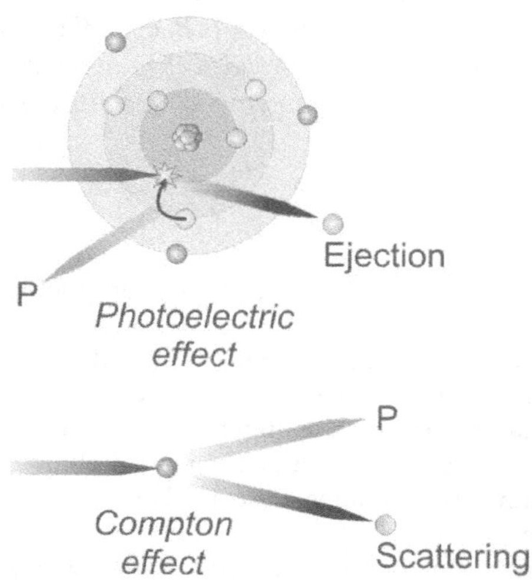

Fig. 1. The two main mechanisms of X-ray (blue line) attenuation are photoelectric effect and Compton effect. Photoelectric effect happens within electronic shells (layers) and consists in electron (colored sphere) ejection with concomittant emission of photon and reorganisation of electrons between shells. Compton effect happens with electrons which are scattered with concomittant emission of photon.

At the energy levels used in diagnostic imaging, Compton effect is almost independent of X-ray photon energy, while photoelectric effect is strongly energy dependent (Sprawls Perry). The probality of photoelectric interaction increases as the energy is nearer to that of the K shell binding. The K edge is the energy level where there is a spike in attenuation, and which corresponds to energy levels just greater than that of the K shell binding. The K edge increases with the atomic number (Table 1)

K Edges and Atomic Numbers of Physiologic Substances and Contrast Agents

Substance	K Edge (keV)	Atomic Number (Z)
Hydrogen	0.01	1
Carbon	0.28	6
Nitrogen	0.40	7
Oxygen	0.53	8
Calcium	4.00	20
Iodine	33.20	53
Barium	37.45	56
Gadolinium	50.20	64

Table 1. Relationships between material atomic number and photon energy (Coursey et al. 2010)

DECT imaging relies on energy dependence of the photoelectric effect and on the variability of K edges. The optimal energies must be just greater than the K edge of substances explored (Coursey et al. 2010); using different energy levels, DECT allows distinguishing materials according to attenuation coefficients at selected energy levels.

Material decomposition (MD) does not identify *stricto sensu* materials. Material attenuation curve is indirectly studied using the linear combination of two other materials (fig.2). Thus given two arbitrary selected basic materials, MD determines how much of each material would be needed to produce the observed measurements at low (65 Kev) energy and high (140 Kev) energy. These last two values correspond to common fixed DECT parameters of energy.

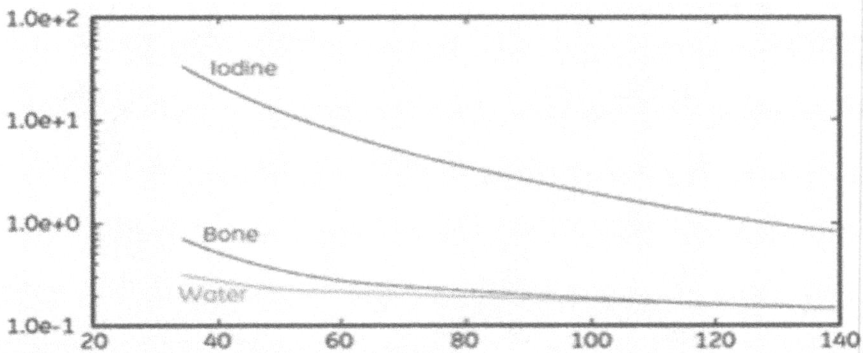

Fig. 2. The bone attenuation curve is a linear combination of iodine and water X-ray; x-axis, photon energy, Kev; y-axis, mass attenuation coefficient, m^2/Kg (from D.A.Langan, (Langan DA 2008)

For medical diagnosis, iodine and water are generally used, because they span the atomic number of the different materials that can be found in clinical practice.

3.2 Pratical consequences

Monochromatic spectral images obtained with DECT imaging are similar to that of a conventional Hounsfield unit image, but with fewer artefacts. This property is particularly useful to demonstrate implanted metallic devices such as coil, clip and electrode. In CT

angiography, it can distinguish between contrast in a vessel and calcification; it also allows removing skull base bone artefacts (Watanabe et al. 2009).
With post-processing, monochromatic energy levels can be chosen within a range from 40 to 140 Kev. At high energy levels, material contrasting is limited, whereas at low energy levels, they are more important. This allows material differenciation and quantitative evaluation of density (Thorsten R C Johnson et al. 2007).

4. Volume helical shuttle and CT brain perfusion

4.1 Principle of Volume Helical Shuttle (VHS)

With the latest generation of multidetector CT scanners, it is possible to cover large volumes of anatomy in a very short time. As a consequence, a thick portion of the brain is explored.
However, when width of coverage increases, it might increase phenomenas such as cone beam artefact (wide cone angle for wide-area detector), heel effect (non-uniform illumination of X-ray of the tube anode for wide-area detector) and scatter of X-ray photons. These inconveniences are reduced by VHS, which is a new adaptative technology enabling the CT table to travel back and forth using continuous periodic table movement during the acquisition (fig.3).

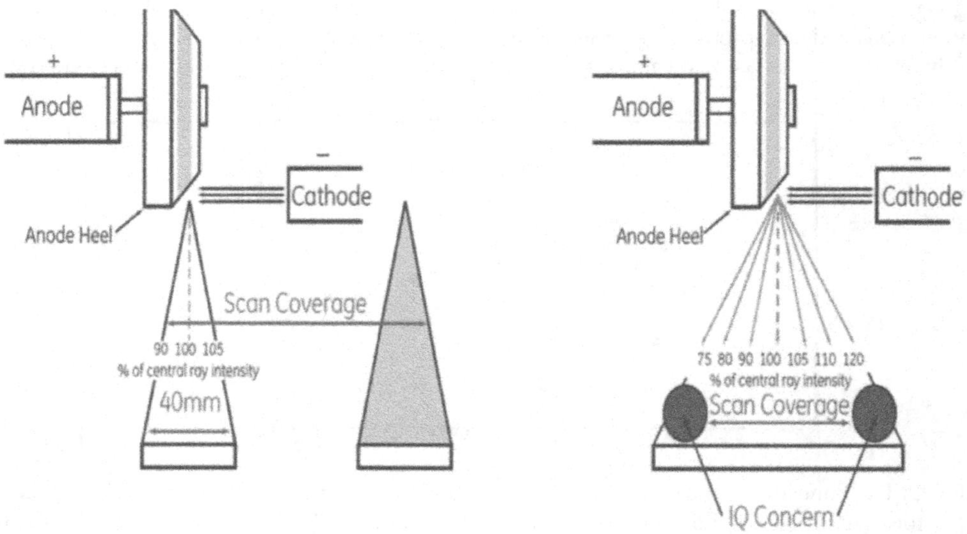

Fig. 3. Volume helical Shuttle (VHS, left) compared to wide-coverage detector axial acquisitions (right): there is no image quality (IQ) concern with VHS, whereas with wide-coverage detetector IQ concerns, as well as heel effect, cone beam artefact and increase photon scaterring, are known (from A. Hagiwara, 2008)

VHS affords minimal overscanning, consequently reducing unnecessary radiation exposure, (fig.4). VHS also improves temporal sampling; for maximum scan coverage of 312.5 mm, the system realizes 20 passes (10 round trips) within 60 sec, with a temporal sampling of 2.9 sec at the center of the volume.

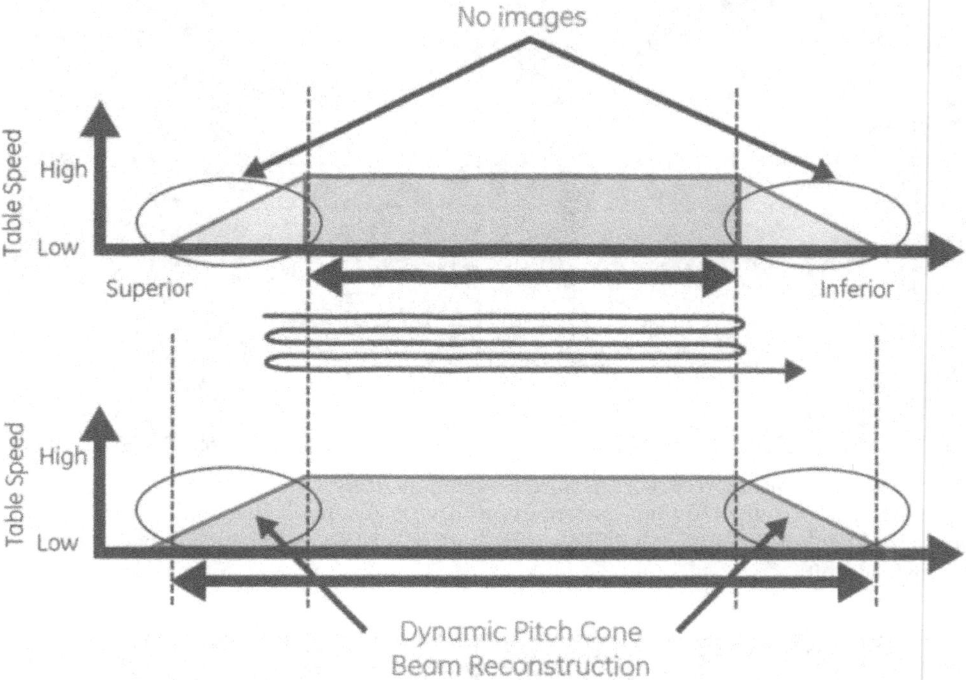

Fig. 4. There is no overscanning with Volume Helical Shuttle (top) conversely to conventional helical scanning (bottom) (from A. Hagiwara, 2008)

4.2 Principle of CT brain perfusion

VHS main application in neuroimagery is CT brain perfusion.

Until today, maximum coverage allowed in a sufficient temporal resolution was of 20-mm thickness for four detector-rows CT, and 80 mm for sixteen detector rows. With VHS technology, the coverage for brain CT perfusion is 120 mm, obtained in less than 48 sec, with a temporal resolution of 0.2 sec.

For many years, CT and MRI have been used for structural information. After the development of perfusion MRI, CT perfusion has been perfected and these two modalities now allow assessment of haemodynamic characteristics in brain tissue.

CT perfusion consists in analysis of the time evolution of contrast agent during the first passage of an intravenous bolus of iodine (Grand et al. 2007) (Hoeffner et al. 2004). Scans are obtained in dynamic mode during the injection. Functional data of brain perfusion are automatically calculated according to the central volume principle, which relates cerebral blood volume (CBV), cerebral blood flow (CBF) and mean transit time (MTT) in the following equation: CBF = CBV/MTT. MTT is given by deconvolution of tissue enhancement curves with reference to an arterial curve, generally obtained in the anterior cerebral artery (fig. 5). For each parenchymal pixel, CBV is calculated as the area under the curve divided by the area under the curve in the arterial ROI. Then, CBF is calculated according to central volume equation.

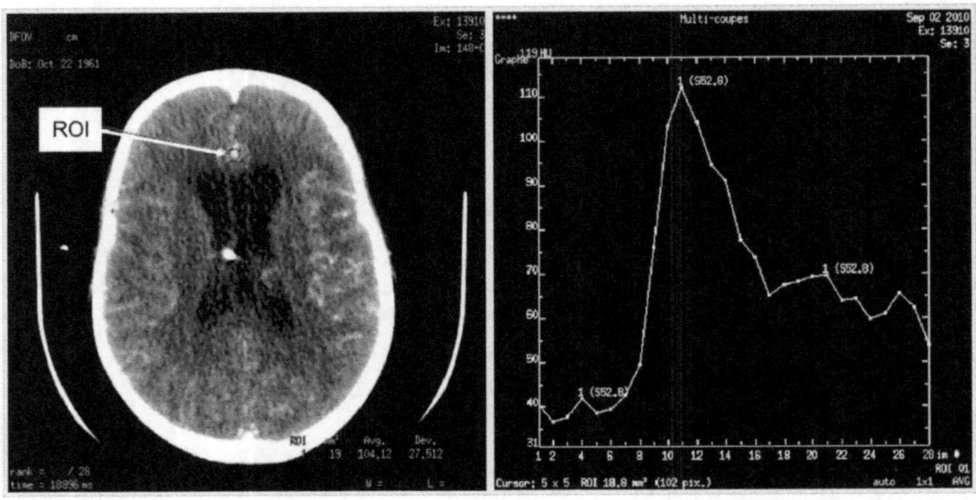

Fig. 5. Time-concentration curve. The anterior cerebral artery is generally choosen as the input artery (ROI, left), and time-concentration curve is generated from data within the ROI pixels (right; in this example the ROI comprises 102 pixels; x-axis, image number; y-axis, Hounsfield unit).

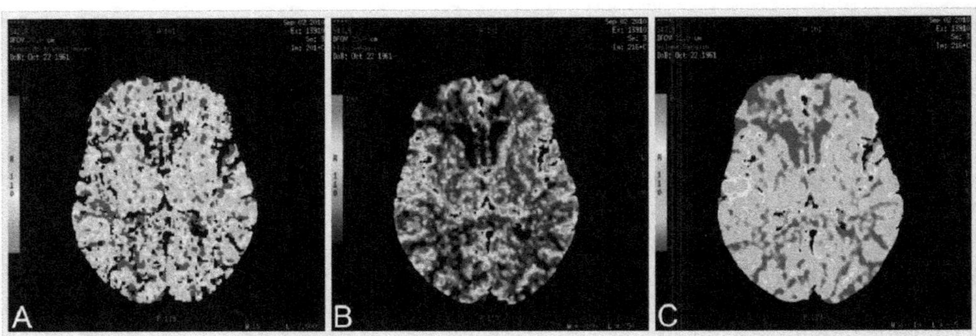

Fig. 6. (A) Mean Transit Time color map, msec, from 0, red, to 15, blue; (B) Cerebral Blood Flow color map, ml/msec, from 0, blue, to 100, red; (C) Cerebral Blood Volume color map, ml, from 0, blue, to 10, red. (Normal data)

A parameter related to vascular dynamics process has also been introduced, namely Permeability Surface Area Product (PS), which evaluates the flow of contrast agent crossing the capillary wall between intravascular and extravascular compartments.

This trans compartment flow is often called blood vessel leakness or blood clearance of contrast agent and is extrapolated from Patlak graphical analysis used for glomerule filtration rate exploration (Dawson 2006). The formula is as follows: PS = P × S; P (permeability) = D / t, with D = diffusion coefficient of contrast agent, and t = thickness of endothelium; S = surface of capillary tree.

PS is expressed in ml / 100 g of tissue / min. A voxel-wise approach leads to PS map (Fig. 7)

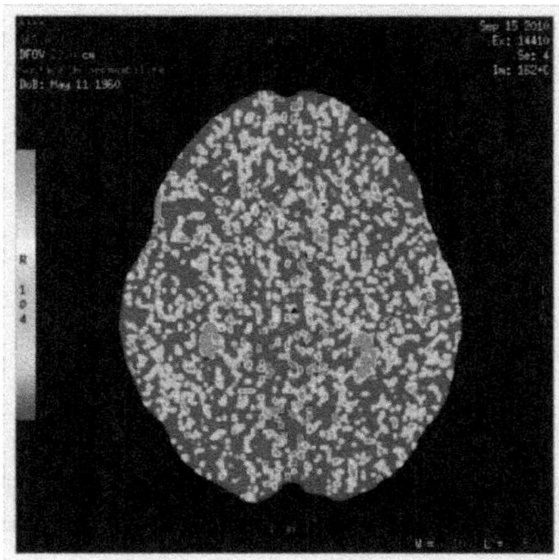

Fig. 7. Permeability Surface Area Product (PS) map, from 0, blue, to 10, red, in ml / 100 g of tissue / min (normal data)

CT perfusion presents some advantages compared with magnetic resonance imaging (MRI) perfusion:

- It allows qualitative and quantitative analysis, by giving absolute values of brain perfusion.
- Patient access is generally easier and CT perfusion is easy to perform; thus CT perfusion can be the initial exploration.
- Spatial resolution is good; voxel size is about 1-2mm.
- Results are obtained in less than 15 mn.

The main limitation of CT perfusion was the thickness of coverage, which is of 20 mm for a 4-detector row and 80 mm for a 16-detector row) (Grand et al. 2007)). VHS now allows coverage of 120 mm of the brain, with a temporal resolution of 1 image every 3 sec.

The main drawbacks are the risk of radiation overexposures and adverse effects due to iodinated contrast agent.

5. Reducing radiation dose in CT neuroimagery: use of adaptative statistical reconstruction algorithm (ASIR)

Since the inception of CT, the number of CT scans per year has dramatically increased (Brenner et Hall 2007). This results from its large availability, speed and diagnostic benefits. The drawback was increased radiation doses, requiring new techniques reducing these doses while improving diagnosis performances.

Reconstruction algorithms currently used such as filtered back projection (FBP) are unable to generate diagnostic quality images if X-ray tube currents decrease because signal-difference-to-noise ratio decreases with low-dose CT.

One alternative is iterative reconstruction technique (McCollough et al. 2009)(Silva et al. 2010) perfected with an adaptative statistical iterative reconstruction technique (ASIR), which limits computing time.

ASIR uses information obtained from the FBP algorithm and then uses matrix algebra to transform the value of each pixel to a new estimate of the pixel value. This new pixel value is then comparated with the ideal value predicted with the noise model. Iterations are

successively performed until final estimated and ideal pixel values converge (Silva et al. 2010)(Hara et al. 2009). It is possible to blend ASIR and FBP images in a range of 10% to 100%(Leipsic et al. 2010)(Flicek et al. 2010) .
Recent studies have demonstrated that ASIR reduces noise and improve signal-difference-to-noise ratio. By applying an appropriate percentage of ASIR, radiation doses are reduced between 23% to 65% (Leipsic et al. 2010)(Flicek et al. 2010)(Sagara et al. 2010)(Prakash et al. 2010).

6. Medical Neuroimaging

6.1 Applications of CT perfusion

6.1.1 Acute stroke

Recent advances in thrombolytic therapy, allowing reperfusion of brain tissue, have fostered the identification of biological parameters witnessing of reversible cell damage within the hypoperfused territory. Restoration of normal cell activity depends on severity of cell damage and on blood supply, particularly oxygen content and cerebro-vascular autoregulation. The tissue tolerance of CBF reduction ranges from 20 ml/100g/min to 6-10 ml/100g/min; below 6-10 ml/100g/min, cell damage and synaptic conduction may be irreversible, leading to infarction; below 20 ml/100g/min, often called the "penumbral flow threshold", damage may be reversible (Zaro-Weber et al. 2009)
One of the challenges is to identify the area where the cerebro-vascular autoregulation is maintained, because of the likelihood to reverse non-lethal cell damage. CT perfusion can determine this penumbra area, defined by normal or elevated CBV, while CBF is decreased and MTT is increased because of hypoperfusion (Max Wintermark et al. 2002).
The infarct core, i.e. area of irreversibility of damaged tissue, is characterized by the loss of cerebro-vascular autoregulation, and defined by decreased CBV, decreased CBF and increased MTT; (Grand et al. 2007)(Hoeffner et al. 2004)(Schramm et al. 2004)(Schaefer et al. 2006)(Mejdoubi, Calviere, et Dumas 2010) (fig.8).

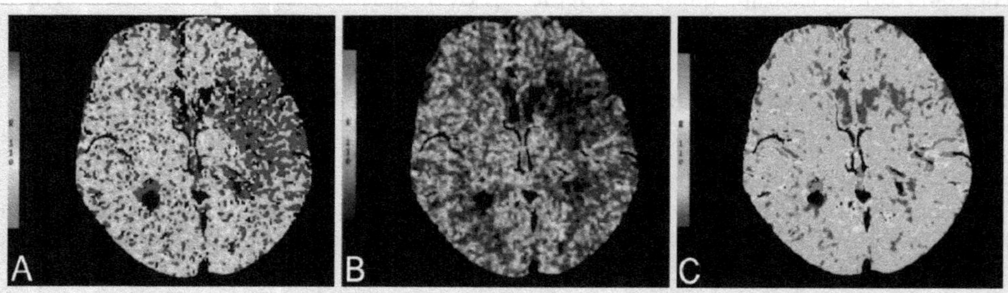

Fig. 8. Recent stroke in the left middle cerebral artery territory. Infarct tissue has elevated MTT (A), decreased CBF (B) and decreased CBV (C). Note the mismatch between the infarct area and the tissue at risk of infarction, which corresponds to the area where CBV is maintained and MTT is increased.

Patients with acute stroke can benefit from reperfusion therapy if undertaken before six hours, if the size of infarct area is less from one third of the middle cerebral artery territory, and if there is a minimal mismatch ratio of 20%, between the infarct core and the penumbra, hence more than 20% of the hypoperfused region could recover (Furtado et al. 2010). In addition, mismatch ratio increases with the z-axis coverage, or thickness, of CT Perfusion (Furtado et al. 2010). Consequently, increasing coverage of CT Perfusion, improves accuracy of functional data; it also prevents missing a lesion by incorrect selection of the tissue block analysis.

The most sensitive criteria of early detection of ischemia seems the relative increase of MTT, compared with controlateral safe hemisphere, higher than 145%, and the most accurate parameter to determine infarcted area seems a CBV value under 2ml/100mg; the mismatch between areas with a CBV lower than 2ml/100mg and areas with increased MTT allows the most accurate delineation of tissue at risk of infarction (Max Wintermark et al. 2006).

Another recent study shows that the risk of hemorrhagic transformation in acute stroke patients is correlated with increased PS (Aviv et al. 2009)

CT angiography (CTA) is usually performed during the same session to determine stroke etiology, intra or extracranial vessel occlusion or dissection, and occlusion location. Conventional CTA images are well known to have poor quality in skull base region (Ma et al. 2010). In DECT acquisitions, value of iodine increases much more than bone or calcium with decreasing of X-ray tube voltage. By varying the values of Kev on Material Decomposition images, skull base bone artefacts are exclude, while keeping good contrast in the lumen of arteries, and vascular calcifications are removed, allowing to insulate the lumen vessel (Thorsten R C Johnson et al. 2007) (Coursey et al. 2010)(Watanabe et al. 2009).

Finally, CT is a reliable and accurate technique to explore patients with acute stroke, combining CT without injection to exclude intracranial haemorrhage, CT Perfusion to evaluate penumbra, and CTA to determine the etiology of ischemia (Grand et al. 2007)(Hoeffner et al. 2004)(Furtado et al. 2010).

However, CT may be insufficient for lacunar or brainstem infarction and also to determine directly cell damage.

6.1.2 Vasospasm

Vasospam is a complication of aneurysmal subarachnoïd hemorrhage that can worsen the prognosis. Severe vasospasm can lead to delayed cerebral ischemia (DCI) and symptomatic vasospasm, this latter can lead to delayed ischemic neurologic deficit (DIND); one can bear in mind that the relationship between vasospasm and DIND is not straightforward (Al-Tamimi et al. 2010)

The diagnosis of vasospasm and DCI stays difficult to establish and often delayed. Currently, the gold standard of arterial vasospam diagnosis is conventional angiography, and the survey of patients relies mainly on clinical examination and transcranial Doppler. Recent studies show that CT Perfusion is useful and reliable to assess vasospasm and DCI, vasospasm induces increased MTT and further decreased CBV (Grand et al. 2007)(Dankbaar et al. 2009)(van der Schaaf et al. 2006)(M Wintermark, N U Ko, et al. 2006).(Max Wintermark et al. 2008). MTT seems the most sensitive parameter to detect regions at risk to vasospam (M Wintermark, N U Ko, et al. 2006) (Pham et al. 2007) (Max Wintermark et al. 2008) (fig.9).

In addition, CT Perfusion is repeatable at regular intervals with reproductible parameters, making it useful in this critical period, while taking into account risk of radiation overexposures and adverse effects due to iodinated contrast agent.

VHS can help to detect directly the vasospasm on the vascular tree during CTA, allowing wider exploration of vascular territories. DEACT reduces artefacts generated by metallic clips or coils enabling better analysis of vessels (fig.10); it also removes bone artefacts.

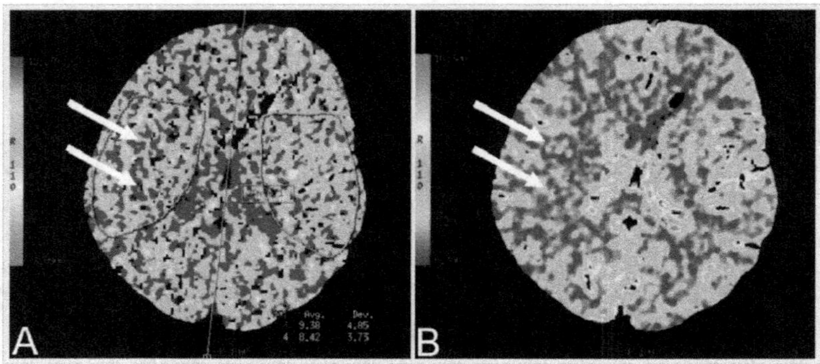

Fig. 9. CT Perfusion performed seven days after intravascular embolisation of anterior communicant artery aneurysm revealed by subarachnoïd hemorrhage: increased MTT (A) associated with decreased CBV (B) in right middle cerebral artery territory (white arrows) is the result of vasospam.

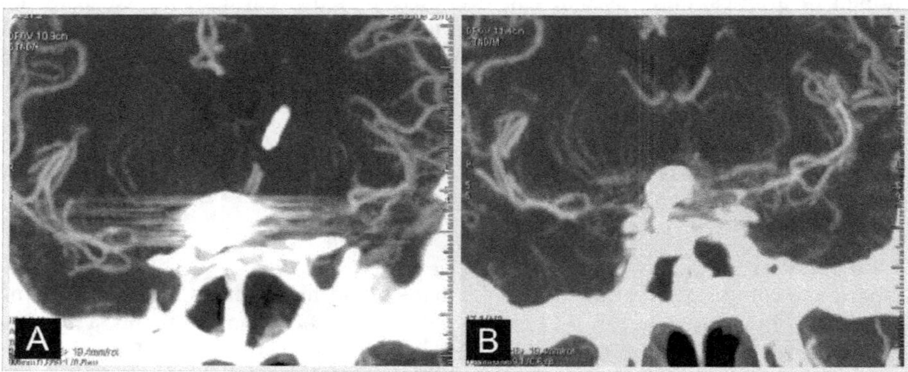

Fig. 10. Using DEACT (B) removes most of artefacts visible on current CT acquisition (A); same patient than in fig. 8.

Compromise must be found when increasing Kev to reduce artefact, because this can lead a false reducing of vascular luminal diameter, mimicking a vasospasm.

6.1.3 Tumors

It is challenging to determine the bio-architecture of brain tumor. Modern non invasive imaging techniques allow estimating many biological parameters, which must be interpreted cautionly and compared with histological findings, which are still the gold standard for tumor classification (Scheithauer, Fuller, et VandenBerg 2008). Among bio-architectural parameters, such as cell proliferation and energetic metabolism, vascularization is of upmost importance since it was demonstrated that it could be an important prognostic factor, nowdays easily accessible with non invasive imaging (Scheithauer, Fuller, et VandenBerg 2008).
However the word vascularisation covers different conditions, such as hypervascularization, neo vascularization whatever the cause (e.g. tumor growth, tumoral

vessels, radionecrosis) and blood brain barrier (BBB) dysfunction up to permanent rupture. Imaging perfusion allows quantifying CBF, CBV, MTT and PS product that could be usefull to show differences between diverse brain tumors and to determine non-invasive prognostic factors.

Thus, for the last few years, studies of MRI perfusion imaging have shown correlation between increasing of regional CBV (rCBF), Permeability Surface-area product (PS) and grading of tumors (Grand et al. 2007)(Hoeffner et al. 2004)(R Jain et al. 2008)(Law et al. 2003)(Ding et al. 2006). CNS lymphomas have intense contrast enhancement with increased PS product whereas CBV remains low (Schramm et al. 2010). In gliomas, perfusion imaging could also be useful to guide the biopsy where there is the greatest increasing of rCBV and PS (Grand et al. 2007) .

Lastly, it can assess the response to treatment (besides the tumoral volume), and differentiate tumor recurrence from radionecrosis(Grand et al. 2007) (see e.g fig.11)

One of the main advantage of CT Perfusion compared with MRI is the quantitative assessment of PS. Poor anatomical definition remains a drawback of this technique, and additional studies are required to validate results; however it seems to be a good alternative or complement to MRI perfusion imaging, especially to obtain quantitative data.

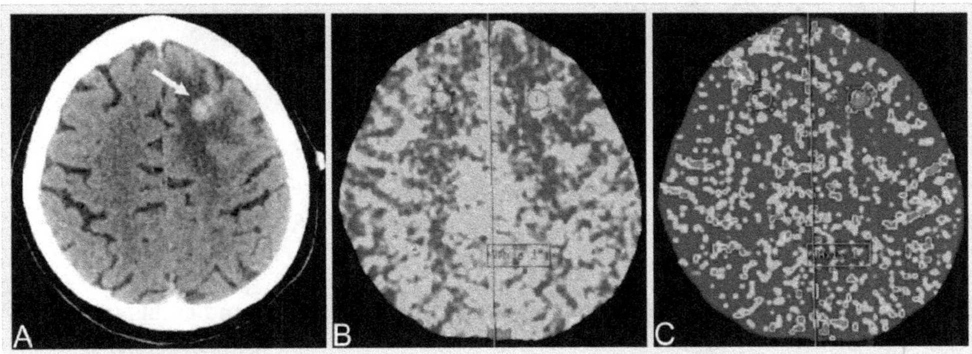

Fig. 11. CT Scan (iodinated contrast injection) performed 2 years after fractionated radiotherapy for a frontal metastasis (A) shows a contrast-enhancing lesion (white arrow); CT perfusion has revealed increased CBV (B) and increased PS (C) favoring tumor recurrence confirmed by histopathological analysis.

6.1.4 Other applications of vascular imaging

CT Perfusion is a non-invasive way to characterize cerebral vascular autoregulation, and could hence be used to adjust and monitor brain oedema therapy following head injury (M Wintermark, Chiolero, et al. 2006). In this indication, VHS is always interesting to study a greater width of cerebral parenchyma.

Time aspect given by perfusion imaging can be used to obtain dynamic images of cerebral blood flow (fig.12)

This technique is not a current practice because of the volume of data lending long reconstruction time. However, it seems interesting in specific indications, such as arterio-veinous malformation for diagnosis and volume survey of vascular nidus after treatment.

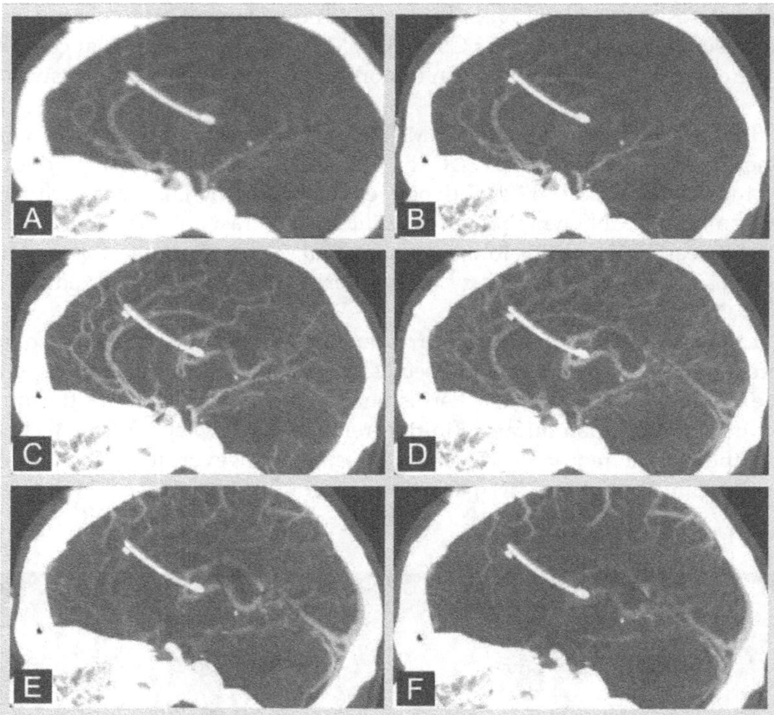

Fig. 12. Dynamic CT acquisitions show the circulation of iodinated contrast agent in the vessels: from arterial time (A) to venous time (F). An intraventricular catheter (white) is visible.

6.2 Analysis of contacts of deep brain stimulation electrodes: a predictable using of spectral CT

Groups performing brain stimulation advocated post-operative imaging, MRI or CT to analyse the anatomic position of each electrod contact (F Caire et al. 2006)(Duffner et al. 2002)(Ferroli et al. 2004)(Lemaire et al. 2007, a) (Pinto et al. 2007)(Vayssiere et al. 2004).
We studied the artefact generated on CT scans by the contacts of the DBS 3389 electrode (Medtronic, Mineapolis, USA) (Hemm et al. 2009). In vitro-study showed that the distal and proximal limits of a lateral black artefact represented the four contacs of the electrode. In vivo-study confirmed that the artefacts are reliable to define the position of the fours contacts. Phantom and patient CT acquisitions showed the presence of three other sorts of artefacts: a white artefact corresponding to the electrode, a lateral black artefact around a part of the electrode due to the large difference in density between the contact and the surrounding tissue, and zones of protuberance of the white artefact, corresponding to the transition from metal to insulation (unlike for MRI, where the biggest artefact correspond to the contact of the electrode). From these observations, three measurements were carried out: height of the lateral black artefact (H), distance between the begining of the white and the lateral black artefact (D), maximal artefact width (W), representing respectively the lengths of the four contacts, the electrode tip and width of the contact zone (fig. 13)

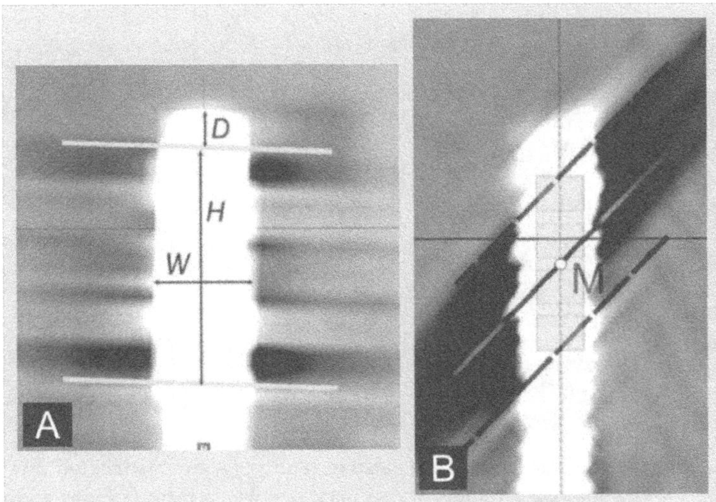

Fig. 13. A. Illustration of the different artefact parameters measured on phantom and patient CT acquisitions; W , maximal width of the white electrode artefact, H height of lateral black artefact along the electrode axis, D, distance between the beginning of the white electrode artefact and the beginning of the lateral black artefact (Hemm et al. 2009). B. After identification of the distal and proximal black artefact boundaries (dotted lines), the location of the four contacts is determined relatively to the point (M) placed in the middle of the distance between the two boundaries (Hemm et al. 2009).

The width of the artefact was nearly twice the theorical electrode diameter because of X-ray diffusion. There was no difference between pseudo-sagittal and pseudo-coronal reconstructions along the electrode axis; however there is a slight influence of the second electrode in the pseudo-coronal direction. Consequently, contact positions analysis relied on (fig.13.B): identification of the end of the distal contact corresponding to the distal boundary of the lateral black artefact, the tip length of approximately 1.2 mm can be used to validate the beginning of this black artefact; identification of the beginning of the proximal contact corresponding to the proximal boundary of the lateral black artefact; calculation of the four contact locations, according to the known electrode geometry.

This study demonstrates that post-operative CT scan in implanted patients is a useful alternative to MRI. In addition, CT offers some advantages over MRI: shorter acquisition time (< 1 min versus 5 min), greater accessibility and lower cost. MRI-CT coregistration allows optimizing post operative data using with the best contact analysis on CT and the best anatomical analysis on MR (Lemaire et al. 2007,b) . There are also safety issues for both techniques: Specific Absorption Rate (SAR) can be a problem for MRI because the presence of a metallic implant carries a potential risk of electrode displacement or of heating under a high magnetic field (Gleason et al. 1992)(Schueler et al. 1999)(Uitti et al. 2002), and CT uses ionising radiations.

Further studies are mandatory to reduce electrode artefacts. First measurements made with DEAC technology seems promising, reducing dramatically artifacts; MRI-CT coregistration and refined electrode analysis suggest that we will have nearly real visualization (fig 14), allowing better understanding of deep brain stimulation mecahnisms.

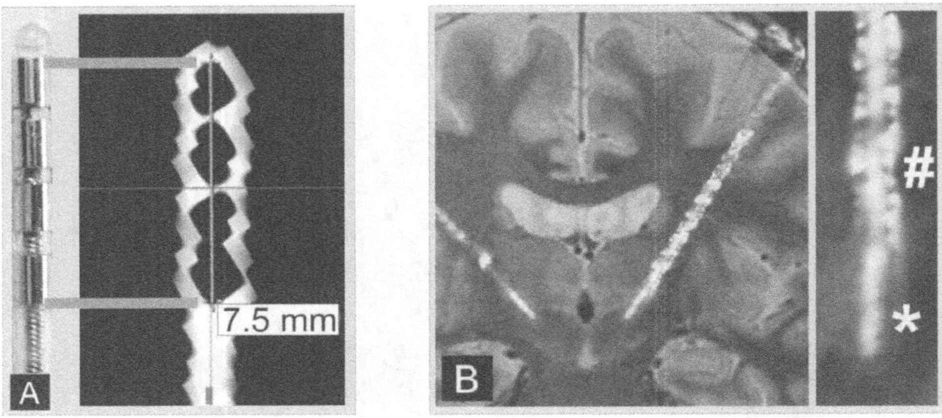

Fig. 13. DEAC monochromatic images are close to reality: (A) reconstructed image along the electrode (DBS 3389), showing artefacts of contacts; B, coregistration of electrode artifact extracted from DEAC images with pre operative MRI, on the right, zoom in of the electrode artifact showing details of the tip (*) and twisted electride wires (#).

6.3 Material decomposition

Multi-Energy CT enables measurement of material density using spectral images, namely Material Decomposition (MD). MD allows separation and characterization of different materials with similar CT density values (Hui et al. 2010). In clinical neuroimaging, this technique can be used for several purposes such as differenciate iodine in the vessel lumen from wall calcifications (Coursey et al. 2010) (Fig.14) and differentiate intracerebral hemorrhage from iodinated contrast (Rajiv Gupta et al. 2010) (fig.15)
Density measurement of products using multi-energy opens prospects in biomedical research. For instance, it is possible to determine physical properties of gels, such as density (mg/cm3) and homogeneity (fig. 16)(Saliege et al. 2010)

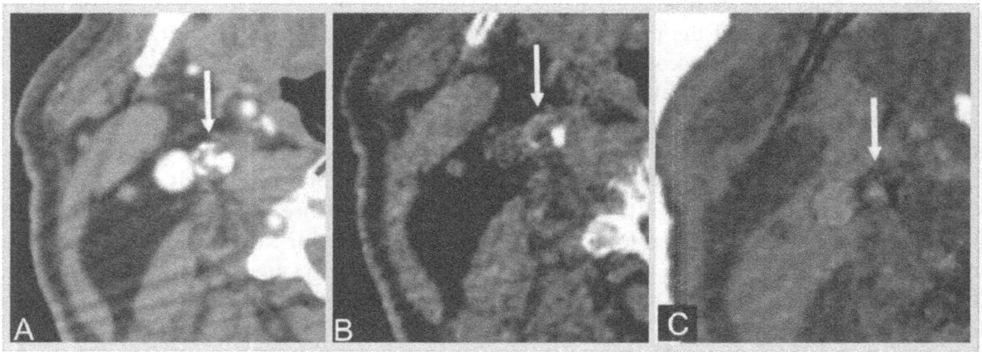

Fig. 14. Carotid (white arrow) CTA: (A) 70 KeV monochromatic image; (B) calcium density windowing; (C) iodine density windowing. Data transformation into effective material densities (MD) improves tissue characterization.

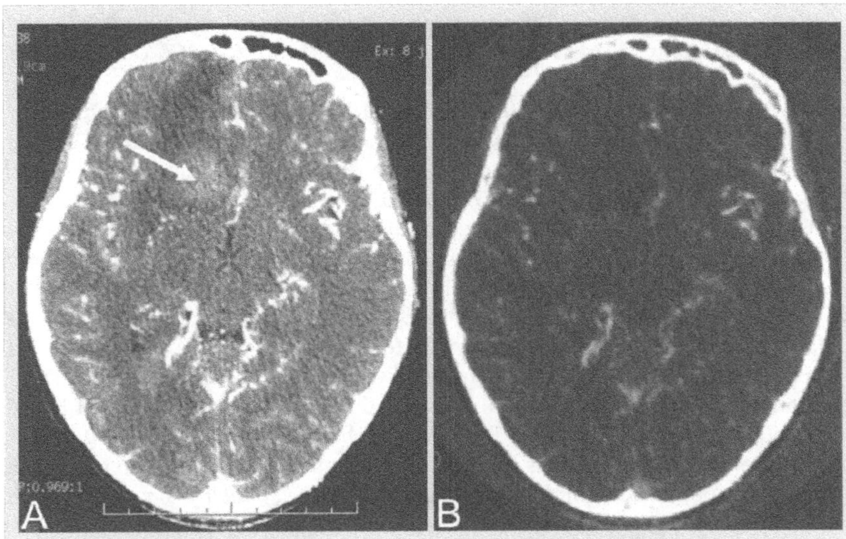

Fig. 15. Hyperdensity due to hemorrhage (white arrow) on mono energy 70 keV images (A) is removed on iodine density image (B).

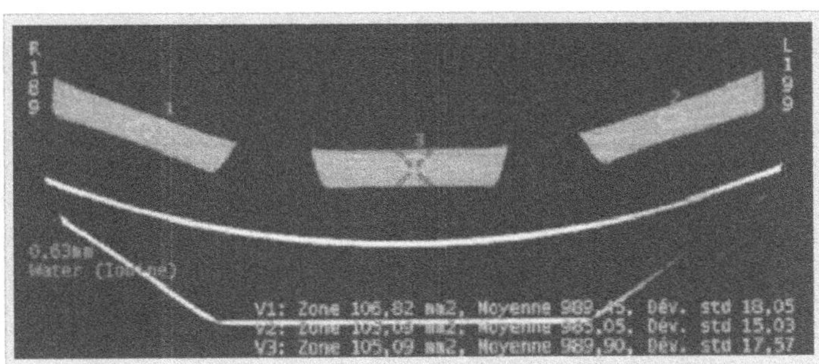

Fig. 16. Measurement of 1.1% agarose gel (3 samples) using post-processing on 65 keV monochromatic image.

7. Conclusion

Most recent advance in medical CT imaging relies on dual-energy and improvement of travelling table system. They enable a more accurate evaluation of tissue density and brain perfusion, with a reduction of artefacts and an increase of cover thickness, retaining moderate radiation dose using suited reconstruction algorithms (ASIR).

8. References

Al-Tamimi, Yahia Z, Nicolas M Orsi, Audrey C Quinn, Shervanthi Homer-Vanniasinkam, et Stuart A Ross. 2010. A review of delayed ischemic neurologic deficit following aneurysmal subarachnoid hemorrhage: historical overview, current treatment, and pathophysiology. *World Neurosurgery* 73, n°. 6 (Juin): 654-667. doi:10.1016/j.wneu. 2010.02.005.

Aviv, Richard I, Christopher D d'Esterre, Blake D Murphy, Julia J Hopyan, Brian Buck, Gabriella Mallia, Vivian Li, Liying Zhang, Sean P Symons, et Ting-Yim Lee. 2009. Hemorrhagic transformation of ischemic stroke: prediction with CT perfusion. *Radiology* 250, n°. 3 (Mars): 867-877. doi:10.1148/radiol.2503080257.

Brenner, David J, et Eric J Hall. 2007. Computed tomography--an increasing source of radiation exposure. *The New England Journal of Medicine* 357, n°. 22 (Novembre 29): 2277-2284. doi:10.1056/NEJMra072149.

Caire, F, Ph Derost, J Coste, J-M Bonny, F Durif, E Frenoux, A Villéger, et J-J Lemaire. 2006. [Subthalamic deep brain stimulation for severe idiopathic Parkinson's disease. Location study of the effective contacts]. *Neuro-Chirurgie* 52, n°. 1 (Février): 15-25.

Coursey, Courtney A, Rendon C Nelson, Daniel T Boll, Erik K Paulson, Lisa M Ho, Amy M Neville, Daniele Marin, Rajan T Gupta, et Sebastian T Schindera. 2010. Dual-energy multidetector CT: how does it work, what can it tell us, and when can we use it in abdominopelvic imaging? *Radiographics: A Review Publication of the Radiological Society of North America, Inc* 30, n°. 4 (Août): 1037-1055. doi:10.1148/rg.304095175.

Dankbaar, Jan Willem, Nicolien K de Rooij, Birgitta K Velthuis, Catharina J M Frijns, Gabriel J E Rinkel, et Irene C van der Schaaf. 2009. Diagnosing delayed cerebral ischemia with different CT modalities in patients with subarachnoid hemorrhage with clinical deterioration. *Stroke; a Journal of Cerebral Circulation* 40, n°. 11 (Novembre): 3493-3498. doi:10.1161/STROKEAHA.109.559013.

Dawson, Peter. 2006. Functional imaging in CT. *European Journal of Radiology* 60, n°. 3 (Décembre): 331-340. doi:10.1016/j.ejrad.2006.06.023.

Ding, Bei, Hua Wei Ling, Ke Min Chen, Hong Jiang, et Yan Bo Zhu. 2006. Comparison of cerebral blood volume and permeability in preoperative grading of intracranial glioma using CT perfusion imaging. *Neuroradiology* 48, n°. 10 (Octobre): 773-781. doi:10.1007/s00234-006-0120-1.

Duffner, F, H Schiffbauer, S Breit, S Friese, et D Freudenstein. 2002. Relevance of image fusion for target point determination in functional neurosurgery. *Acta Neurochirurgica* 144, n°. 5 (Mai): 445-451. doi:10.1007/s007010200065.

Ferroli, Paolo, Angelo Franzini, Carlo Marras, Elio Maccagnano, Ludovico D'Incerti, et Giovanni Broggi. 2004. A simple method to assess accuracy of deep brain stimulation electrode placement: pre-operative stereotactic CT + postoperative MR image fusion. *Stereotactic and Functional Neurosurgery* 82, n°. 1: 14-19. doi:10.1159/000076655.

Flicek, Kristina T, Amy K Hara, Alvin C Silva, Qing Wu, Mary B Peter, et C Daniel Johnson. 2010. Reducing the radiation dose for CT colonography using adaptive statistical iterative reconstruction: A pilot study. *AJR. American Journal of Roentgenology* 195, n°. 1 (Juillet): 126-131. doi:10.2214/AJR.09.3855.

Furtado, A D, B C Lau, E Vittinghoff, W P Dillon, W S Smith, T Rigby, L Boussel, et M Wintermark. 2010. Optimal brain perfusion CT coverage in patients with acute middle cerebral artery stroke. *AJNR. American Journal of Neuroradiology* 31, n°. 4 (Avril): 691-695. doi:10.3174/ajnr.A1880.

Gleason, C A, N F Kaula, H Hricak, R A Schmidt, et E A Tanagho. 1992. The effect of magnetic resonance imagers on implanted neurostimulators. *Pacing and Clinical Electrophysiology: PACE* 15, n°. 1 (Janvier): 81-94.

Grand, S, V Lefournier, A Krainik, P Bessou, I Tropres, S Chabardes, D Hoffmann, et J-F Le Bas. 2007. [MR and CT perfusion imaging of the brain: principles and clinical applications]. *Journal De Radiologie* 88, n°. 3 (Mars): 444-471.

Gupta, Rajiv, Catherine M Phan, Christianne Leidecker, Thomas J Brady, Joshua A Hirsch, Raul G Nogueira, et Albert J Yoo. 2010. Evaluation of Dual-Energy CT for Differentiating Intracerebral Hemorrhage from Iodinated Contrast Material Staining. *Radiology* (Août 2). doi:10.1148/radiol.10091806. http://www.ncbi.nlm.nih.gov/pubmed/20679449.

Hagiwara A. 2008. Volume Helical Shuttle- A technical description. GE internal scientific publication.

Hara, Amy K, Robert G Paden, Alvin C Silva, Jennifer L Kujak, Holly J Lawder, et William Pavlicek. 2009. Iterative reconstruction technique for reducing body radiation dose at CT: feasibility study. *AJR. American Journal of Roentgenology* 193, n°. 3 (Septembre): 764-771. doi:10.2214/AJR.09.2397.

Hemm, Simone, Jérôme Coste, Jean Gabrillargues, Lemlih Ouchchane, Laurent Sarry, François Caire, François Vassal, et al. 2009. Contact position analysis of deep brain stimulation electrodes on post-operative CT images. *Acta Neurochirurgica* 151, n°. 7 (Juillet): 823-829; discussion 829. doi:10.1007/s00701-009-0393-3.

Hoeffner, Ellen G, Ian Case, Rajan Jain, Sachin K Gujar, Gaurang V Shah, John P Deveikis, Ruth C Carlos, B Gregory Thompson, Mark R Harrigan, et Suresh K Mukherji. 2004. Cerebral perfusion CT: technique and clinical applications. *Radiology* 231, n°. 3 (Juin): 632-644. doi:10.1148/radiol.2313021488.

Hui P, Li J, Zhou C, Yu S, Lo G, Wang X, Cao H, Guo Y, Shen Y, 2010. Material decomposition with spectral imaging on HDCT: Phantom experiments.ECR 2010 C-2990. European Society of Radiology - European Congress of Radiology, Vienna, March 4-8, 2010

Jain, R, S K Ellika, L Scarpace, L R Schultz, J P Rock, J Gutierrez, S C Patel, J Ewing, et T Mikkelsen. 2008. Quantitative estimation of permeability surface-area product in astroglial brain tumors using perfusion CT and correlation with histopathologic grade. *AJNR. American Journal of Neuroradiology* 29, n°. 4 (Avril): 694-700. doi:10.3174/ajnr.A0899.

Johnson, Thorsten R C, Bernhard Krauss, Martin Sedlmair, Michael Grasruck, Herbert Bruder, Dominik Morhard, Christian Fink, et al. 2007. Material differentiation by dual energy CT: initial experience. *European Radiology* 17, n°. 6 (Juin): 1510-1517. doi:10.1007/s00330-006-0517-6.

Langan DA. 2008. Gemstone Spectral Imaging. GE internal scientific publication.

Law, Meng, Stanley Yang, Hao Wang, James S Babb, Glyn Johnson, Soonmee Cha, Edmond A Knopp, et David Zagzag. 2003. Glioma grading: sensitivity, specificity, and predictive values of perfusion MR imaging and proton MR spectroscopic imaging compared with conventional MR imaging. *AJNR. American Journal of Neuroradiology* 24, n°. 10 (Décembre): 1989-1998.

Leipsic, Jonathon, Troy M Labounty, Brett Heilbron, James K Min, G B John Mancini, Fay Y Lin, Carolyn Taylor, Allison Dunning, et James P Earls. 2010. Adaptive statistical iterative reconstruction: assessment of image noise and image quality in coronary CT angiography. *AJR. American Journal of Roentgenology* 195, n°. 3 (Septembre): 649-654. doi:10.2214/AJR.10.4285.

Lemaire, Jean-Jacques, Jérôme Coste, Lemlih Ouchchane, François Caire, et al. 2007.a. Brain mapping in stereotactic surgery: a brief overview from the probabilistic targeting to the patient-based anatomic mapping. *NeuroImage* 37 Suppl 1: S109-115. doi:10.1016/j.neuroimage.2007.05.055.

Lemaire, Jean-Jacques, Jérôme Coste, Lemlih Ouchchane, Simone Hemm, Philippe Derost, Miguel Ulla, Séverine Siadoux, Jean Gabrillargues, Franck Durif, et Jean Chazal. 2007.b. MRI anatomical mapping and direct stereotactic targeting in the subthalamic region: functional and anatomical correspondence in Parkinson's disease. *International Journal of Computer Assisted Radiology and Surgery* 2, n°. 2 (7): 75-85. doi:10.1007/s11548-007-0124-2.

Ma, Rui, Cheng Liu, Kai Deng, Shao-juan Song, Dao-ping Wang, et Ling Huang. 2010. Cerebral artery evaluation of dual energy CT angiography with dual source CT. *Chinese Medical Journal* 123, n°. 9 (Mai): 1139-1144.

McCollough, Cynthia H, Andrew N Primak, Natalie Braun, James Kofler, Lifeng Yu, et Jodie Christner. 2009. Strategies for reducing radiation dose in CT. *Radiologic Clinics of North America* 47, n°. 1 (Janvier): 27-40. doi:10.1016/j.rcl.2008.10.006.

Mejdoubi, M, L Calviere, et H Dumas. 2010. [Value of CT perfusion for the diagnosis of early middle cerebral artery stroke]. *Journal De Radiologie* 91, n°. 5 (Mai): 555-560.

Pham, M, A Johnson, A J Bartsch, C Lindner, W Müllges, K Roosen, L Solymosi, et M Bendszus. 2007. CT perfusion predicts secondary cerebral infarction after aneurysmal subarachnoid hemorrhage. *Neurology* 69, n°. 8 (Août 21): 762-765. doi:10.1212/01.wnl.0000267641.08958.1b.

Pinto, Serge, Jean-François Le Bas, Laura Castana, Paul Krack, Pierre Pollak, et Alim-Louis Benabid. 2007. Comparison of two techniques to postoperatively localize the electrode contacts used for subthalamic nucleus stimulation. *Neurosurgery* 60, n°. 4 (Avril): 285-292; discussion 292-294. doi:10.1227/01.NEU.0000255353.64077.A8.

Prakash, Priyanka, Mannudeep K Kalra, Subba R Digumarthy, Jiang Hsieh, Homer Pien, Sarabjeet Singh, Matthew D Gilman, et Jo-Anne O Shepard. 2010. Radiation dose reduction with chest computed tomography using adaptive statistical iterative reconstruction technique: initial experience. *Journal of Computer Assisted Tomography* 34, n°. 1 (Janvier): 40-45. doi:10.1097/RCT.0b013e3181b26c67.

Rutherford, R A, B R Pullan, et I Isherwood. 1976. Measurement of effective atomic number and electron density using an EMI scanner. *Neuroradiology* 11, n°. 1: 15-21.

Sagara, Yoshiko, Amy K Hara, William Pavlicek, Alvin C Silva, Robert G Paden, et Qing Wu. 2010. Abdominal CT: comparison of low-dose CT with adaptive statistical iterative reconstruction and routine-dose CT with filtered back projection in 53 patients. *AJR. American Journal of Roentgenology* 195, n°. 3 (Septembre): 713-719. doi:10.2214/AJR.09.2989.

Saliege M, Boyer-Grand A, Lemaire JJ, Chopineau J, Sautou V, Gabrillargues J, Coste A, Sakka L, Coste J, Tixier F, Martin C, Achim V. 2010. Agarose gels : model of artificial brain in neurosurgery.Therapeutic drug monitoring (TDM), ESCP10LYON-1860. Société Française de Pharmacie Clinique - European Symposium of Clinical Pharmacy (SFPC-ESCP), Lyon, Octobre 22-23, 2010.

van der Schaaf, Irene C, Birgitta K Velthuis, Marieke J H Wermer, Nanne J Frenkel, Charles B L M Majoie, Theo D Witkamp, Gerard de Kort, Nicole J Freling, et Gabriel J E Rinkel. 2006. Multislice computed tomography angiography screening for new aneurysms in patients with previously clip-treated intracranial aneurysms: Feasibility, positive predictive value, and interobserver agreement. *Journal of Neurosurgery* 105, n°. 5 (Novembre): 682-688. doi:10.3171/jns.2006.105.5.682.

Schaefer, P W, L Roccatagliata, C Ledezma, B Hoh, L H Schwamm, W Koroshetz, R G Gonzalez, et M H Lev. 2006. First-pass quantitative CT perfusion identifies thresholds for salvageable penumbra in acute stroke patients treated with intra-arterial therapy. *AJNR. American Journal of Neuroradiology* 27, n°. 1 (Janvier): 20-25.

Scheithauer, Bernd W, Greg N Fuller, et Scott R VandenBerg. 2008. The 2007 WHO classification of tumors of the nervous system: controversies in surgical neuropathology. *Brain Pathology (Zurich, Switzerland)* 18, n°. 3 (Juillet): 307-316. doi:10.1111/j.1750-3639.2008.00179.x.

Schramm, Peter, Peter D Schellinger, Ernst Klotz, Kai Kallenberg, Jochen B Fiebach, Sonja Külkens, Sabine Heiland, Michael Knauth, et Klaus Sartor. 2004. Comparison of perfusion computed tomography and computed tomography angiography source images with perfusion-weighted imaging and diffusion-weighted imaging in patients with acute stroke of less than 6 hours' duration. *Stroke; a Journal of Cerebral Circulation* 35, n°. 7 (Juillet): 1652-1658. doi:10.1161/01.STR.0000131271.54098.22.

Schramm, Peter, Argyro Xyda, Ernst Klotz, Volker Tronnier, Michael Knauth, et Marius Hartmann. 2010. Dynamic CT perfusion imaging of intra-axial brain tumours: differentiation of high-grade gliomas from primary CNS lymphomas. *European Radiology* (Mai 22).
doi:10.1007/s00330-010-1817-4. http://www.ncbi.nlm.nih.gov/pubmed/20495977.

Schueler, Beth A., Todd B. Parrish, Jyh-Cherng Lin, Bruce E. Hammer, Brian J. Pangrle, E. Russell Ritenour, John Kucharczyk, et Charles L. Truwit. 1999. MRI compatibility and visibility assessment of implantable medical devices. *Journal of Magnetic Resonance Imaging* 9, n°. 4 (4): 596-603. doi:10.1002/(SICI)1522-2586(199904)9:4<596::AID-JMRI14>3.0.CO;2-T.

Silva, Alvin C, Holly J Lawder, Amy Hara, Jennifer Kujak, et William Pavlicek. 2010. Innovations in CT dose reduction strategy: application of the adaptive statistical iterative reconstruction algorithm. *AJR. American Journal of Roentgenology* 194, n°. 1 (Janvier): 191-199. doi:10.2214/AJR.09.2953.

Sprawls Perry. Interaction of Radiation with Matter. In *The Physical Principles of Medical Imaging*. 2 éd. Sprawls Educational Foundation. Online textbook.

Uitti, Ryan J, Yoshio Tsuboi, Robert A Pooley, John D Putzke, Margaret F Turk, Zbigniew K Wszolek, Robert J Witte, et Robert E Wharen. 2002. Magnetic resonance imaging and deep brain stimulation. *Neurosurgery* 51, n°. 6 (Décembre): 1423-1428; discussion 1428-1431.

Vayssiere, Nathalie, Niels van der Gaag, Laura Cif, Simone Hemm, Regis Verdier, Philippe Frerebeau, et Philippe Coubes. 2004. Deep brain stimulation for dystonia confirming a somatotopic organization in the globus pallidus internus. *Journal of Neurosurgery* 101, n°. 2 (Août): 181-188. doi:10.3171/jns.2004.101.2.0181.

Watanabe, Yoshiyuki, Kensuke Uotani, Tetsuro Nakazawa, Masahiro Higashi, Naoaki Yamada, Yoshiro Hori, Suzu Kanzaki, Tetsuya Fukuda, Toshihide Itoh, et Hiroaki

Naito. 2009. Dual-energy direct bone removal CT angiography for evaluation of intracranial aneurysm or stenosis: comparison with conventional digital subtraction angiography. *European Radiology* 19, n°. 4 (Avril): 1019-1024. doi:10.1007/s00330-008-1213-5.

Wintermark, M, R Chiolero, G Van Melle, J P Revelly, F Porchet, L Regli, P Maeder, R Meuli, et P Schnyder. 2006. Cerebral vascular autoregulation assessed by perfusion-CT in severe head trauma patients. *Journal of Neuroradiology. Journal De Neuroradiologie* 33, n°. 1 (Février): 27-37.

Wintermark, M, N U Ko, W S Smith, S Liu, R T Higashida, et W P Dillon. 2006. Vasospasm after subarachnoid hemorrhage: utility of perfusion CT and CT angiography on diagnosis and management. *AJNR. American Journal of Neuroradiology* 27, n°. 1 (Janvier): 26-34.

Wintermark, Max, William P Dillon, Wade S Smith, Benison C Lau, Saadia Chaudhary, Songling Liu, Melissa Yu, et al. 2008. Visual grading system for vasospasm based on perfusion CT imaging: comparisons with conventional angiography and quantitative perfusion CT. *Cerebrovascular Diseases (Basel, Switzerland)* 26, n°. 2: 163-170. doi:10.1159/000139664.

Wintermark, Max, Adam E Flanders, Birgitta Velthuis, Reto Meuli, Maarten van Leeuwen, Dorit Goldsher, Carissa Pineda, et al. 2006. Perfusion-CT assessment of infarct core and penumbra: receiver operating characteristic curve analysis in 130 patients suspected of acute hemispheric stroke. *Stroke; a Journal of Cerebral Circulation* 37, n°. 4 (Avril): 979-985. doi:10.1161/01.STR.0000209238.61459.39.

Wintermark, Max, Marc Reichhart, Jean-Philippe Thiran, Philippe Maeder, Marc Chalaron, Pierre Schnyder, Julien Bogousslavsky, et Reto Meuli. 2002. Prognostic accuracy of cerebral blood flow measurement by perfusion computed tomography, at the time of emergency room admission, in acute stroke patients. *Annals of Neurology* 51, n°. 4 (Avril): 417-432.

Zaro-Weber, Olivier, Walter Moeller-Hartmann, Wolf-Dieter Heiss, et Jan Sobesky. 2009. The performance of MRI-based cerebral blood flow measurements in acute and subacute stroke compared with 15O-water positron emission tomography: identification of penumbral flow. *Stroke; a Journal of Cerebral Circulation* 40, n°. 7 (Juillet): 2413-2421. doi:10.1161/STROKEAHA.108.540914.

14

Synchrotron Radiation Micro-CT Imaging of Bone Tissue

Zsolt-Andrei Peter[1] and Françoise Peyrin[2,3]
[1]*Université Paris Ouest Nanterre La Défense, IUT de Ville d'Avray, Département GTE*
[2]*Creatis, CNRS UMR 5220; INSERM U630; Université de Lyon; INSA Lyon*
[3]*European Synchrotron Radiation Facility*
France

1. Introduction

The evaluation of bone fragility remains an open question that is all the more important given that the prevalence of osteoporosis is increasing in industrial countries with the ageing of the population and its greater sedentarity. This disease, which affects one in three menopausal women, is responsible of fractures and vertebral compression that can lead to invalidity. Osteoporosis is a "silent disease": 40% of women and 13% of men after 50 years old are concerned with and 24% of aged patients die one year after a hip fracture. Thus this disease represents a major cost for public health.

The diagnosis of bone fragility and the associated therapeutic decision are currently based on the measurement of bone mineral density (BMD) using dual X-ray absorptiometry (DXA) techniques. However, although BMD is an important determinant of bone fragility, it doesn't provide a sufficient prediction of fracture risk (estimated between 60% and 70%) and it appears necessary to develop new methods for bone strength evaluation.

Bone quality changes that occur during aging and osteoporosis are receiving increasing interest. Among bone quality factors, the role of bone micro-architecture which refers essentially to the organization of the trabecular network has been widely demonstrated.

The quantification of bone micro-architecture should make possible to improve the prediction of bone mechanical resistance. Although bone architecture was conventionally evaluated by histomorphometry, new non-destructive techniques derived from medical imaging are increasingly used for the assessment of bone tissue.

In this chapter, we shall concentrate on X-ray imaging techniques, and in particular on 3D X-ray microtomography (micro-CT) which is progressively supplanting standard histomorphometry for the analysis of bone micro-architecture. This technique is non destructive, avoids sample preparation and provides three-dimensional images with a high and isotropic spatial resolution in the three spatial directions.

Using synchrotron radiation (SR) coupled to micro-CT instead of standard X-ray beams possesses additional advantages in terms of image quality and signal to noise ratio. Thanks to the properties of synchrotron radiation, this modality enables to study simultaneously bone microstructure and bone mineralization.

As clinicians expect more than images, objective measures of bone architecture and quantification techniques based on these images have been developed. The availability of

3D micro-CT images makes it possible to measure model independent parameters of bone micro-architecture, and thus to obtain reliable information on the geometry and topology of the bone structures as well as its connectivity, orientation, and anisotropy.
In the following we shall first present basic notions in bony biology. Then we shall briefly describe the evolution of bone imaging by means of X-ray based techniques, and detail the powerful synchrotron radiation micro-CT tool for imaging bone tissue. We shall then present image processing techniques to extract quantitative measurement from micro-CT images. After addressing the segmentation of bone from background and the separation of trabecular from cortical bone, we shall review specific methods to analyze trabecular and cortical bone. On the one hand, methods allowing the morphometric and topologic quantification of the trabecular network will be presented. On the other hand, new methods allowing the quantification of cortical bone from SR micro-CT images will be described. Then, examples of applications of SR micro-CT in bone research will be reviewed. We shall then conclude by some perspectives opened by this modality for the investigation of bone tissue.

2. Bone tissue

Bone achieves several functions in the organism; it has a multiscale structure exhibiting different levels of organization. At the microstructural scale, it is possible to distinguish cortical and cancellous (trabecular) bone being, respectively, a dense external shell and a porous inner material made of thin trabeculae (hundred of micrometers). Figure 1 a) illustrates a 3D SR micro-CT image of a mice tibia bone obtained by our group at the ESRF (voxel size : 5µm) with a zoom on the cortical (b) and trabecular (c) structures.
The trabecular or spongy bone constitutes 70% of the axial (or central) skeleton in humans, and can be seen as a honeycomb of vertical and horizontal bars called trabeculae. It is within this region that human red marrow is almost exclusively located.
The cortical or compact bone constitutes 80% of the total human skeleton, located primarily in the peripheral skeleton. It plays a major role in bone strength and bone fragility depends on its micro-structure. Human cortical bone is mainly organized in osteons and includes a complex network of canals: the mainly longitudinally oriented Havers canals and perpendicular to it, the Volkmann canals.
A fundamental process in bone biology is remodeling which replaces old bones with new one and allows bone to adapt its properties to mechanical constraints. All along our life, bone is constantly remodeled, which means that it is sequentially resorbed and reconstructed. The surface-to-volume ratio is much higher in trabecular than cortical bone and accordingly bone remodeling has a greater effect on trabecular bone because it has an annual turnover rate of about 25% in trabecular and 2-3% in cortical bone. After bone reconstruction, its mineral concentration in localized regions increases progressively. Thus bone tissue can be seen as an arrangement of bone modeling units (BMU) with different degrees of mineralization.
At the cellular scale, bone tissue includes micrometric or submicrometric porosities such as micro-cracks, osteocyte lacunae, and canalicules. The composition of bone tissue itself is a mixture of collagen, water and mineral (hydroxyapatite (HA) crystals). The collagen and mineral phases are complementary in the sense that they respectively provide toughness and stiffness.

If the general organization of bone microstructure is well described in an anatomy handbook, its particular organization for a given bone may vary with aging, disease, or therapy. The main particularity of bone as a material is to be able to adapt itself to mechanical constraints. This adaptation is the consequence of complex biological processes which are not fully elucidated but which result in modifications at all levels, from the arrangement of mineralized particles to that of its micro and macro structure.

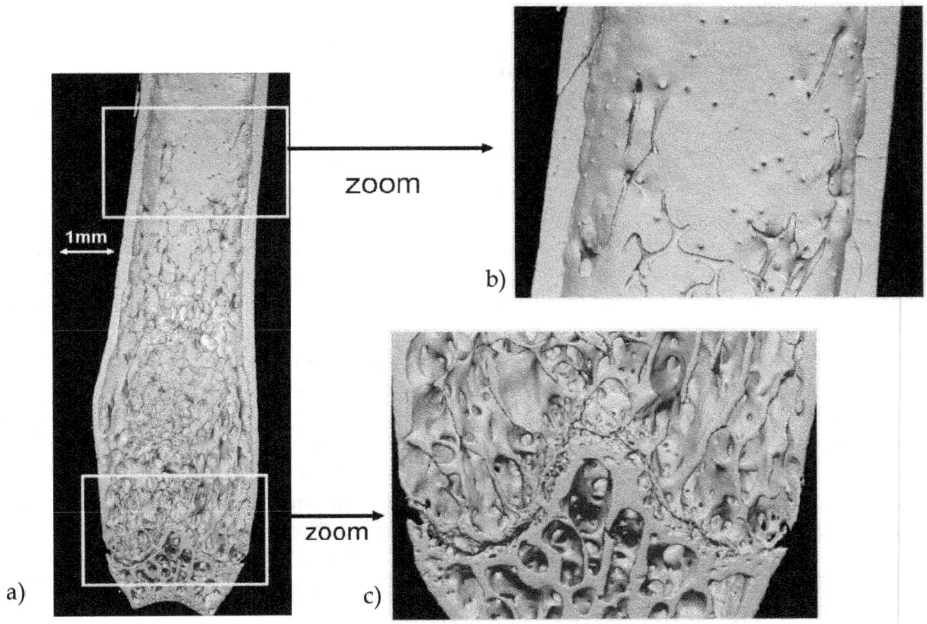

Fig. 1. a) SR micro-CT image of a mice bone; b) zoom on the cortical envelope; c) zoom on the trabecular part of the bone

Among the different means of investigating bone, imaging techniques may provide various types of information at different scales. While spatial resolutions between 5-10 µm are appropriate to study bone microstructure, a submicrometric resolution is necessary to examine the ultra-structural level and a nanometric resolution is required to get information about the crystalline structure.

3. X-ray based imaging techniques of bone

X-ray radiography is the oldest and simplest medical imaging technique. Although it does not directly produce a three-dimensional image of bone structure, different groups have suggested coupling it with texture analysis techniques to assess bone architecture (Cortet, B. et al., 1995). Research in this area involves the optimization of radiographic imaging together with texture analysis. When using flat panel detectors, the choice of spatial resolution has been shown to be a key issue. Texture analysis consists in extracting characteristic parameters of the arrangement of more or less regular patterns that constitute the bone image. Fractal approaches have been particularly exploited (Benhamou, C.L. et al.,

2001), but other statistical or structural approaches are also appropriate (Apostol, L. et al., 2006). Nevertheless these techniques have inherent limitations since they only allow studying 2D projections of the 3D bone microstructure.

X-ray Computerized Tomography (CT) avoids the overlay problem encountered in radiography by providing slices within the structure. Since its discovery, the technology of X-ray CT has considerably evolved and recent spiral scanners are well suited to the acquisition of fast serial sections. CT and particularly Quantitative CT (QCT) are increasingly used to measure BMD since it measures a volumetric density instead of an areal density as in standard DXA (Engelke, K. et al., 2009). CT has also been proposed to quantify in vivo trabecular texture to evaluate osteoporosis (Chevalier, F. et al., 1992), (Laval-Jeantet, A.M. et al., 1993), (Mundinger, A. et al., 1993). The typical spatial resolutions vary between 300 μm and 500 μm in the cutting plane for a slice thickness which is generally between 1 mm and 2 mm. The partial volume effect in these images is important given the size of the trabeculae (estimated at a few hundred micrometers) compared to the spatial resolution. It is manifested by the disappearance of the finest trabeculae or the grouping of the closest trabeculae, and can only provide indicators (Bousson, V. et al., 2000), (Bousson, V. et al., 2001). New peripheral CT systems such as the Xtreme C (from Scanco) can now provide 3D images of the bone micro-architecture at the human extremities (tibia or radius) at very high spatial resolution (~100 μm).

Even higher spatial resolution can be achieved in vitro with 3D microtomography (micro-CT) for the three-dimensional analysis of bone microarchitecture. A pioneer work in this area was that of Feldkamp (Feldkamp, L.A. et al., 1989) who was the first to develop a cone-beam micro-CT to acquire three-dimensional images of the bone with an isotropic spatial resolution of 70 μm. That technique possesses several advantages over histomorphometry: first, it is non-destructive, thus it does not compromise the sample for other testing methods (for instance biomechanical testing) and then it provides a 3D characterization able to render the complex organization of the bone tissue. This technique has received a considerable success and many commercial cone-beam micro-CT systems are now available for the analysis of bone samples (Cooper, D.M. et al., 2006).

Micro-CT can be improved by using X-ray beams extracted from synchrotron radiation. In fact, synchrotron sources permit to use a monochromatic X-ray beam while maintaining a high flux. Thus Synchrotron Radiation (SR) micro-CT provides three-dimensional images of bone structure at high or very high resolution of a few micrometers in relatively short exposure times. The feasibility of three-dimensional synchrotron microtomography to image bone samples was first demonstrated by Engelke (Engelke, K. et al., 1989). Bonse (Bonse, U. et al., 1994) presented three-dimensional images of iliac crest biopsies with a cubic voxel size of 8 μm. Kinney showed the possibility of acquiring in vivo three-dimensional synchrotron microtomography on rats at 9 μm (Kinney, J.H. et al., 1995). A three-dimensional synchrotron microtomography was developed at the European Synchrotron Radiation Facility (ESRF) in Grenoble (France), to study bone architecture (Salome, M. et al., 1999), and will be described in the following section.

4. Synchrotron Radiation (SR) micro-CT imaging technique

In this section we will briefly present the physical properties of the synchrotron radiation sources and the major advantages of coupling it to micro-CT. In particular, we will describe the SR micro-CT setup available at the ESRF, on beamline ID19, which is very well adapted to image bone tissue.

4.1 Synchrotron radiation sources

Electromagnetic waves are emitted when a charged particle is submitted to acceleration. In a circular accelerator such as a synchrotron or a storage ring, electrons are deviated by magnetic fields. This deviation is due to the radial force which attracts the electrons towards the center or the ring, and we call "synchrotron radiation" the light emitted by these electrons. Its wide spectrum reaches the X-ray range, it has a very high intensity and a continuous spectrum, spanning the whole range from infra-red (wavelength between 2.5 to 25µm) to X-rays (wavelength between 0.1 to 3Å), which is reached only when the energy of the electrons is high enough (of the order of several billion electronvolts - GeV). This wide range of wavelengths will allow studying different properties of materials at different scales and tiny features, e.g. bonds in molecules, nanoscale objects etc., but also lets to follow for example chemical reactions on a very short time scale.

The storage ring in a synchrotron facility includes different types of magnets and insertion devices connected to the beamline. Beamlines are located all around the storage ring and are optimized for a given technique.

The most important advantage of synchrotron radiation over a laboratory X-ray source is its brilliance. A synchrotron source like the ESRF (Figure 2 a)) has a brilliance that is more than a billion times higher than a laboratory source. It belongs to third generation sources, like APS (Chicago, USA) and Spring'8 (Himeji, Japan). The Sincrotrone Trieste (Trieste, Italy), SLS (Zürich, Switzerland), ALS (Berkeley, USA), SOLEIL (Orsay, France) also belong to third generation sources but have a lower critical energy.

4.2 SR micro-CT setup

The use of synchrotron X-rays compared to laboratory X-ray sources has several advantages in micro-CT. A first major property is the very high intensity of the X-ray beam, which allows improving the signal to noise ratio (SNR) in the images while reducing acquisition times. In 3D CT, the necessary number of photons is proportional to the fourth power of the voxel size to keep the same noise level, and then the high photon flux permits measurements at high spatial resolution. A second major property offered by synchrotron sources is the possibility to perform tomography with a monochromatic X-ray beam for a selected energy. Monochromaticity is a basic assumption in the theory of tomographic reconstruction which avoids beam hardening artifacts that can occur with a polychromatic standard X-ray tube. On a SR micro-CT setiup, the energy of the X-ray beam is tunable, and can be optimized for a given sample or a series of samples. Finally, unlike in most commercialized system using cone-beam sources, it is possible to implement parallel beam acquisition. This mode of acquisition has the advantage to allow exact tomographic reconstruction and thus to avoid typical cone-beam artefacts with conventional systems.

In three-dimensional (3D) SR micro-CT, hundreds of two-dimensional (2D) projection radiographs of the specimen are taken at several different angles. The accuracy of the CT image is dependent on the number of parallel beam projections and the number of data points in each projection. Each radiograph is a projection of the linear absorption distribution in the sample along the direction of X-ray beam onto the plane perpendicular to the direction of the X-ray beam propagation. Thus, SR micro-CT images represent maps of the linear absorption coefficient within the sample for a given energy.

An important limitation in high resolution micro-CT, which is inherent to the principle of CT, is the limited size of the sample. An important issue is the choice of spatial resolution versus overall sample size. Indeed, since the number of pixels of the detector is fixed, the higher the spatial resolution, the smaller the field of view. Moreover, during data acquisition, the sample must completely fit into the field of view to avoid local tomography, compromising quantitative reconstruction.

During data acquisition, a number of parameters have to be selected: energy of the X-ray beam, exposure time per projection, number of projection, number of frames. Ideally, the energy should be chosen such that the specimens absorb 85-90% of the incident radiation to obtain the best signal to noise ratio in the reconstructed image. In a homogeneous sample, absorbing 90% of the incident radiation means that the product between the sample thickness and the linear attenuation coefficient associated to the X-ray wavelength corresponds to 2.3. The exposure time and the number of projection will directly impact the signal to noise ratio in the reconstructed image.

Throughout the acquisition, the sample is sequentially rotated over a total angular range of 180°. Typically, several hundreds equiangular radiographic images of the sample are acquired (corresponding to approximately 8-16 GBytes of data per sample with a 2048x2048 detector). In addition, dark current and reference images are recorded with the same exposure time at different moments of each scan, to perform flat field corrections. This set of 2D images is then processed through a tomographic reconstruction algorithm to get the three-dimensional image of the sample. Tomographic image reconstruction consists in solving an inverse problem to estimate an image from its line integrals on different directions, in 2D, and the problem is theoretically equivalent to the inversion of the Radon transform of the image. In practice, there are two major classes of reconstruction algorithms that use fundamentally different approaches to accomplish this conversion: the first are the transform-based methods using analytic inversion formulae, and the other are series expansion methods based on linear algebra. The conventional method used in practice is the Filtered backprojection algorithm (FBP) which belongs to the first class of methods.

An SR micro-CT setup has been implemented on beamline ID19, one of the two long beamlines (145 m) of the ESRF (Salome, M. et al., 1999). The experimental scheme and a photo of this particular micro-CT setup are represented on Figure 2 b) and c).

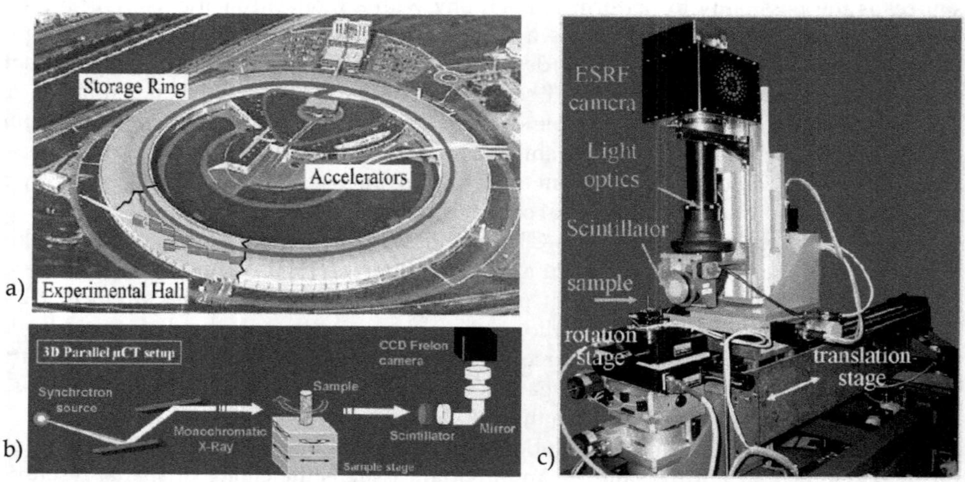

Fig. 2. a) the ESRF in Grenoble; b) and c) the SR micro-CT setup at the ID19 beamline (ESRF)

A wide SR parallel beam (up to 40mmx14 mm) with an energy ranging from 10 to 80 keV is available. A double crystal monochromator sets to diffract in the symmetrical Bragg reflection geometry, selects the appropriate energy from the white SR beam emerging from the storage ring. The sample is mounted on a goniometer including high resolution translations and rotations to position the sample and to rotate it in the beam. A two-dimensional detector records the beam transmitted through the sample. The distance between the sample and detector must be as small as possible to avoid phase contrast effects due to the coherence of the beam (Cloetens, P. et al., 1997). The two-dimensional detector is based on a two-dimensional charge coupled device (CCD) Fast REadout LOw Noise (FRELON) camera developed by the ESRF detector group (2048 x 2048 CCD chip, 14 bit dynamic range) (Labiche, J.-C. et al., 2007). This camera records the light image converted from a scintillator screen, after optical magnification. The optical system is modular and can be used with different objectives to adapt the field of view and the spatial resolution to the sample under investigation. Typically, pixel sizes of 10.13 μm, 6.65 μm, down to 0.28 μm may be used (Weitkamp, T. et al., 2010).

4.3 Comparison between micro-CT and SR micro-CT in bone research

As already mentioned, SR micro-CT presents a number of advantages over standard micro-CT because it allows quantitative imaging with high SNR in smaller acquisition times. SR micro-CT is thus often used as a reference technique to evaluate emerging imaging modalities.

SR and standard micro-CT have previously been compared to assess trabecular bone microarchitecture in a large subset of human bone specimens (Chappard, C. et al., 2006). In that work SR micro-CT images with a voxel size of 10.13 μm were reconstructed from 900 2D radiographic projections (with angular step of 0.2°), while standard micro-CT images with a voxel size of 10.77 μm were reconstructed from 205, 413 and 825 projections obtained using angular steps of 0.9°, 0.45° and 0.23°, respectively. The results show that streak-like artifacts occurred with standard micro-CT as a result of reconstruction artifacts, geometrical blurring, and beam hardening. These streak-like artifacts appear on histograms as an intermediate grey level between bone and background and therefore tend to reduce image contrast. Although systematic differences were noted between SR micro-CT and standard micro-CT images, correlations between the techniques were high and the differences would generally not change the discrimination between the studied groups. In conclusion, standard micro-CT was shown to provide a reliable 3D assessment of human bone when working with 0.23° or 0.45° rotation step, but not with 0.9° rotation step, thus highlighting the importance of acquisition conditions in practical study.

Another fundamental property of SR micro-CT in bone studies is the possibility to observe differences in mineralization within the bone phase and therefore to access another factor of bone quality. The differences observed in gray levels are related to various stages of mineralization associated with bone remodeling. The accuracy of the system was evaluated by using solutions mimicking hydroxyapatite, the main component of bone, at different known concentrations (Nuzzo, S. et al., 2001). This property is related to the monochromaticity of the beam but also to the high SNR of SR micro-CT images, and makes it possible to quantify the local degree of mineralization in bones. The method was validated and compared with quantitative microradiography (Nuzzo, S. et al., 2002b). It is therefore possible to quantify the degree of mineralization of bone in three-dimensions simultaneously to the bone architecture. This technique was applied to study the effects of a treatment for osteoporosis with etidronate on paired iliac crest biopsies (Nuzzo, S. et al., 2002a).

5. 3D analysis of SR micro-CT bone images

After tomographic reconstruction, 3D renderings of obtained data may be made by electronically stacking up the slices. These 3D volumes may be also sectioned in arbitrary ways, zoomed and rotated to better locate individual details. While the 2D slice images and 3D renderings are very useful for making qualitative observations of an internal concrete structure, the real benefit is the quantitative information that can be extracted from the 3D datasets.

The development of new 3D image analysis techniques is mandatory to fully exploit the wealth of information provided by SR micro-CT. We will thus review original image processing methods which are intimately related to the particular features of the available images. In this respect, the segmentation of the phases of interest is crucial since it will determine the accuracy of any quantitative analysis. The analysis of huge 3D images (between 2 and 16 GBytes per sample) involves the additional need to develop fast and automatic 3D image processing algorithms in order to study a statistically significant amount of data.

5.1 Segmentation of bone from background

With SR micro-CT, the segmentation of bone from background is much easier than with standard micro-CT due to the high SNR and high contrast in the image. In addition, parallel beam SR micro-CT avoids cone beam artifacts encountered in most standard micro-CT systems and resulting in various blurring effects. Thus it results that the gray level histogram of a SR micro-CT is typically bimodal, with two well defined peaks, one corresponding to background and the other to bone. Note that this property is deteriorating rather quickly with the spatial resolution of the image.

The segmentation of the bone phase can thus be appropriately done by simple thresholding based on standard techniques such as Otsu method. In SR micro-CT, the choice of the threshold will be less sensitive than in standard micro-CT, where this method is known to generate isolated particles and disconnection in the trabecular network. When processing a whole series of samples acquired in the same conditions, it is generally better to use the same threshold for all samples.

5.2 Separation of cortical and trabecular bone in a composite sample

To be biologically relevant, the extraction of quantitative parameters must be done separately on the trabecular and cortical envelops. This task cannot be simply performed by thresholding gray levels since both bone structures are in the same range of attenuation.

In previous work, we proposed an automatic method to separate both cortical and trabecular bone in those bone samples that contained the two components (Martín-Badosa, E. et al., 2003b). To this aim, we used the fact that the cortical envelope, as being the external shell surrounding the trabecular bone, is much more compact than the trabecular bone. Thus, a customized algorithm for identification of the cortical envelope based on geometrical considerations was developed. The process was mainly based on an iterative filling procedure. The exterior region was scanned until bone was reached and filled with a constant gray level value. Then, the same procedure was used to label the cortical region with a different gray-level value, starting from the exterior cortical border and stopping when darker regions were reached.

5.3 3D analysis of trabecular bone

5.3.1 Quantification of trabecular microarchitecture

The typical analysis of trabecular bone involves the computation of quantitative morphometric parameters calculated from the binarized images.

A first possible approach is to reproduce those parameters which are conventionally used in histomorphometry and are calculated slice by slice on the volume data (Peyrin, F. et al., 2000). This method, although based on a two-dimensional calculus, provides parameters which are measured throughout the volume and capture the variability of parameters both on the slice level and on the direction of analysis.

A second approach is to use a 3D version of the mean intercept length (MIL) method (Hipp, J.A. & Simmons, C.A., 1997), which was initially proposed for 2D images. For random directions in 3D space, the number of intercepts of a set of parallel test lines with the bone structure is computed and normalized by the total length of test lines. Then, a number of morphometric parameters are derived from the MIL measurements based on the hypothesis that the bone network is organized in a parallel plate model (Parfitt, A.M. et al., 1983): Trabecular Bone Volume fraction (BV/TV in %, where TV stands for total bone sample volume), Bone Surface on Bone Volume ratio (BS/BV in mm^{-1}), Trabecular Thickness (Tb.Th in mm), Trabecular Number (Tb.N in mm^{-1}), and Trabecular Separation (Tb.Sp in mm). The nomenclature used for quantifying bone microarchitecture in trabecular (and cortical) bone has been standardized in a reference paper of Parfitt (Parfitt, A.M. et al., 1987).

However, these so-called derived architectural parameters have the drawback to rely on a geometrical model of bone structures which is obviously not completely appropriate in all situations. This is particularly the case when comparing normal and pathological data since it may not be known if observed differences are real or are due to an inappropriate model.

Fortunately, the availability of 3D images makes it possible to avoid such assumptions, allowing the proposal of new model independent morphometric parameters.

A definition of local thickness on three-dimensional images proposed in the work (Hildebrand, T. & Rüegsegger, P., 1997a) evaluates the thickness at any point of the bone structure, which is a direct or model-independent definition requiring no prior assumption. A theoretical local thickness is defined at each point of the volume as the diameter of the maximal sphere centered in that point. We proposed a method for computing the local thickness of 3D discrete images based on discrete geometry (Martín-Badosa, E. et al., 2003b). A medial axis of the bone structure, defined by the centers of maximal balls, is derived from the local maxima of a 3D discrete distance map. The discrete thickness map is then obtained by propagating the sorted values of the diameter of the maximal balls to the entire balls. We typically use a 3D chamfer distance which provides a good approximation of the Euclidian distance (Apostol, L. et al., 2006). Figure 3 a) shows a 3D rendering of a human trabecular bone (voxel size : 10 µm) and its associated thickness map (Figure 3 b)). This method provides a thickness value at each point of the bone volume, and thus makes available the distribution of thickness over the entire volume. Statistical results such as the histogram of thickness, and the mean, median, and standard deviation of the distribution can be computed.

5.3.2 Topological and geometrical classification of the trabecular bone

Three-dimensional images may also be used to get information on the orientation and anisotropy of the structure, as well as on the topology of the bone network (Martín-Badosa, E. et al., 2003b). Orientation and anisotropy may be obtained from the MIL method by fitting the points defined by each direction and the normalized number of intersections in this direction, by an ellipsoid in 3D space (Hipp, J.A. & Simmons, C.A., 1997). The degree of anisotropy (DA) is estimated by the ratio of the largest to the smallest axis value. The main orientation of the ellipsoid gives an estimate of the orientation of the structure.

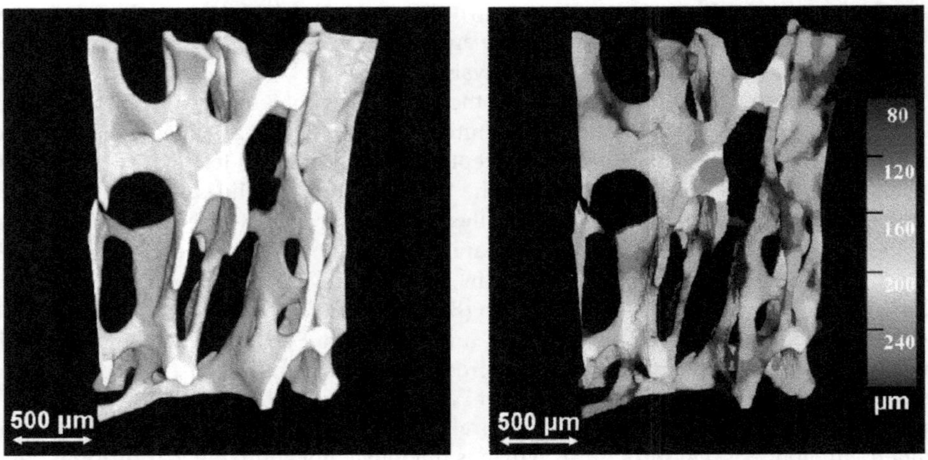

(a) (b)

Fig. 3. a) 3D SR micro-CT image of a human trabecular bone volume; b) the associated thickness map

In terms of topological parameters, the connectivity of the structure is often quantified using the number of Euler-Poincaré. A method for computing it on discrete three-dimensional images is described in the work of Odgaard (Odgaard, A. & Gundersen, H.J.G., 1993) and the result is often normalized to bone volume which is called Euler density. If the structure contains only one connected component, the Euler density decreases when the connectivity increases. Other studies have suggested the use of a skeleton to extract three-dimensional topological parameters, like the number of branches, number of connections (Pothuaud, L. et al., 2002). However, in three dimensions, there are different types of skeletons, wireframe or surface, and these methods have a high sensitivity to noise especially for high resolution images (Peyrin, F. et al., 1998b).

The assessment of the type of trabecular structure as being plate-like or rod-like was introduced by Hildebrand with the Structure Model Index (SMI) (Hildebrand, T. & Rüegsegger, P., 1997b). This parameter was a major advance in the characterization of trabecular bone since it is known that with age or disease, there is conversion of plate trabeculae into rods. The SMI thus provides relevant information about the plateness or rodness of the structure. Technically, the SMI involves the computation of the bone surface and its derivative and is based on a model.

However, while the SMI is a global parameter, it can also be of interest to characterize locally the geometry of trabeculae ("plate"-like or "rod"-like). First works in this area were done by analyzing the skeleton of the image and applied to in vivo MRI images (Wehrli, F.W. et al., 2001). Nevertheless, this method was restricted to the analysis of the skeleton, which can be noisy when dealing with SR micro-CT images at high resolution. To overcome this problem, a new method was introduced in order to characterize locally all voxels of the 3D image and not only the skeleton (Bonnassie, A. et al., 2003). This technique uses an original idea of making a local topological analysis in the neighbourhood of each point in order to classify the voxels of the bone structure (Peyrin, F. et al., 2007). This approach is based again on three-dimensional medial axis transformation for describing geometrical shapes in three-dimensional images. For 3D images, the medial axis, which is composed of both curves and medial surfaces, provides a simplified and reversible representation of structures. The local topological analysis method works in three main steps:

1. the voxels of the medial axis are classified in four classes: boundary, branching, regular and arc points.
2. the reversibility of the medial axis is used to propagate the classification to the whole object.
3. the boundary points are eliminated.

From this decomposition, it is possible to count the percentage of branch, plate and rod points in the bone volume, respectively denoted NV/BV, PV/BV, and RV/BV, as well as the thickness of each structure of interest (Peyrin, F. et al., 2010). As an illustration, Figure 4 shows the application of this method to a trabecular bone volume obtained by SR micro-CT at the ESRF (voxel size : 10µm). The labelled volume is shown on Figure 4 b), and on the zoomed image one can see the highly reliable classification of the original volume's voxels.

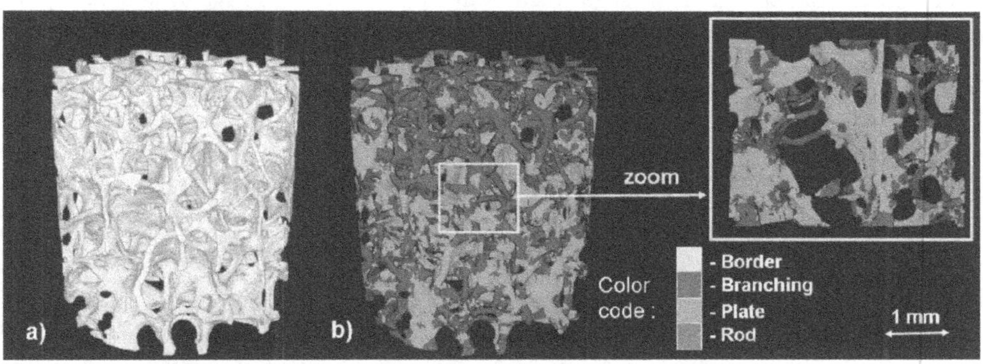

Fig. 4. a) human trabecular bone; b) local topological classification

5.4 Analysis of cortical bone

Although less studied than trabecular bone, the investigation of cortical bone is also raising increasing interest The possibility offered by SR micro-CT to tune the energy higher than for trabecular bone is an important asset to get quantitative images of cortical bone. Figure 5 a) shows the 3D rendering of a typical cortical bone sample imaged from SR micro-CT (voxel size : 10 µm), illustrating its compact structure compared to that of trabecular bone presented above.

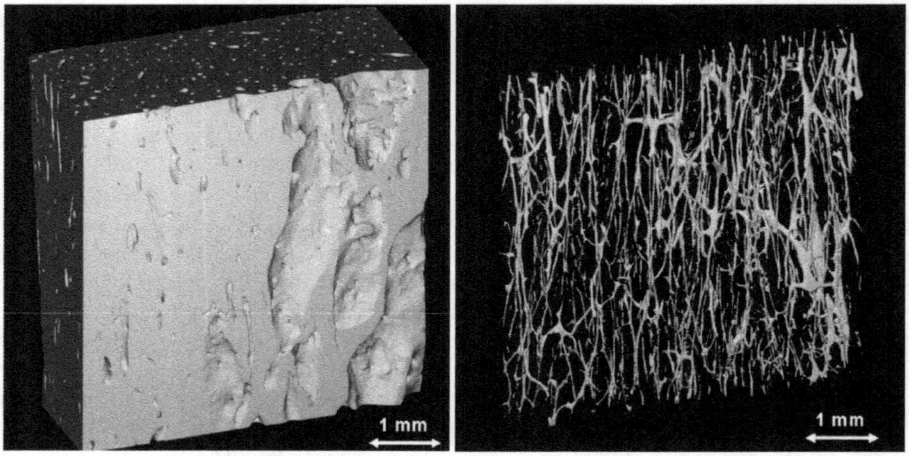

(a) (b)

Fig. 5. a) 3D rendering of the cortical bone (6x6x6 mm^3 sample) imaged with SR micro-CT (voxel size : 10 μm); b) porous network of a) limited to 300 μm thickness corresponding to the arrangement of Havers and Volkman canals

5.4.1 Extraction of the canal network from the cortical bone

The filled cortical bone envelop, can typically be obtained by using mathematical morphology tools, including opening and closing operations (Bousson, V. et al., 2004). The pore network can be then easily segmented from the SR micro-CT image by subtracting the porous cortical volume to the cortical envelop, as demonstrated in Figure 5 b).

As described in section 2, the pore network in cortical bone including the so-called Havers and Volkman canals is of great interest to characterize cortical bone. This network which is extremely dense can be characterized by using the same types of parameters than those used for the quantification of the trabecular bone network (see section 5.3.1). The porosity can be evaluated as the ratio of the pore volume to the filled cortical envelop (Cooper, D.M. et al., 2007).

5.4.2 Segmentation of remodeling regions

Compared to standard micro-CT, we already pointed out that SR micro-CT has the ability to provide the mineral concentration in bone tissue, also called the degree of mineralization of bone (DMB). The quantification of the DMB provides important information about the metabolism of bone and is typically only studied by 2D methods.

However, even if the Bone Mineral Units (BMUs) can be observed in the SR micro-CT slices (see Figure 6a)), their automatic detection is challenging since the contrast between osteons and interstitial bone may be very weak and close to the standard deviation of noise.

So far, the quantification of ancient versus new bone from SR micro-CT images had only been addressed by simple thresholding (Borah, B. et al., 2006) and global parameters such as the mean and standard deviation calculated on the entire bone phase were used to characterize the DMB. Although this method may give an approximate value of the respective volume of the two phases, it is obviously not sufficient to identify each osteon.

In a previous work, we addressed this problem and proposed a segmentation scheme associated to a denoising process (Peter, Z. et al., 2008). While there are many general segmentation approaches which perform well in various applications, a number of them fail when they are used to separate low-contrast features. Several approaches, such as K-means or a region growing method using the energy model of Mumford and Shah (Dibos, F. & Koepfler, G., 2000) were tested to segment osteons. The later is based on the minimization of an energy term incorporating a constraint on the curvature. Although these methods seemed attractive, the results showed over-segmentations: false detections appeared in bone background and a remodeling zone corresponding to a physiological entity could be split in many sub-regions. Thus we designed a customized method based on a region growing segmentation scheme associated to a denoising process using wavelets. The first step of the method was to improve the signal to noise ratio of the image by using a denoising method which preserves high frequency features and contours. Then, we developed customized region growing methods, which use some prior biological knowledge and whose principles will be recalled in the following section.

Denoising

Despite their exceptional quality, SR micro-CT images are generally corrupted by photonic Poisson or Gaussian noise and ring artifacts, related to image formation process. These may influence to some extent the treatment, because the structures of interest are generally small and with low contrast. To avoid the degradation of the spatial resolution, a non linear denoising method is preferred.

In this class, wavelet based denoising has been showed efficient in many applications (Mallat, S., 1997). Basically, the noisy image is transformed into the wavelet domain, then the wavelet coefficients are subjected to soft or hard thresholding, and in the last step the result is inverse-transformed. If W denote the wavelet transform (and w the set of the wavelet coefficients), then the whole denoising process with a threshold t, amounts to a non-linear operator T_η :

$$T_\eta = W^{-1} \circ \eta_t \circ W \tag{1}$$

where $\eta_t(w) = \mathrm{sgn}(w)(|w| - t)_+$ for the soft thresholding, and $\eta_t(w) = w\ 1_{\{|w|>t\}}$ for the hard thresholding.

The application of this method yields some oscillations which are especially pronounced in the vicinity of discontinuities and rapid changes (Donoho, D. & Coifman, R. R., 1995). These "pseudo-Gibbs" oscillations are caused by the fact that only a subset of the full set of basis elements has been used for the reconstruction after the thresholding. In contrast to the classical Gibbs-phenomena associated with Fourier analysis, the "pseudo-Gibbs-phenomena" are much better behaved, much better localized and much more moderate in oscillation; nevertheless they can yield incorrect results in the subsequent segmentation.

These artifacts exhibited by denoising with traditional wavelet transforms are due to the lack of translation invariance of the wavelet basis. The main idea of the "second generation denoising" method, also called "translation invariant (TI) wavelet denoising", proposed in (Donoho, D. & Coifman, R. R., 1995), is the following: for a range of shifts, one shifts the data, denoises the shifted data and then unshifts the denoised data. Doing this for each of a

range of shifts, and averaging the several results so obtained, produces a reconstruction subject to far weaker Gibbs phenomena.
For a signal $(x_t : 0 \le t < n)$, let S_h denote the circulant shift by $h \in \mathrm{N}$, $(S_h x)_t = x_{(t+h) \bmod n}$. This operator is unitary, and hence invertible: $S_{-h} = (S_h)^{-1}$. In term of operators, the idea of shifting to avoid artifacts is the following: given an analysis technique T_η, calculate the shifted version $\widetilde{T}_\eta$, for a range H of shifts (all n for instance) and average over the several results so obtained:

$$\widetilde{T}_\eta\left(x;(S_h)_{h\in H}\right) = Aver_{h\in H} S_{-h}\left(T_\eta\left(S_h(x)\right)\right). \tag{2}$$

Hard thresholding combined with translation invariance give both good visual quantitative characteristics (Donoho, D. & Coifman, R. R., 1995).

Segmentation

Among the different possible approaches to image segmentation, we proposed to use a customized region growing taking into account biological prior information. According to bone physiology, osteons in cortical bone are located around pores and are relatively elliptic although their shapes may vary (see for instance the darker zones around the black pores on Figure 6 a)). The method proceeds as follows.
First, the original image (Figure 6 a)) is binarized using a threshold which enables to keep as much pores as possible (Figure 6 c)). The contours are detected by a simple gradient method and the exterior contour is eliminated. The pore contours (Figure 6 b) are then obtained and tracked to get closed and 1 pixel-thick contours. Then a connected component analysis is performed in order to label each pore contour. This image is then used to initialize the region growing process. The number of connected pore sets the number of regions in the image.
The simple region growing method proceeds as follows. For each region, labeled by l, a neighbor pixel $\mathbf{x} = (x, y)$ is labeled in the region if :

$$|I(\mathbf{x}) - m(l)| < \alpha\sigma(l) \tag{3}$$

where $I(\mathbf{x})$ is the image gray level, $m(l)$ and $\sigma(l)$ are the current mean and standard deviation of the region, and α is a parameter. The direct application of this algorithm gives poor results, but using denoising schemes like TI wavelets prior to segmentation considerably improved the quality of the segmentation. On Figure 6 f) we can check the localization and the shape of detected remodeling zones, superimposed to the original image. Although some remodeling zones are missing, a majority of them are detected at the good location. However the application of this method shows a number of problems. First, some regions are missing: looking in more details to the image, it appeared that some remodeling zones aren't really homogeneous due to phase contrast which is inherent to SR micro-CT imaging and creates a contrast which behaves as a second derivative at the boundaries. This phase contrast is almost invisible but may also compromise the growing of some regions. Second, leakage in ring artifacts frequently occurs, leading to false detection.
Therefore we proposed a second segmentation strategy including shape constraints to overcome this inconveniency. To this aim, we exploited the additional biological prior that remodeling zones are formed around the pores, they follow roughly the shape of the

contours and their thickness is also almost isotropic around each pore. This physiological sketch led us to use the distance map *dist* associated to the image. The different steps of the method are illustrated in Figure 6. We calculate the distance map of the binarized image (see Figure 6 d)). The brightness ("hotness") of each pixel in the distance map is the distance to the nearest boundary, so in our case, to the nearest pore. The hotter a pixel is, it is farther from a pore. The maxima lines of the distance map give the best estimate of the separation lines between two different remodeling regions. The maxima of the distance map correspond to the boundaries of the watershed image (see Figure 6 e)).

The regions to be segmented are initialized, as previously, by the contours of the pores, but now assuming that the remodeling regions are entirely included in the polygon-like zones (the so-called "catchment basins") delimitated by the watershed boundaries around each pore. Each remodeling zone is segmented separately starting from the initial contours. For each label l, the segmented remodeling zone is constructed by agglomerating pixels at increasing distances satisfying a given criterion while being still included in the corresponding watershed zone (catchment basin) C_l. The final segmentation of each remodeling zone can be expressed by:

$$R_l = \{I(x,y) / (x,y) \in C_l \text{ and } dist(x,y) \le d_l\} \quad (4)$$

and the overall segmentation result by applying this method is represented on Figure 6 e).

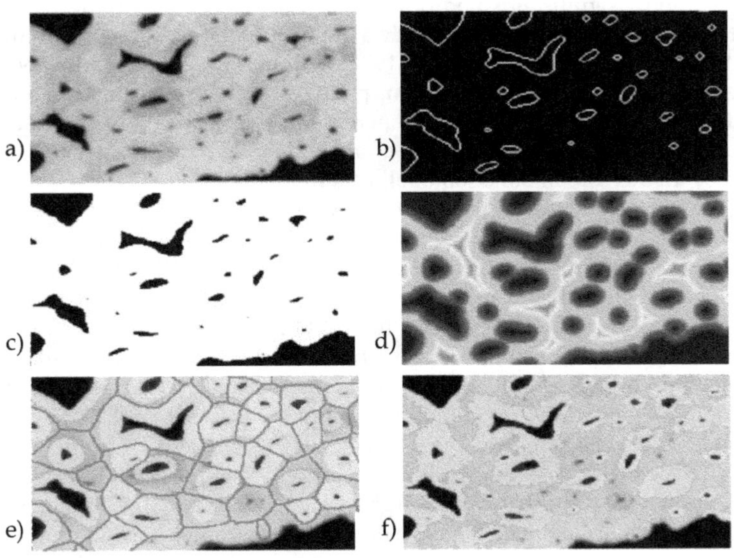

Fig. 6. a) Region of Interest on the original cortical bone slice : the remodeling regions appear in darker gray levels around the black pores; b) the contours of the pores; c) the binarized image associated to a); d) the distance map image (coded with the "jet" colorbar) obtained from c); e) location of remodeling regions: overlay of the areas segmented with the shape constraint method (in green) and the boundaries of watershed image (in red) on the original image on a); f) the initial segmentation of the osteons, obtained by homogeneity guided region growing.

Different criteria may be used to define the maximum distance d_l, corresponding to the thickness of the remodeling zones. We used the maximization of the derivative of the mean gray level value of the pixels at a given distance from the pore. Roughly speaking, this distance is supposed to identify the change in the image contrast and it corresponds to the boundary of the remodeling zones.

The results presented in Figure 6 e) show that the segmentation is closely related to the shape of the pores and is no more influenced by the ring artifacts since it is purely related on the maximal thickness of the zone. However, this method can also slightly under-estimate those remodeling regions whose boundary is irregular around the pore.

6. Application of the SR micro-CT in bone research

Applications of SR micro-CT in bone research have been performed at different synchrotrons in the world (SSL (Swiss Light Source), ALS, in Lawrence Berkeley National Laboratory Berkeley National (USA), Japan, ESRF). In most studies, the important property of SR micro-CT to provide the degree of mineralization of bone was exploited. We shall only mention a few of these studies, either related to animal models or to human bone.

SR micro-CT has first been used to study the effects of treatment of osteoporosis with etidronate by analyzing biopsies from osteoporotic patients before and after one or two years of treatment. The results showed an increased degree of mineralization with the treatment without significant modification of the micro-architecture, which was in agreement with what was expected with a biphosphonate treatement (Nuzzo, S. et al., 2002a) (Meunier, P.J. & Boivin, G., 1997). A more recent study focused on the characterization of subchondral bone in patients with osteoarthritis and osteoporosis (Chappard, C. et al., 2006). A significant increase in the thickness of trabeculae in patients with osteoarthritis and a lower degree of mineralization were observed, which can be interpreted by an increase in bone remodeling activity.

With the development of studies on animal models for therapeutics or genetics, imaging of small animals, and particularly mice, has become a major issue. In this field, SR micro-CT offering higher spatial and density resolution is also particularly attractive. It was used to assess significant differences in micro-architecture and mineralization between two strains of mice (Martín-Badosa, E. et al., 2003a). In addition these two strains showed a different response to a model of osteoporosis by hind-limb suspension (Martín-Badosa, E. et al., 2003a). The properties of SR micro-CT were particularly exploited to study the mineralization in genetically modified mice and in treated mice with bone metabolic diseases (Yao, W. et al., 2006), (Balooch, G. et al., 2007). SR micro-CT at the micrometer scale permitted to study the role of insulin like growth factor-I (IGF-I) in regulating bone mineralization in fetal bone structure (Burghardt, A.J. et al., 2007). While most studies were performed after animal sacrifice, the feasibility of imaging mice bone in vivo with SR micro-CT was also demonstrated (Kinney, J.H. et al., 1998), (Bayat, S. et al., 2005).

7. Conclusions and future works

The development of micro-CT in bone research was first driven by the need for having a highly precise means of reconstructing the complex architecture of bone tissue at a high resolution. During the last decade, it has become a standard tool for the evaluation of bone micro-architecture. By exploiting the physical properties of synchrotron light, Synchrotron micro-CT overpasses standard micro-CT. Its major advantage is to allow the simultaneous analysis of bone morphometry and bone mineralization.

The quantitative exploitation of SR micro-CT images has also driven the development of new image analysis techniques that have been briefly recalled in this chapter. Specific developments were designed to extract morphometric, topologic and geometric parameters on the trabecular network. Work is also in progress to analyze the osteonal system in cortical bone, including the pore network and the remodeling zones. The methods developed so far have already been applied in a number of studies on human or animal bone. A limitation is that SR micro-CT techniques cannot be used *in vivo* on humans (due to the high X-ray dose received by the samples (Salome, M. et al., 1999)), but only *ex vivo* on extracted bone biopsies.

A first perspective in SR micro-CT is to push the resolution limit at the nanometer level, which is currently an active research topic at the international level. This opens interesting opportunities and can help to visualize in particular unrevealed features of bone ultra-structure. The feasibility of visualizing osteocyte lacunae in human vertebra imaged at two scales (6.7 and 1.4 μm) was demonstrated in an earlier work (Peyrin, F. et al., 1998a). Nevertheless, relatively few micro-CT studies have so far been conducted on bone ultrastructure in humans (Hengsberger, S. et al., 2003) and mice (Schneider, P. et al., 2007). We have also presented recently new methods for extracting three-dimensional characteristics of osteocyte lacunae and micro-cracks (Peyrin, F., 2009), (Larrue, A. et al., 2007). This subject with the development of new nano-CT systems is becoming a hot topic to characterize the osteocyte system which has a fundamental role in bone biology.

A second perspective in SR micro-CT is to exploit phase contrast imaging which is also raising increasing interest. While different experimental procedures allow obtaining phase contrast, the coherence properties of the ESRF beam makes it possible to implement phase contrast by simple propagation. Phase contrast imaging allows to image samples with low absorption and to enhance very small differences in attenuation. Different acquisition strategies may be used. The "edge enhancement" mode consists in making a scan with the detector not just after the sample but at a given distance. The "holotomographic" mode consists in recording several scans (in general two to four) placing the detector at different distances from the sample. In this case, the phase map is obtained by tomographic reconstruction after a so-called "phase retrieval" algorithm, processing the radiographs acquired at these different distances for each angle. The phase retrieval methods which were initially proposed for low absorbing samples have recently been extended to absorbing samples (Langer, M. et al., 2008), and open interesting perspectives to quantify simultaneously the bone tissue and the organic matrix.

A third perspective, is the development of new image analysis methods to provide smart solutions to image segmentation and analysis in this domain, which also requires multidisciplinary vision on bone research. These new techniques should be inspired from recent theoretical developments in fields like mathematics or image processing (engineering). It is mandatory to integrate improvements in data backup solutions but also of new techniques in speeding up computer calculations. The complex processing algorithms should be parallelized in order to manage huge 3D image volumes of about 16 Gbytes/volume. The advances concerning the GPU (Graphics Processing Unit) and their compatibility with widely used scientific softwares could make possible to manipulate easier 3D renderings, which is very important when working with 3D image volumes representing such a complex and multiscale structures like the bone tissue.

All these improvements together raise exciting perspectives to acquire novel knowledge on bone tissue, bone strength and the physiopathology of bone.

8. References

Apostol, L.; Boudousq, V.; Basset, O.; Odet C.; Yot, S.; Tabary, J.; Dinten, J.M.; Boller, E.; Kotzki, P.O. & Peyrin, F. (2006). Relevance of 2D radiographic texture analysis for the assessment of 3D bone micro-architecture. *Med. Phys.*, Vol. 33, N°. 9, p. 3546-3556.

Balooch, G.; Yao, W.; Ager, J.W.; Balooch, M.; Nalla, R.K.; Porter, A.E.; Ritchie, R.O. & Lane, N.E. (2007). The aminobisphosphonate risedronate preserves localized mineral and material properties of bone in the presence of glucocorticoid. *Arthritis Rheum.*, Vol. 56, N°. 11, p. 3726-3737.

Bayat, S.; Apostol, L.; Boller, E.; Brochard, T. & Peyrin, F. (2005). In vivo imaging of bone micro-architecture in mice with 3D synchrotron radiation microtomography. *Nucl. Instrum. Meth. Phys. Res. A (Elsevier)*, Vol. 548, p. 247-252.

Benhamou, C.L.; Poupon, S.; Lespessailles, E.; Loiseau, S.; Jennane, R.; Siroux, V.; Ohley, W. & Pothuaud, L. (2001). Fractal analysis of radiographic trabecular bone texture and bone mineral density: two complementary parameters related to osteoporotic fractures. *J. Bone Miner. Res.*, Vol. 16, N°. 4, p. 697-704.

Bonnassie, A.; Peyrin, F. & Attali, D. (2003). A new method for analyzing local shape in three-dimensional images based on medial axis transformation. *IEEE Transactions on Systems, Man and Cybernetics, PART B-CYBERNETICS*, Vol. 33, N°. 4, p. 700-705.

Bonse, U.; Busch, F.; Günnewig, O.; Beckmann, F.; Pahl, R.; Delling, G.; Hahn, M. & Graeff, W. (1994). 3D computed X-ray tomography of human cancellous bone at 8 μm spatial resolution and 10-4 energy resolution. *Bone and Mineral*, Vol. 25, p. 25-38.

Borah, B.; Dufresne, T.E.; Ritman, E.L.; Jorgensen, S.M.; Liu, S.; Chmielewski, P.A.; Phipps, R.J.; Zhou, X.; Sibonga, J.D. & Turner, R.T. (2006). Long-term risedronate treatment normalizes mineralization and continues to preserve trabecular architecture: sequential triple biopsy studies with micro-computed tomography. *Bone*, Vol. 39, N°. 2, p. 345–352.

Bousson, V.; Bergot, C.; Meunier, A.; Barbot, F.; Parlier-Cuau, C.; Laval-Jeantet, A.M. & Laredo, J.-D. (2000). CT of the middiaphyseal femur: Cortical bone mineral density and relation to porosity. *Radiology*, Vol. 217, p. 179-187.

Bousson, V.; Meunier, A.; Bergot, C.; Vicaut, E.; Rocha, M.A.; Morais, M.H.; Laval-Jeantet, A.-M. & Laredo, J.-D. (2001). Distribution of intracortical porosity in human midfemoral cortex by age and gender. *J. Bone Miner. Res.*, Vol. 16, N°. 7, p. 1308-1317.

Bousson, V.; Peyrin, F.; Bergot, C.; Hausard, M.; Sautet, A. & Laredo J.D. (2004). Cortical bone of the human femoral neck : three-dimensional appearance and porosity using synchrotron radiation. *J. Bone Miner. Res.*, Vol. 19, N°. 5, p. 794-801.

Burghardt, A.J.; Wang, Y.; Elalieh, H.; Thibault, X.; Bikle, D.; Peyrin, F. & Majumdar, S. (2007). Evaluation of fetal bone structure and mineralization in IGF-I deficient mice using synchrotron radiation microtomography and Fourier transform infrared spectroscopy. *Bone*, Vol. 40, N°. 1, p. 160–168.

Chappard, C.; Peyrin, F.; Bonnassie, A.; Lemineur, G.; Brunet-Imbault, B.; Lespessailles, E. & Benhamou, C.L. (2006). Subchondral bone micro-architectural alterations in osteoarthritis: a synchrotron micro-computed tomography study. *Osteoarthritis Cartilage*, Vol. 14, N°. 3, p. 215–223.

Chevalier, F.; Laval-Jeantet, A.M.; Laval-Jeantet, M. & Bergot, C. (1992). CT image analysis of the vertebral trabecular network in vivo. *Calcified Tissue International*, Vol. 51, p. 8-13.

Cloetens, P.; Pateyron-Salomé, M.; Buffière, J.; Peix, G.; Baruchel, J.; Peyrin, F. & Schlenker, M. (1997). Observation of microstructure and damage in materials by phase sensitive radiography and tomography. *J. Appl. Phys.*, Vol. 81, p. 5878–5886.

Cooper, D.M.; Thomas, C.D.; Clement, J.G. & Hallgrímsson, B. (2006). Three-dimensional microcomputed tomography imaging of basic multicellular unit-related resorption spaces in human cortical bone. *Anat. Rec. A Discov. Mol. Cell. Evol. Biol.*, Vol. 288, N°. 7, p. 806-816.

Cooper, D.M.; Turinsky, A.; Sensen, C. & Hallgrimsson, B. (2007). Effect of voxel size on 3D micro-CT analysis of cortical bone porosity. *Calcif. Tissue Int.*, Vol. 80, N°. 3, p. 211-219.

Cortet, B.; Cohn, D.; Dubois, P.; Delcambre, B. & Marchandise, X. (1995). Les differentes methodes d'analyse quantitative de la structure osseuse trabeculaire. *Rev. Rhum. [French edition]*, Vol. 62, p. 841-855.

Dibos, F. & Koepfler, G. (2000). Global total variation minimization. *SIAM Journal on Numerical Analysis*, Vol. 37, p. 646-664.

Donoho, D. & Coifman, R. R. (1995). Translation Invariant De-Noising. *Wavelets and Statistics, A. Antoniadis and G. Oppenheim, Eds. New York: Springer-Verlag*, p. 125--150.

Engelke, K.; Lohmann, M.; Dix, W.R. & Graeff, W. (1989). A system for dual energy microtomography of bones. *Nuclear Instruments and Methods in Physics Research*, Vol. 274, p. 380-389.

Engelke, K.; Mastmeyer, A.; Bousson, V.; Fuerst, T.; Laredo, J.D. & Kalender W.A. (2009). Reanalysis precision of 3D quantitative computed tomography (QCT) of the spine. *Bone*, Vol. 44, N°. 4, p. 566-572.

Feldkamp, L.A.; Goldstein, S.A.; Parfitt, A.M.; Jesion, G. & Kleerekoper, M. (1989). The direct examination of three-dimensional bone architecture in vitro by computed tomography. *J. Bone Miner. Res.*, Vol. 4, p. 3-11.

Hengsberger, S.; Enstroem, J.; Peyrin, F. & Zysset, P. (2003). How is the indentation modulus of bone tissue related to its macroscopic elastic response? A validation study. *J. Biomech.*, Vol. 36, N°. 10, p. 1503- 1509.

Hildebrand, T. & Rüegsegger, P. (1997a). A new method for the model independent assessment of thickness in three-dimensional images. *J. Microsc.*, N°. 185, p. 67-75.

Hildebrand, T. & Rüegsegger, P. (1997b). Quantification of bone microarchitecture with the Structure Model Index. *Comp. Meth. Biomech. Biomed. Eng.*, Vol. 1, p. 15-23.

Hipp, J.A. & Simmons, C.A. (1997). Method-based differences in the automated analysis of the three-dimensional morphology of trabecular bone. *J. Bone Miner. Res.*, Vol. 12, p. 942-947.

Kinney, J.H.; Lane, N.E. & Haupt, D. L. (1995). In vivo, Three-dimensional microscopy of trabecular bone. *J. Bone Miner. Res.*, Vol. 10, p. 264-270.

Kinney, J.H.; Ryaby, J.T.; Haupt, D.L. & Lane, N.E. (1998). Three-dimensional in vivo morphometry of trabecular bone in the OVX rat model of osteoporosis. *Technol. Health Care*, Vol. 6, N°. 5-6, p. 339-350.

Labiche, J.-C.; Maton, O.; Pascarelli, S.; Newton, M.A.; Ferre, G.C.; Curfs, C.; Vaughan, G.; Homs, A. & Carreiras, D.F. (2007). The FReLoN camera as a versatile X-ray detector for time resolved dispersive EXAFS and diffraction studies of dynamic problems in materials science, chemistry, and catalysis. *Rev. Sci. Instrum.*, N°. 091301.

Langer, M.; Cloetens, P.; Guigay, J.P. & Peyrin, F. (2008). Quantitative comparison of direct phase retrieval algorithms in in-line phase tomography. *Med. Phys.*, Vol. 35, p. 4556-4566.

Larrue, A.; Rattner, A.; Laroche, N.; Vico, L. & Peyrin, F. (2007). Feasibility of micro-crack detection in human trabecular bone images from 3D synchrotron microtomography. *Proc. IEEE Eng. Med. Biol. Soc.*, p. 3918-3921.

Laval-Jeantet, A.M.; Chevalier, F.; Bergot, C., Laval-Jeantet, M.; Peyrin, F. & Houssard, J.P. (1993). La structure trabéculaire vertébrale en tomodensitométrie. *Architecture et resistance mecanique osseuses, Marcelli, C; Sebert, J.L., Eds. Paris : Masson*, p. 82-91.

Mallat, S. (1997). *A Wavelet Tour of Signal Processing*, San Diego, CA: Academic Press.

Martín-Badosa, E.; Amblard, D.; Nuzzo, S.; Elmoutaouakkil, A.; Vico, L. & Peyrin, F. (2003a). Excised bone structures in mice: imaging at three-dimensional synchrotron radiation micro CT. *Radiology*, Vol. 229, N°. 3, p. 921-928.

Martín-Badosa, E.; Elmoutaouakkil, A.; Nuzzo, S.; Amblard, D.; Vico, L. & Peyrin, F. (2003b). A method for the automatic characterization of bone architecture in 3D mice microtomographic images. *Computerized Medical Imaging and Graphics*, Vol. 27, N°. 6, p. 447-458.

Meunier, P.J. & Boivin, G. (1997). Bone Mineral Density Reflects bone mass but also the degree of mineralization of bone: therapeutic implications. *Bone*, Vol. 21, p. 373-377.

Mokso, R.; Cloetens, P.; Maire, E.; Ludwig, W. & Buffière, J.-Y. (2007). Nanoscale zoom tomography with hard X rays using Kirkpatrick–Baez optics. *Appl. Phys. Lett.*, Vol. 90, N°. 144104.

Mundinger, A.; Wiesmeier, B.; Dinkel, E.; Helwig, E.; Beck, A. & Schulte-Moenting, J. (1993). Quantitative image analysis of vertebral body architecture-improved diagnosis in osteoporosis based on high-resolution computed tomography. *Br. J. Radiol.*, Vol. 66, p. 209-213.

Nuzzo, S.; Lafage-Proust, M.H.; Martin-Badosa, E.; Boivin, G.; Thomas, T.; Alexandre, C. & Peyrin, F. (2002a). Synchrotron Radiation Microtomography Allows the Analysis of Three-Dimensional Micro-architecture and Degree of Mineralization of Human Iliac Crest Biopsies: Effects of Etidronate Treatment. *J. Bone Miner. Res.*, Vol. 17, N°. 8, p. 1372-1382.

Nuzzo, S.; Peyrin, F.; Cloetens, P.; Baruchel, J. & Boivin G. (2002b). Quantification of the degree of mineralization of bone in three dimension using Synchrotron Radiation Microtomography. *Med. Phys.*, Vol. 19, N°. 11, p. 2672-2681.

Nuzzo, S.; Peyrin, F.; Martín-Badosa, E.; Lafage-Proust, M.H. & Boivin, G. (2001). Assessment of Bone Mineral Content from 3D Synchrotron Radiation Microtomography Images. *IEEE Transactions On Nuclear Science*, Vol. 48, N°. 3(Pt2), p. 859 -863.

Nuzzo, S.; Peyrin, F.; Martín-Badosa, E.; Lafage-Proust, M.H. & Boivin, G. (2003). Quantitative analysis of mineral bone variation in 3D Synchrotron Radiation Microtomography images. *J. Bone Miner. Res.*, Vol. 18, N°. 4, p. 760-768.

Odgaard, A. & Gundersen, H.J.G. (1993). Quantification of connectivity in cancellous bone, with special emphasis on 3D reconstructions. *Bone*, Vol. 14, p. 173-182.

Parfitt, A.M.; Drezner, M.K.; Glorieux, F.H.; Kanis, J.A.; Malluche, H.; Meunier, P.J.; Ott, S.M. & Recker, R.R. (1987). Bone Histomorphometry: Standardization of Nomenclature, Symbols, and Units. *J. Bone Miner. Res.*, Vol. 2, N°. 6, p. 595-610.

Parfitt, A.M.; Mathews, C.H.; Villanueva, A.R.; Kleerekoper, M.; Frame, B. & Rao, D.S. (1983). Relationships between surface, volume, and thickness of iliac trabecular bone in aging and in osteoporosis. Implications for the microanatomic and cellular mechanisms of bone loss. *J. Clin. Invest.*, Vol. 72, N°. 4, p. 1396-1409.

Peter, Z.; Bousson, V.; Bergot, C. & Peyrin F. (2008). A constrained region growing approach based on watershed for the segmentation of low contrast structures in bone micro-CT images. *Pattern Recognition*, Vol. 41, N°. 7, p. 2358-2368.

Peyrin, F. (2009). Investigation of bone with synchrotron radiation imaging: from micro to nano. *Osteoporos. Int.*, Vol. 20, N°. 6, p. 1057-1063.

Peyrin, F.; Attali, D.; Chappard, C. & Benhamou, C.L. (2010). New geometric parameters for the description of three-dimensional bone structures from very high resolution microtomography images. *Med. Phys.*, Vol. 37, N°. 8, p. 4364-4376.

Peyrin, F.; Peter, Z.; Larrue, A.; Bonnassie, A. & Attali, D. (2007). Local geometrical analysis of 3D porous network based on medial axis: application to bone micro-architecture microtomography images. *Image Analysis & Stereology*, Vol. 26, N°. 3, p. 179-185.

Peyrin, F.; Salome, M., Cloetens, P., Laval-Jeantet, A.M.; Ritman, E. & Rüegsegger, P. (1998a). Micro-CT examinations of trabecular bone samples at different resolutions : 14, 7 and 2 micron level. *Technology and Health Care*, Vol. 6, p. 391-401.

Peyrin, F.; Salome, M.; Dupont, F.; Laval-Jeantet, A.M.; Cloetens, P. & Baruchel, J. (1998b). 3D Synchrotron Radiation microtomography imaging : characterisation of bone architecture. *Image and Multidimensional Digital Signal Processing. Proceedings of IEEE SP society. Niemann, H.; Seidel, H.P.; Girod, B., Eds.; Alpbach, Austria*, p. 55-58.

Peyrin, F.; Salome, M.; Nuzzo, S.; Cloetens, P.; Laval-Jeantet, A.M. & Baruchel, J. (2000). Perspectives in three-dimensional analysis of bone samples using synchrotron radiation microtomography. *Cell. Mol. Biol.*, Vol. 46, p. 1089-1102.

Pothuaud, L.; Laib, A.; Levitz, P.; Benhamou, C.L. & Majumdar, S. (2002). Three-dimensional-line skeleton graph analysis of high-resolution magnetic resonance images: a validation study from 34-µm-resolution microcomputed tomography. *J. Bone Miner. Res.*, Vol. 17, N°. 10, p. 1883-1895.

Salome, M.; Peyrin, F.; Cloetens, P.; Odet, C.; Laval-Jeantet, A.M.; Baruchel, J. & Spanne, P. (1999). A synchrotron radiation microtomography system for the analysis of trabecular bone samples. *Med. Phys.*, Vol. 26, N°. 10, p. 2194 - 2204.

Schneider, P.; Stauber, M.; Voide, R.; Stampanoni, M.; Donahue, L.R. & Müller, R. (2007). Ultra-structural properties in cortical bone vary greatly in two inbred strains of mice as assessed by synchrotron light based micro- and nano-CT. *J. Bone Miner. Res.*, Vol. 22, N°. 10, p. 1557–1570.

Wehrli, F.W.; Gomberg, B.R.; Saha, P.K.; Song, H.K.; Hwang, S.N. & Snyder, P.J. (2001). Digital topological analysis of in vivo magnetic resonance microimages of trabecular bone reveals structural implications of osteoporosis. *J. Bone Miner. Res.*, Vol. 16, N°. 8, p. 1520-1531.

Weitkamp, T.; Tafforeau, P.; Boller, E.; Cloetens, P.; Valade, J.-P.; Bernard, P.; Peyrin, F.; Ludwig, W.; Helfen, L. & Baruchel, J. (2010). Status and evolution of the ESRF beamline ID19. *Proc ICXOM20, Karlsruhe, Germany, 2009, in X-RAY OPTICS AND MICROANALYSIS, PROCEEDINGS Book Series AIP Conference Proceedings*, Vol. 1221, p. 33-38.

Yao, W.; Balooch, G.; Balooch, M.; Jiang, Y.; Nalla, R.K.; Kinney, J.; Wronski, T.J. & Lane, N.E. (2006). Sequential treatment of ovariectomized mice with bFGF and risedronate restored trabecular bone microarchitecture and mineralization. *Bone*, Vol. 39, N°. 3, p. 460–469.

Part 5

CT Imaging and Analysis for Non-Medical Applications

15

Usability of CT Images of Frontal Sinus in Forensic Personal Identification

Ertugrul Tatlisumak, Mahmut Asirdizer and Mehmet Sunay Yavuz
Celal Bayar University
Turkey

1. Introduction

Forensic personal identification is a fundamental topic of forensic sciences and technologies to identify lived subjects, recently deceased bodies and human remains often at a crime scene by using several appropriate techniques.

Throughout human history, many different methods were used for personal identification. The most commonly used method was relying on one's memory to identify the distinguishing features and characteristics of other humans, such as their outward appearance or the sound of their voice before the introduction of computer technology (Michael & Michael, 2006). In Ancient Egypt and China, criminals and victims of several medico-legal events was often identified through visual characteristics such as sex, human height, body weight, deformation of the body, tattoos, old scars or caste marks and clothing, etc. In the forensic personal identification, progressions based on science accelerated in 19th century. Italian Cesarè Lombroso (1835-1909) had studied on body structures of prison inmates and had claimed that criminals have particular physiognomic attributes or deformities. In 1823, known first documentation of fingerprints were defined in a thesis by Johannes Evangelists Purkinje (1787-1869), a Czech anatomist and physiologist. French Police Officer Alphonse Bertillon (1853-1914) created first anthropometric scientific system based on physical measurements for identifying criminals in 1880. Sir Francis Galton (1822-1911) was an English inventor, devised a method for classifying fingerprints that proved useful in forensic science and he wrote first book about fingerprints in 1892 (Soysal & Eke, 1999). In November 1895, the detection of electromagnetic radiation in a wavelength range - today known as x-rays or Röntgen rays - by Wilhelm Conrad Röntgen (1845-1923), a German physicist, marked an era in forensic science as well as in clinical diagnosis. The discovery of ABO blood group system by Karl Landsteiner (1868-1943), an Austrian biologist and physician, in 1901 and rhesus blood system by Landsteiner and Alexander Solomon Wiener (1907-1976), American Scientist, in 1937, and description of Coombs test by British immunologists Robin Coombs (1921-2006), et al., blood samples was used to be a unique profile that could be used for personal identification in legal and criminal areas. At 9:05 am on Monday 10 September 1984, Sir Alec John Jeffreys (1950-....), British geneticist, looked at the X-ray film image of a deoxyribonucleic acid (DNA), then he developed techniques for DNA fingerprinting and DNA profiling, which provided a significant contribution for forensic personal identification in all over the world (Soysal & Eke, 1999).

Although the development of new techniques, forensic imaging studies have continued to increase until now and has not lost its importance especially in difficult cases of DNA analysis—for example, relatives, twins, or cases of poorly conserved remains (Cameriere et al., 2008).

In the last years of 20th century and first decade of 21st century, the use of radiological techniques improved and became widespread by the creation of computerized tomography (CT), magnetic resonance imaging (MRI), multislice computed tomography (MSCT) and ultrasound (USG). These creations provided opportunity for developing newer techniques in the forensic sciences.

In this chapter, we aimed to present the usage of radiographic technique especially CT images in forensic sciences, morphological structure of frontal sinus, usability of CT images of frontal sinus in forensic personal identification, and techniques for forensic personal identification by using CT images of frontal sinus.

2. Usage of radiographic techniques in forensic sciences

Historically, early application of x-ray in forensic sciences was introduced in 1896 - just one year following the x-ray discovery - by Prof. Arthur Schuster (1851-1934) of Owens College, Manchester in England, to demonstrate the presence of lead bullets inside the head of a victim (Eckert & Garland, 1984).

It was expressed that, Schüller from Vienna proposed the possibility of utilizing by comparison of radiological images of the frontal sinuses with plates formerly taken for identification purposes in 1921 and the first complete radiological identification by using pneumatic cells of the skull was described by Culbert & Law, in 1927 (Culbert & Law, 1927; Gruber & Kameyama, 2001; Carvalho et al., 2009).

Today, forensic scientists have regularly used radiographic images as part of the autopsy procedures and clinical forensic applications.

2.1 Usage of radiographic techniques in autopsy procedure

Radiological techniques are part of autopsy techniques and they have been fairly common used in modern forensic facilities. The stage at which radiology is implemented during autopsy varies according to the individual circumstances, but usually it is be after the external examination and prior to the dissection (Kahana & Hiss, 1999).

Radiological techniques may provide important clues to determine the manner of death. In the autopsy procedure, radiography is best and earliest method of demonstrating air embolism to the heart, brain or vascular tree and forensics can be alerted in advance to the presence of pneumothorax, pneumoperitonium, pneumopericardium, pneumomediastinum or abnormal air collections associated with abscess, obstruction or paralytic dysfunction (Brogdon, 1998).

Whilst, the identification of some fractures, fracture sequels, baro-traumas and soft tissue injuries present some difficulties, the determination of them by radiological techniques may be relatively easy. Radiological determination of manner of death in medico-legal cases by using CT, MRI, MSCT and USG was defined to be *"virtopsy (virtual autopsy) technique"*.

Virtopsy has been proposed as an alternative to conventional autopsy in cases when the next of kin oppose the necroscopy and as a complementary tool for better visualization of postmortem findings such as fractures, especially pelvic and extremity fractures; visceral and vascular injuries and pathologies like intracranial hemorrhages, cerebral contusions and edema, splenomegaly, aneurysms, air and fat embolism, hemothorax and pneumothorax, pneumonia, aspiration of foreign bodies, food or blood, subcutaneous emphysema, myocardial infarction, some tumors (Kahana & Hiss, 2005; Poulsen & Simonsen, 2007).

Bullet or bullet fragments in death related firearms, bomb fragments or shrapnel in death related bombings and glass or metallic fragments in death related traffic or air-craft accidents, animals, plants or minerals, which embedded, aspirated or injected, in several deaths, etc., can be determined and exerted, to be presented as evidence in court, by using x-rays and other radiological techniques during medico-legal autopsy applications (Brogdon, 1998; Gruber & Kameyama, 2001; Carvalho et al., 2009). It was reported that CT data and the 3-D reconstruction could provide valuable information in the forensic assessment of patients with gunshot wounds for determination of firing distance (Stein et al., 2000).

The angiographic techniques including corpuscular radiopaque material such as menninge (a red lead oxide), barium sulfate, bismuth chloride, potassium iodide, corn syrup; oily liquids such as iodized oil, propyliodone, mixture of diesel oil and paraffin oil; hydro-soluble preparations such as diatrizoate meglumine, diatrizoate sodium, ioxithalamate; casts such as mixtures of lead, bismuth, and cadmium, celluloid and celloidin, nylon, neoprene latex, polyester resin, vinyl and silicon rubber; and their special mixtures was defined very useful for postmortem investigation of cardiovascular system (Grabherr et al., 2007) (Fig-2).

The usage of radiological techniques in postmortem applications allows creating of permanent records of autopsy findings for reevaluation, comparison in personal identification and submission to be evidence to courts (Swift & Rutty, 2006).

Also, radiological techniques allow forensic personal identification of the ripped, lacerated, carbonized, macerated, putrefied or skeletonized corpses (Gruber & Kameyama, 2001; Carvalho et al., 2009) and in mass disasters (Kahana & Hiss, 1999; Swift & Rutty, 2006).

2.2 Usage of radiographic techniques in clinical forensic applications

The importance of radiological techniques in clinical forensic application is widely recognized for definition type, severity, healing degree and mechanism of injuries (Kahana & Hiss, 2005; Swift & Rutty, 2006). It was defined that some skull fractures can not be diagnosed on conventional CT; they can be distinguished with the use of plain x-rays (Yavuz et al., 2001).

Radiological examinations play significant role in differential diagnosis to non-accidental fractures from accidental fractures (Asirdizer & Zeyfeoglu, 2005); in determination of radiological evidence of physical child abuse (Asirdizer & Zeyfeoglu, 2005; Kahana & Hiss, 2005; Yavuz et al., 2008), torture (Vogel et al., 2007) and medical malpractice cases (Ulucay et al., 2010); localization and type of bullets remained within body (Brogdon, 1998).

Also, radiological techniques have been used by aim of personalization and age determination of victims or defendants in criminal cases and persons in civil litigations (Brogdon, 1998; Kahana & Hiss, 1999; Kahana & Hiss, 2005).

2.3 Usage of radiographic techniques in forensic personal identification

In forensic personal identification, forensic scientists have benefited from the variations of normal anatomical structures in radiographs and they compared shapes, contours, distinctive trabecular patterns, healed fractures, deformities, abnormal calcifications or other pathological features of several bones in radiographs, which taken to determine the identity, with previously existent radiographs (Jablonski & Shum, 1989). Also, they take into account

the absence or replacing of some anatomical structures, and the presence of metallic materials such as prosthesis.
Among radiographs used for forensic personal identification, there were several parts of skull (Bodey et al., 2003; Teke et al., 2007), ribs (Rejtarová et al., 2004), hip (Varga & Takács, 1991), dental, chest and abdominal areas (Kahana & Hiss, 1999). Identification of human remains by comparison of antemortem and postmortem radiographs of frontal sinuses is a well established procedure among forensic scientists and even some of the authors claim to use them as a substitute for fingerprints and frontal sinuses in particular have always been assumed to be different in every person (Yoshino et al., 1987; Harris et al., 1987; Kullman et al., 1990). Computerized tomography is an advanced and new technique and in literature there are only a few reports on identification of unknown bodies using CT scans of frontal sinus (Reichs, 1993; Riepert et al., 2001; Tatlisumak et al., 2007; Pfaeffli et al., 2007; Blau et al., 2008; Uthman et al., 2010).

3. Morphological structure of frontal sinus

3.1 The location of frontal sinus

The frontal sinuses are a part of paranasal sinuses and they located in the frontal bone above each eye (Fig-1). They make an important contribution to normal forehead and glabellar contour.

3.2 The development of frontal sinus

According to classical knowledge based on x-rays, frontal sinus is not apparent at birth and development begins during the second year of life (Yoshino et al., 1987; Quatrehomme et al., 1996; Kirk et al., 2002). However, CT studies show that frontal sinus begins development in

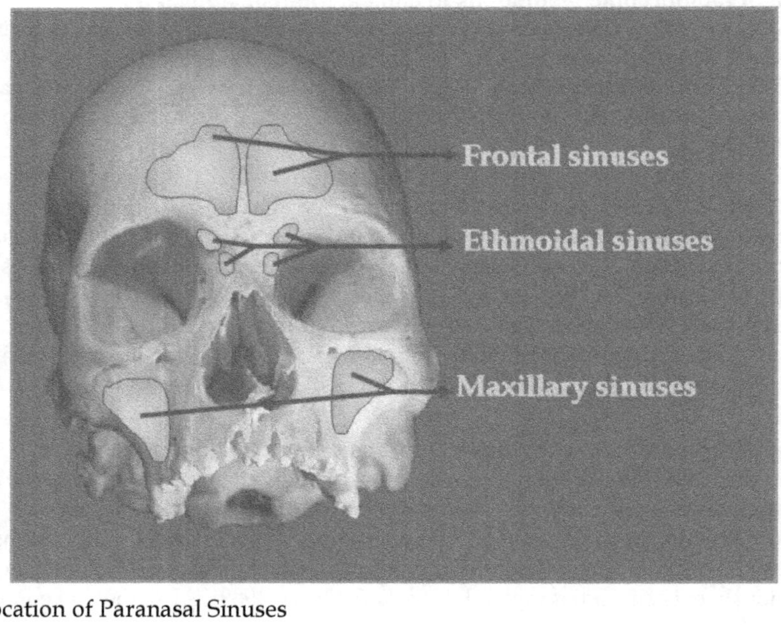

Fig. 1. Location of Paranasal Sinuses

the region of frontal recess of the frontal nasal meatus in a fetus aging 4th months of gestation. In the latter weeks of the fetal life, the frontal recess of the middle nasal meatus transforms upwards into an oval thin-walled space corresponding to the developing frontal sinus. It adheres to the ethmoidal labyrinth, integrating with it (Miller & Amedee, 1998; Porowski et al., 1999).

The frontal sinus rarely is visible on radiographs earlier than the second year of life. The sinus invades the frontal bone by about 5 years of age and slowly grows to reach an adult size in late adolescence (Miller & Amedee, 1998).

Whilst it is widely accepted that the development of the frontal sinus is complete by about 20 years of age and remains stable until further enlargement of the chambers can occur from bone resorption during the advanced ages (Yoshino et al., 1987; Quatrehomme et al., 1996; Kirk et al., 2002); Tatlisumak et al., reported that, the highest values of measurements of frontal sinus were at the 31–40 age group in both sexes and there were a tendency to decrease with aging (Tatlisumak et al, 2008). Also, McLaughlin et al., suggested that the frontal sinus continued to expand until the age of 40 years because of mechanical stresses of mastication and growth hormone levels (McLaughlin et al., 2001).

3.3 Morphological structure of frontal sinus

The frontal sinus is a triangular, pyramid-shaped (its apex is superior and its base is inferior) cavity extending between the anterior and posterior tables of the ascending portion of the frontal bone (Clemente, 2004). The structure of frontal sinus can be variable from person to person and its sizes might be different in different populations (Miller & Amedee, 1998; Tatlisumak et al., 2008). Yoshino et al. described 20,000 types of frontal sinus (Yoshino et al., 1987). Although, Miller and Amedee reported that height of frontal sinus was between 5 and 66 mm, and its width between 17 and 49 mm (Miller & Amedee, 1998); the maximum and minimum sizes of frontal sinus were defined variable by several scientists in several populations.

Usually, there was a complete intersinus septum between both frontal sinuses. The anterior wall of frontal sinus is the strongest of the sinus walls and its thickness can reach to 12 mm. In the entire sinus wall, there were diploë, although the diploë is minimal in the posterior wall and floor of sinus (inferior wall). The posterior wall is a plate of thin, compact bone (1-2 mm) whose upper part is vertical. It separates the frontal sinus from the anterior cranial fossa and can extent to lesser wing of sphenoid bone. The floor of the sinus also functions as the supraorbital roof in the lateral side and naso-etmoid floor in the medial side. The drainage ostium is located in the posteromedial portion of the sinus floor. The frontal infundibulum is a more narrow area within the sinus that leads to the ostium. The frontal sinus-ostium-frontal recess complex is shaped like an hourglass. The size of the bottom half depends on the dimensions of the frontal recess (Miller & Amedee, 1998; Clemente, 2004).

3.4 Functions of frontal sinus

The functions of frontal sinuses which are a part of paranasal sinuses greatly resemble to paranasal sinus functions. The functional significance of paranasal sinuses remains largely unknown. The sinuses have been believed to play numerous roles, but no substantive

laboratory studies have confirmed any of these hypothetical functions (Miller & Amedee, 1998).
Prevailing theories suggest that the paranasal sinuses perform: (a) humidifying and warming inspired air, (b) assisting in regulation of intranasal pressure, (c) increasing the surface area of the olfactory membranes, (d) lightening the skull to maintain proper head balance or assist in flotation, (e) imparting resonance to the voice, (f) absorbing shock to the head, (g) contributing to facial growth, (h) existing as evolutionary remains of useless air spaces, (i) secreting of immunoglobulin, interferon and lysozyme (Miller & Amedee, 1998; Wang & Berke, 1998). Also, Qian et al described a role of frontal sinus in nitric oxide output (Qian et al, 2005).
The complete function of the paranasal sinuses is probably not described by a single theory but is instead most likely a combination of several of the foregoing theories (Miller & Amedee, 1998).

4. Usage of radiology of frontal sinus in forensic personal identification

Some of the features of frontal sinus morphology make it most convenient part of the skeleton for forensic identification (Fig-2 & Fig-3). Firstly, it presents highly variable nature and shows variation even among the monozygotic twins (Yoshino et al., 1987; Quatrehomme et al., 1996; Cox et al., 2009). This empirically accepted variability was proven

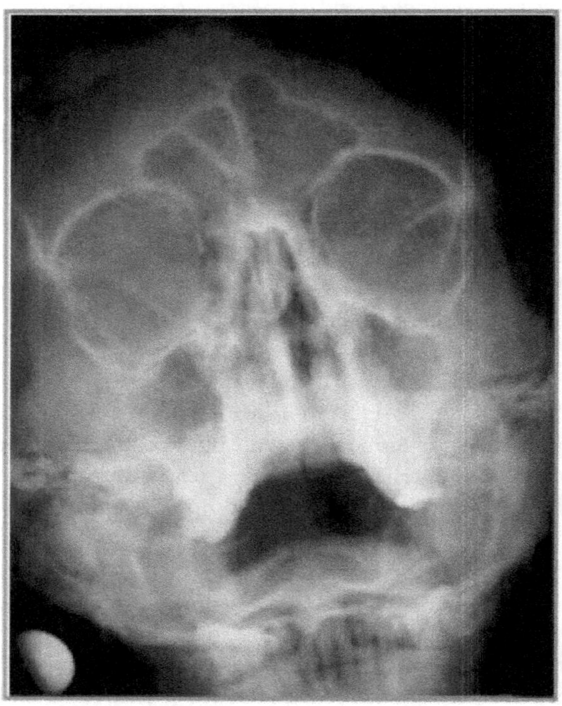

Fig. 2. Appearance of Frontal Sinus in an x-ray

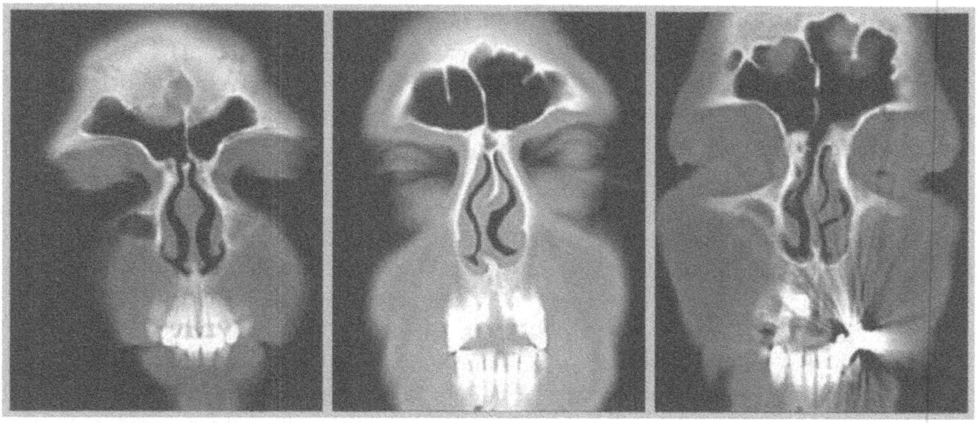

Fig. 3. Appearance of Several Frontal Sinuses in CTs

mathematically using Elliptical Fourier analysis by Christensen (Christensen, 2005). Second feature is its relatively stable structure during adult life (Cox et al., 2009). But changes in the dimensions of the frontal sinus throughout the adult life were shown by the investigators (McLaughlin, et al., 2001; Tatlisumak et al., 2008). Therefore, writers of this text is suggesting that the radiographs not older than ten years are more reliable for the identification purposes. Thirdly, the resiliency of the frontal sinus makes it useful for forensic purposes. It has very strong walls and preserved intact in human remains (Marlin, et al., 1991; Nambiar, et al., 1999; Fairgrieve, 2008) Fourthly, paranasal sinus radiographs are taken commonly for diagnostic purposes and almost everybody has one in his/her health folder (Tatlisumak, et al., 2007; Cox, et al., 2009).

Radiographic comparison permits the matching of unique anatomical features and has the advantage of making possible the matching of external and internal bony anatomy, therefore increasing by several-fold the potential number of points of correspondence available for identification (Jablonski & Shum, 1989).

In the presence of an antemortem radiograph, it can be compared with a postmortem one and personal identification of a human remain can be made. It is a widely accepted procedure in forensic sciences. Comparison of the antemortem and postmortem radiographs of the frontal sinus can be made by superimposition or coding systems. Superimposition is accepted as a reliable method (Yoshino, et al., 1987; Riberio Fde, 2000; Kirk, et al., 2002; Nambiar, et al., 1999; Marlin, et al., 1991). But there are some disadvantages: Data can not be stored and the evaluation should be made again and again for every case and both radiographs should be in hands for comparison. To overcome this problem, systems were proposed for coding frontal sinuses (Yoshino, et al., 1987; Tatlisumak, et al., 2007; Cameriere, et al., 2008). But none of them is perfect and there is always a possibility of false positive results (Tatlisumak, et al., 2007; Tang, et al., 2009).

These systems are still are far from being as useful as fingerprints. Today, discrimination of the most of the radiographs by using simple features and applying pattern matching for the remaining ones is seen logical as an algorithm (Tatlisumak, et al., 2007).

Computerized tomography is a significant advance in radiology and it is becoming increasingly available and replacing gradually the conventional radiographs (Haglund &

Fligner., 1993; Tatlisumak, et al., 2007). Computerized tomography is a suitable imaging method in the identification of unknown human remains and presents alot of advantages as compared with conventional radiographs. Firstly, it gives the opportunity of avoiding the superimposition of structures beyond the plane of interest and allowing the visualization of small differences of density (Reichs, 1993; Jackowski, et al., 2008; Carvalho, et al., 2009). Secondly, the images can be easily manipulated and internal points that should be evaluated can be shown by images segmentation. Thirdly, Craniometric points can be precisely located and measurements can be more accurately performed than on conventional radiographs. Volumes and areas can be determined. Fourtly, the film includes a description of the technical details and knowledge about the patient which can be very useful for the identification process (Jackowski, et al., 2008; Carvalho, et al., 2009).

There are several studies in the literature presenting successful identification using CT images of frontal sinus (Reichs, 1993; Haglund & Fligner., 1993; Smith, et al., 2002; Tatlisumak, et al., 2007). It is expected that forensic scientists will make more identification in the future by using CT scans. The identification technique by conventional radiography was based on the comparison to ante-mortem images of frontal sinuses recorded in clinics and radiology departments with post-mortem radiographic images obtained in autopsy rooms or during autopsy procedure.

5. References

Michael, K. & Michael, M.G. (2006). The proliferation of identification techniques for citizens throughout the ages, In: *The Social Implications of Information Security Measures on Citizens and Business*, (Eds., K. Michael & M.G. Michael), pp.7-26, University of Wollongong, Centre for eBusiness Application Research (CeBAR), ISBN: 1-74128-118-0, NSW-Australia

Soysal, Z. & Eke, M. (1999). The history and development of forensic medicine in the world, In: *Forensic Medicine, Volume: 1*, (Eds. Z. Soysal & C. Cakalir), pp. 1-29, Printing House and Film Center of Istanbul University, ISBN: 975-404-540-2, Istanbul-Turkey

Cameriere, R.; Ferrante, L.; Molleson, T. & Brown, B. (2008). Frontal sinus accuracy in identification as measured by false positives in kin groups. *Journal of Forensic Sciences*. Vol. 53, No. 6, p. 1280-1282, ISSN: 0022-1198

Eckert, W.G. & Garland N. (1984). The history of the forensic applications in radiology. *The American Journal of Forensic Medicine and Pathology*. Vol. 5, No. 1, p. 53–56, ISSN: 0195-7910

Culbert, W.L. & Law, F.M. (1927). Identification by comparison of roentgenograms of nasal accessory sinuses and mastoid processes. *The Journal of American Medical Association*. Vol. 88, No. 21, p. 1634-1636, ISSN: 0098-7484

Gruber, J. & Kameyama, M.M. (2001). The role of radiology in forensic dentistry. *Pesquisa Odontológica Brasileira*. Vol. 15, No. 3, p. 263-268, Print ISSN: 1517-7491

Carvalho, S.P.M.; Alves da Silva, R.H.; Lopes-Júnior, C. & Peres, A.S. (2009). Use of images for human identification in forensic dentistry. *Radiologia Brasileira*. Vol. 42, No. 2, p. 125-130, ISSN: 0100-3984

Kahana, T. & Hiss, J. (1999). Forensic Radiology. *The British Journal of Radiology*. Vol. 72, No. 854, p. 129-133, ISSN: 0007-1285

Brogdon, B.G. (1998). Scope of forensic radiology. In: *Forensic Radiology*, (Ed., B.G. Brogdon), pp. 35-52, CRC Press LLC, ISBN: 0-8493-8105-3, Boca Raton, Florida-USA

Kahana, T. & Hiss, J. (2005). Forensic Radiology. In: *Forensic Pathology Reviews, Volume-3*, (Ed., M. Tsokos), pp. 443-460, Humana Press, ISBN: 1-59259-416-1, Totowa, New Jersey-USA.

Poulsen, K. & Simonsen J. (2007). Computed tomography as routine in connection with medico-legal autopsies. *Forensic Science International*. Vol. 171, No. 2-3, p. 190-197, ISSN: 0379-0738

Stein, K.M.; Bahner, M.L.; Merkel, J.; Ain, S. & Mattern, R. (2000). Detection of gunshot residues in routine CTs. *International Journal of Legal Medicine*. Vol. 114, No. 1-2, p. 15-18, ISSN: 0937-9827

Grabherr, S.; Djonov, V.; Yen, K.; Thali, M.J. & Dirnhofer, R. (2007). Postmortem angiography: review of former and current methods. *American Journal of Roentgenology*. Vol. 188, No. 3, p. 832-838, ISSN: 0361-803X

Swift, B. & Rutty G.N. (2006). Recent advances in forensic radiology, In: *Forensic Pathology Reviews, Volume-4*, (Ed., M. Tsokos), pp. 355-404, Humana Press Inc, ISBN: 1-59259-921-4, Totowa, New Jersey-USA

Yavuz, M.S.; Asirdizer, M.; Cetin Agirbas, A. & Altinkok, M. (2001). The importance of cranial x-ray to diagnoses linear skull fractures cannot be seen by CT. *Clinical Forensic Medicine*. Vol. 1, No. 2, p. 81-88, ISSN: 1302-9908

Asirdizer, M. & Zeyfeoglu, Y. (2005). Femoral and tibial fractures in a child with myelomeningocele. *Journal of Clinical Forensic Medicine*. Vol. 12, No. 2, p. 93-97, ISSN: 1353-1131

Yavuz, M.S.; Buyukyavuz, I.; Savas, C.; Ozguner, I.F.; Kupeli, A. & Asirdizer M. (2008). A battered child case with duodenal perforation. *Journal of Forensic and Legal Medicine*. Vol. 15, No. 4, p. 259-262, ISSN: 1752-928X

Vogel, H.; Schmitz-Engels, F. & Grillo, C. (2007). Radiology of torture. *European Journal of Radiology*. Vol. 63, No. 2, p. 187-204, ISSN: 0720-048X

Ulucay, T.; Dizdar; M.G.; Yavuz M.S. & Asirdizer, M. (2010). The importance of medico-legal evaluation in a case with intraabdominal gossypiboma. *Forensic Science International*. Vol. 198, No. 1-3, p. e15-e18, ISSN: 0379-0738

Jablonski, N.G. & Shum B.S.F. (1989). Identification of unknown human remains by comparison of antemortem and postmortem radiographs. *Forensic Science International*. Vol. 42, No. 3, p. 221-230, ISSN: 0379-0738

Bodey, T.E.; Loushine, R.J. & West, L.A. (2003). A retrospective study evaluating the use of the panoramic radiograph in endodontics. *Military Medicine*. Vol. 168, No. 7, p. 528-529, ISSN: 0026-4075

Teke, H.Y.; Duran, S.; Canturk, N. & Canturk, G. (2007). Determination of gender by measuring the size of the maxillary sinuses in computerized tomography scans. *Surgical and Radiological Anatomy*. Vol. 29, No. 1, p. 9-13, ISSN: 0930-1038

Rejtarová, O.; Slízová, D.; Smoranc, P.; Rejtar, P. & Bukac, J. (2004). Costal cartilages—a clue for determination of sex. *Biomedical Papers*. Vol. 148, No. 2, p.241-243, ISSN: 1213-8118

Varga, M. & Takács, P. (1991). Radiographic personal identification with characteristic features in the hip joint. *American Journal of Forensic Medicine and Pathology*. Vol. 12, No. 4, p. 328-331, ISSN: 0195-7910

Yoshino, M.; Miyasaka, S.; Sato, H. & Seta, S. (1987). Classification system of frontal sinus patterns by radiography: Its application to identification of unknown skeletal remains. *Forensic Science International*. Vol. 34, No. 4, p. 286-299, ISSN: 0379-0738

Harris, A.M.; Wood, R.E.; Nortjé, C.J. & Thomas, C.J. (1987). The frontal sinus: Forensic fingerprint? A pilot study. *Journal of Forensic Odonto-Stomatology*. Vol. 5, No. 1, p. 9-15. ISSN: 0258-414X

Kullman, L.; Eklund, B. & Grundin, R. (1990). Value of the frontal sinus in identification of unknown persons. *Journal of Forensic Odonto-Stomatology*. Vol. 8, No. 1, p. 3-10. ISSN: 0258-414X

Reichs, K.J. (1993). Quantified comparison of frontal sinus patterns by means of computed tomography. *Forensic Science International*. Vol. 61, No. 2-3, p. 141-168, ISSN: 0379-0738

Riepert, T.; Ulmcke, D.; Schweden, F. & Nafe, B. (2001). Identification of unknown dead bodies by X-ray image comparison of the skull using the X-ray simulation program FoXSIS. *Forensic Science International*. Vol. 117, No. 1-2, p. 89-98, ISSN: 0379-0738

Tatlisumak, E.; Yilmaz Ovali, G.; Aslan, A.; Asirdizer, M.; Zeyfeoglu, Y. & Tarhan, S. (2007) Identification of unknown bodies by using CT images of frontal sinus. *Forensic Science International*. Vol. 166, No. 1, p. 42-48, ISSN: 0379-0738

Pfaeffli, M.; Vock, P.; Dirnhofer, R.; Braun, M.; Bolliger, S.A. & Thali, M.J. (2007). Post-mortem radiological CT identification based on classical ante-mortem X-ray examinations. *Forensic Science International*. Vol. 171, No. 2-3, p. 111-117, ISSN: 0379-0738

Blau, S.; Robertson, S. & Johnstone, M. (2008). Disaster victim identification: new applications for postmortem computed tomography. *Journal of Forensic Sciences*. Vol. 53, No. 4, p. 956-961, ISSN: 0022-1198

Uthman, A.T.; Al-Rawi, N.H.; Al-Naaimi, A.S.; Tawfeeq, A.S. & Suhail, E.H. (2010). Evaluation of frontal sinus and skull measurements using spiral CT scanning: an aid in unknown person identification. *Forensic Science International*. Vol. 197, No. 1-3, p. 124e1-124e7, ISSN: 0379-0738

Quatrehomme, G.; Fronty, P.; Sapanet, M.; Gre´vin, G.; Bailet, P. & Ollier, A. (1996). Identification by frontal sinus pattern in forensic anthropology. *Forensic Science International*. Vol. 83, No. 2, p. 147-153, ISSN: 0379-0738

Kirk, N.J.; Wood, R.E. & Goldstein, M. (2002). Skeletal identification using the frontal sinus region: A retrospective study of 39 cases. *Journal of Forensic Sciences*. Vol. 47, No. 2, p. 318-323, ISSN: 0022-1198

Miller, A.J. & Amedee, R.G. (1998). Sinus anatomy and function. In: *Head and Neck Surgery-Otolaryngology, 5th edition*, (Eds., B.J. Bailey & K.H. Calhoun), pp. 457–461, Lippincott-Raven, ISBN: 0-78175-561-1 Philadelphia-USA

Porowski, L.; Skórzewska, A.; Radziemski, A. & Szpakowska-Rzymska, I. (1999). Development of frontal sinus in human fetuses as seen in computerized tomography. *Folia Morphologica*. Vol. 58, No. 3, p. 215-221, ISSN: 0015-5659

Tatlisumak, E.; Ovali, G.Y.; Asirdizer, M.; Aslan, A.; Ozyurt, B.; Bayindir, P. & Tarhan, S. (2008). CT study on morphometry of frontal sinus. *Clinical Anatomy*. Vol. 21, No. 4, p. 287-293, ISSN: 0897-3806

McLaughlin, R.B. Jr.; Rehl, R.M. & Lanza, D.C. (2001). Clinically relevant frontal sinus anatomy and physiology. *Otolaryngologic Clinics of North America*. Vol. 34, No. 1, p. 1-22, ISSN: 0030-6665

Clemente, M.P. (2004). Surgical anatomy of paranasal sinus, In: *Sinus Surgery: Endoscopic and Microscopic Approaches, 1st edition*, (Eds., H.L. Levine & M.P. Clemente), pp. 1-56, Thieme Medical Publisher, ISBN: 0-86577-972-3, New York-USA.

Wang, M.B. & Berke, G.S. (1998). Paranasal sinus endoscopy, In: *Endoscopy of the Central and Peripheral Nervous System*, (Eds., W.A. King; J.G. Frazee & A.A.F. De Salles), pp. 147-154, Thieme Medical Publisher, ISBN: 0-86577-690-3, New York-USA.

Qian, W.; Makitie, A.A.; Witterick, I. & Haight, J.S. (2005). A comparison between nitric oxide output in the nose and sinuses: A pilot study in one volunteer. *Acta Oto-Laryngologica*. Vol. 125, No. 10, p. 1080-1085, ISSN: 0001-6489

Christensen, A.M. (2005). Assessing the variation in individual frontal sinus outlines. American Journal of Physical Anthropology. Vol. 127, No. 3, pp. 291-295, ISSN: 1096-8644

Cox, M; Malcolm, M. ; Fairgrieve, S.I. (2009). A new digital method for the objective comparison of frontal sinuses for identification. *Journal of Forensic Sciences*. Vol. 54, No. 4, p. 761-772, ISSN: 0022-1198

Marlin, D.C.; Clark, M.A.; Standish, S. M. (1991). Identification of human remains by comparison of frontal sinus radiographs: a series of four cases. *Journal of Forensic Sciences*. Vol. 36, No. 6, p. 1765-1772, ISSN: 0022-1198

Nambiar, P.; Naidu, M.D. ; Subramaniam, K. (1999). Anatomical variability of the frontal sinuses and their application in forensic identification. *Clinical Anatomy*. Vol. 12, No. 1, p. 16-19, ISSN: 0897-3806

Fairgrieve, S.I. (2008). Forensic cremation: recovery and analysis. CRC Press, ISBN: 0-84939-189-X, Boca Roton

Ribeiro Fde A. (2000). Standardized measurements of radiographic films of the frontal sinuses: an aid to identifying unknown persons. *Ear, Nose and Throat Journal*. Vol. 79, No. 1, pp. 26-33, ISSN: 0145-5613

Tang, J.P.; Hu, D.Y.; Jiang, F.H.; Yu, X.J. (2009). Assessing forensic applications of the frontal sinus in a Chinese Han population. *Forensic Science International*. Vol. 183, No. 1-2, p. 104e1-104e3, ISSN: 0379-0738

Haglund, W.D.; Fligner, C.L. (1993). Confirmation of human identification using computerized tomography (CT). *Journal of Forensic Sciences*. Vol. 38, No. 3, p. 708-712, ISSN: 0022-1198

Jackowski, C.; Wyss, M., Persson, A.; Classens, M.; Thali, M.J. & Lussi, A. (2008). Ultra-high-resolution dual-source CT for forensic dental visualization-discrimination of ceramic and composite fillings. *International Journal of Legal Medicine.* Vol. 122, No. 43, p. 301-307, ISSN: 0937-9827

Smith, D.R; Limbird, K.G. & Hoffman, J.M. (2002). Identification of human skeletal remains by comparison of bony details of the cranium using computerized tomographic (CT) scans. *Journal of Forensic Sciences*. Vol. 47, No. 5, p. 1-3, ISSN: 0022-1198

Enhancing Product Development through CT Images, Computer-Aided Design and Rapid Manufacturing: Present Capabilities, Main Applications and Challenges

Andrés Díaz Lantada and Pilar Lafont Morgado
Mechanical Engineering Department - Universidad Politécnica de Madrid
c/ José Gutiérrez Abascal 2, 28006 Madrid
Spain

1. Introduction

1.1 Historical perspective of product development methodologies

It is difficult to find the origins of what we call "systematic design". To offer but one example, anyone studying the diagrams and sketches of Leonardo da Vinci can hardly fail to observe the depth of his analysis and how he systematically used variations to suggest possible solutions and be able to compare them (Taddei, Kaiser, König, 2006, Bautista, 2007). Up to the Industrial revolution, product design and development work was essentially linked to art and craft and only with the gradual mechanization of processes halfway through the 19th Century did a need begin to emerge to optimize the use of materials and perform detailed studies on strength, stiffness, wear, friction, assembly and maintenance (Reuleaux, 1875).

However, it was not until the 20th Century that a systematic evaluation of these parameters was put forward as a way of gradually reaching an optimal solution. (Erkens, Wörgebauer). Just before the Second World War a need was beginning to be noticed to rationalize product design processes but progress in this direction was hampered by the following factors:

- An absence of effective methods for representing abstract ideas.
- The widespread belief that design was an art and not a technical activity that could be carried out methodically and not just through creativity.

A large-scale use of systematic design methodologies would have to wait for these limitations to be overcome and for the introduction of a more widespread use of automation and the appearance of more modern data processing procedures.

Modern ideas on systematic development were given an enormous boost by relevant figures (Kesselring, 1951, 1954, Tschochner, 1954, Matousek, 1957 or Niemann, 1950, 1965, 1975), whose revolutionary ideas continue to suggest ways of solving and dealing with specific tasks related to machine and product design processes (Kaiser, König, 2006). During the 40s and the 50s Kesserling put forward a method based on successive approaches where each approach optimized different variables in line with technical and economic criteria. He also proposed several principles like "minimal production costs", "minimal weight and volume", "minimal loss" and "optimal functionality and operability". On the other hand, in the 50s Tschochner emphasized the importance of four basic design factors: the principles of functionality, material, shape and size, similar to what Matousek would later do, but emphasizing the need to consider: the principles of functionality, material, manufacture and geometry. Niemann's approach designed in the 60s and 70s consisted in starting out design by defining a general outline for the product with the main sizes to be worked on in greater depth. To this end, the overall design continued to be divided into different parts that could be developed in parallel. The optimal solution was finally reached by a systematic variation of all the possible solutions.

These progressive approaches towards ever more systematic methodologies for product design were mainly performed by university lecturers who had learned the fundamentals of design and development during their practical class contacts with increasingly complex products. They realized that not only was it possible to apply more mathematical concepts, physical principles, information theory-based methods and systematic design, but that with the gradual increase in the division of work it was becoming indispensable. Their designs were evidently strongly influenced by the industries they worked for, but many of their principles suitably modified can be adapted to numerous cases of design in other sectors. The currently accepted principles for effectively carrying out new product development are based on the ideas of the foregoing authors, as well as on the series of design steps that subsequently set apart important researchers (Hansen, 1956, Wächtler, 1967 o Kuhlenkamp, 1971). In general terms, these researchers talk of "pre-studies", "defining the basic principle", "basic design" and "detailed design" as the main stages. They are also listed in "design guidelines" written by organizations like the "VDI - Verein Deutscher Ingenieure" or the "ISO - International Organization for Standardization" in reference to global testing and quality management.

1.2 Stages of a product's systematic development process

The outcomes of previous research, satisfactorily proven through numerous developed products, led to a slightly modified work structure (Roozenburg, Eeckels, 1995, Pahl, Beitz, 1996, Ulrich, Eppinger, 2007) which included: planning, conceptual design, basic engineering and detailed engineering, although a clear dividing line cannot always be set between these stages.

Defining objectives and planning.- This broadly consists of the strategic decision taken by a company, university or research centre as to which products or ideas must be developed to satisfy the new social needs, taking account of the scientific-technological and socio-economic circumstances of the time. To set about a product idea that will be successful the state of the market has to be fully understood and especially customers and their needs. Thus, market and customer requirements become the major stimuli for developing new products. However, these stimuli frequently have other origins, the most important of which are politics, the appearance of new technologies, processes, materials, discoveries or research results and environmental issues. Neither should the role played by internal stimuli be underestimated (arising in the company, university or technology centre itself) when it comes to making a decision about a new product. Among these internal stimuli are new ideas or outcomes related to research activity and the implementation of new means of production as well as production being made more rational and diversified. Depending on the stimuli mentioned, the main tasks to be included in the "defining objectives and planning" stage are:

- Situation analysis.- By carrying out an in-depth study of the company and its products, together with market analysis and other possible information sources, a thorough analysis can be reached of the starting out point.
- Drawing up search strategies.- By bearing in mind the companies' aims, strengths and weaknesses, as well as market gaps and needs, certain areas or promising fields can be discovered where ideas can be sought to be applied.
- Finding product ideas.- From the search in the chosen field for new applications, functions, principles of functionality, geometries, materials, energy management methods and other alternatives, a set of product ideas can be found.
- Choosing product ideas.- Depending on the company's aims and market needs, the set of ideas found are evaluated in order to choose the most attractive product idea.
- Defining the product to be developed.- By evaluating the different alternatives against a list of requirements a product proposal or definition is reached together with some initial objectives concerning costs, prices and schedules.

Conceptual design.- This is the stage where a decisive global principle is reached or a basis for reaching a satisfactory solution based on identifying crucial problems and choosing the right functional principles that in combination will attain the set objective. If this stage is to be properly tackled a series of prerequisites must be fulfilled linked to a correct conclusion of the previous stage. The objective must therefore be clearly stated and, in principle, be technically and financially viable. In addition, the designer must be informed of the needs of this conceptual design stage and the existence of possible solutions that allow proceeding directly to the design or basic engineering stage. The scope and depth required for the conceptual design stage must also be pre-established. Related to the above, the main tasks included in this stage are listed below:

- Abstraction for identifying basic problems.- The decisive designs and principles based on traditional methods cease to provide optimum responses in the face of scientific-technological advances concerning technologies, materials or procedures, which when used in combination usually provide the key to more effective new solutions. On the other hand, every industry, company or research centre has countless experiences, which, although valuable, can lead to prejudice and hinder the creative process. For this reason, particularly at the outset of a new product design, designers must make an effort of abstraction and distance themselves from the influences of conventional ideas and focus on analysing the list of requirements and setting out the fundamental problem or problems in an objective manner.
- Setting functional frameworks.- Having set out the basic problem to be solved, a global function must be obtained based on energy flows, mass and signals so that a relationship between the inputs to, and outputs from the plant, machine, part or object to be designed can be established. This global function can then be divided into less complex sub-functions and a lower level of abstraction, all of which can be individually dealt with to facilitate the search for solutions. Combining and relating these sub-functions leads to the so-called functional framework. It is advisable to draw up several functional frameworks depending on whether it is wished to optimize costs, functionalities, quality, development time or other factors.

- Designing functional frameworks.- After establishing the different functional frameworks the principles of functionality for each of the sub-functions need to be sought. When they have been found, they should be properly interconnected to produce all the different possible functional frameworks that fulfil the global function. In line with the different preferences (cost, timeframe, quality and others) a table of choices can be made to choose the most suitable functional frameworks.
- Obtaining the decisive principle.- By taking the functional frameworks the different decisive principles to be evaluated can be obtained based on the different techno-economic criteria and preliminary calculations that can lead to the choice of the most adequate decisive principle (proposal for a preliminary solution or product concept) that can be worked on.

Basic engineering.- When the decisive principle has been arrived at it is time to specify the underlying ideas behind this preliminary proposal for a solution or product concept. During the basic engineering stage (also often called basic design) the design engineers have the task of defining the basic shapes and geometries that characterize the product, and must also choose the preliminary materials and appropriate manufacturing processes. It is at this stage when technical, technological and economic considerations become of vital importance. In other words the mission of this stage is to provide a definitive general outline of the product to be developed, on which an effective analysis can be performed concerning: function, duration, manufacture, assembly, functionality, costs and safety.

Unlike the conceptual design stage, the basic engineering stage is subject to numerous checks, which means the work of analysis and synthesis constantly alternate and complement each other. An enormous effort also needs to be made regarding the compilation of information to make it easier to evaluate solutions, identify errors and continuously optimize.

The complexity of this stage is also greater because many actions have to be performed simultaneously. Sub-tasks need to be repeated when high levels of information are reached and because any change in an area or sub-area has repercussions on all the rest. For these reasons, it is impossible to set a series of steps to be strictly adhered to that will ensure the basic engineering will come to a successful conclusion. However, the following approach may be followed in general terms:

- Choose the requirements that are crucially important in the basic engineering stage.
- Make scale drawings with the existing spatial constraints and evaluate the required free spaces.
- Draw up a basic outline to decide which components will be required to fulfil the main functions.
- A preliminary design of the parts and components that fulfil these main functions.
- Draw up a basic outline to decide which components will fulfil the remaining secondary functions.
- Draw up the preliminary designs of parts and components that fulfil these secondary functions.
- Evaluate the designs using both technical and economic criteria.
- Decide the overall preliminary design.
- Optimize the chosen design, eradicating any weak points that may have arisen during evaluation.
- Make proposals for improvement and checking if cost and quality objectives are met.

- Prepare a basic preliminary parts and documentation list for production and assembly. This documentation comprises the starting point for the detailed engineering stage.

During the basic engineering stage it is very useful to use check lists to ensure that when designing the different parts intended for the main product functions, all the various aspects have been taken into account. Of these aspects the most important are:

- Function.
- Principle of functionality.
- Design.
- Safety.
- Regulations.
- Ergonomics.
- Manufacturing.
- Quality control.
- Assembly.
- Transport.
- Operation.
- Fault detection.
- Recycling.
- Maintenance.
- Cost.
- Timescale.

Alongside this stage as part of the work to compare designs and check geometries and functionalities, it is very useful to produce prototypes that will aid decision-making and help reduce the number of design iterations and minimize both the timescales and costs associated with product development. Currently a distinction is made between virtual prototypes, the result of computer-aided design, simulation, calculation and manufacturing programs ("CAD-CAE-CAM" programs) and physical prototypes that coincide with the traditional concept of "original product sample for testing and checking".

The appearance of support "software" for engineering design work and its gradual incorporation into industry since the end of the 80s, together with growing operational and calculating capacity, have caused major changes to the way design processes are carried out. Information exchange has become easier enabling countless effects in combination to be taken into account using multivariable simulations and enabling forecasts to be made concerning the influence of parameters such as the material or the manufacturing process on the end quality of a part or product. All these "software" tools can be included in a set of computer tools for managing the life-cycle of a product or "PLM programs - Product Lifecycle Management" (Stark, 2004, Saaksvuori, 2008). These capabilities enable a company to effectively manage and develop their products and related services throughout their economic life. All companies also need to manage the communications and information with their customers ("CRM tools or programs - Customer Relationship Management"), with their suppliers (programs called "SCM - Supply Chain Management") and company resources (programs referred to as "ERP - Enterprise Resource Planning").

These three groups of software programs together with the PLM programs complete the four cornerstones of the information technology infrastructure that enable the main needs of a company to be addressed. More directly linked to product development in line with the approach taken here, PLM tools that include the following types of software programs come to the fore for performing tasks like:

- PPM - Product and Portfolio Management.- These are programs aimed at helping determine the optimal combination or sequence for the projects proposed for the company to successfully achieve it objectives in accordance with its economic and technological strategy and actual market requirements. These tools help analyse resources, costs, investment, production schedules and how one project affects another.
- CAD – Computer-Aided Design.- These programs support design engineers, architects and other design professionals in their work, which is to make their designs a reality. They usually have 2D and 3D drawing systems for creating files or have all the information on a product's geometry and its different parts, as well as its plans. Changes can be made, symmetries are included, scale designs and numerous operations that can help make changes to the design.
- CAE – Computer-Aided Engineering.- These computer programs allow simulating designs that have usually been made with CAD programs, and apply kinematic, dynamic, thermal or fluid mechanics considerations to the geometries designed and, above all, the chosen materials. They allow analysing how changes will affect the product or its parts and help optimize the number of prototypes or tests required.
- CAM – Computer-Aided Manufacturing.- These programs lend support to prototype manufacturing work and end products by converting the information on part geometry from a CAD program into a code that can be understood by numerical control, manufacturing or rapid prototyping machines. On occasions it has a similar mission to CAE programs, letting part quality be simulated according to the manufacturing process used as well as allowing a study on geometries and materials.
- PDM – Product Data Management.- These are programs focused on facilitating the records and paperwork of the processes to create modify and revise any of the parts of a product. The information stored ranges from specifications, CAD file diagrams, plans, manufacturing documents, assembly documents, tenders, test specifications and quality control, as well as financial reports.

In recent years the boundaries between these types of software are shrinking with the ever more frequent appearance of packs that combine different modules to provide a global response to all the aforementioned needs. As explained, these technologies can provide assistance at every product design stage as well as production start-up, market placement and after-sales services, up to the product's life-end. The benefits of using them become obvious at the basic engineering stage where their use is even more justified in the detailed engineering stage where the amount of information handled increases rapidly, as will be explained further on.

Regarding prototypes, the industrial importance acquired over the last decade by the so-called "manufacturing and rapid prototyping technologies" should be emphasized. These technologies enable physical parts to be directly obtained in a short time (hours or a few days) from the designs made with the help of a computer using "CAD-CAE-CAM" programs. They are of great help in optimizing design iterations, help the early detection of errors and speed up production start-up. They are usually either based on "Layer Manufacturing Technologies" (like Laser Stereolithography or Selective Laser Sintering) or on material elimination manufacturing processes (high speed numerical control machining). The different technologies available mean that prototypes can be obtained in a wide range of metal, ceramic and polymeric materials with remarkable precision (Freitag, Wohlers, 2003, Kucklick, 2006, Lafont, Lorenzo Yustos, Díaz Lantada, 2007, 2008).

Depending on the objective and the similarity to the end product, the physical prototypes are usually divided into the three following levels:

- Level "A" prototypes (commonly called "A-samples").- These are demonstration prototypes for analysing shapes, geometries and other more subjective aspects (like aesthetics, visual impact or ergonomics) related to the product under development.
- Level "B" prototypes (commonly called "B-samples").- These are functional prototypes intended for checking the behaviour of different product parts and their functionalities. Although they are generally made of non-final materials, these tests are usually performed with limits on certain applications.
- Level "C" prototypes (commonly called "C-samples").- These are prototypes with similar materials and behaviour to the end product although the manufacturing methods used to obtain them do not coincide with the methods used in production. These level "C" prototypes are usually manufactured for final checks, to prepare production start-up and for obtaining official approval as part of the detailed engineering stage which will be dealt with further on.

However, the end of the basic engineering stage and the beginning of the detailed engineering stage cannot be precisely delimited as there is always some overlap that is to the benefit of the overall process.

Detailed engineering.- Once the final basic design has been obtained, work must be begun on the requirements of the shape, properties, size and tolerances of the different parts. The final choice of manufacturing and assembly must also be done as well as final cost evaluation.

The outcome of this stage is the definitive technical specifications of the product: a list of functionalities, production plans and the specifications including the instructions for assembly, disassembly and operation.

Based on this information or technical documentation, production start-up can be undertaken as well as the placing of the product on the market. According to the above, detailed engineering work can be divided into the following:

- Finalizing the end design.- The different parts are fully defined by means of plans or 3D geometry CAD files, and materials, tolerances, adjustments and other details are specified.
- Parts integration.- By means of full comprehensive plans or CAD assembly files which define the product as a whole.
- Finalizing paperwork.- For an unambiguous definition of the product and be able to launch production.
- Final checks.- As to compliance with general regulations and company standards. Precision of size and tolerances, the availability of standard or catalogue parts and other checks.

The basic and detailed engineering stages can often be brought together in one single design stage with a global focus where the level of detail is gradually added. The ever more generalized use of CAD-CAE-CAM technologies and the already mentioned PLM tools has promoted this gradual fusion between stages, which also simplifies any information exchange between the agents involved in product design.

In this chapter we will concentrate on the advantages and novel possibilities that CT imaging technologies have helped to introduce into the area of product design and development. We will analyse in the following sections the novel possibilities of CT-aided product development, as a complement to the aforementioned "CAD-CAE-CAM" and rapid prototyping tools, and the implications of computed tomography in all the stages of product lifecycle. The main application fields and some case studies will be provided, so as to give a wider panorama of the related advantages.

2. New possibilities: CT-aided product development

The remarkable advances of the last decades in the different systems of medical image acquisition (mainly computerized tomography, Doppler echography, magnetic resonance and positron emission tomography) have considerably increased the diagnostic capability of these systems as well as the reliability of the diagnoses based on these data and the ensuing decisions made regarding the therapy to be applied.

Computerized Axial Tomography (CAT- Scan) resulted from the research of two teams. One team led by Dr. Alan McLeod Cormack (who disclosed the theoretical formulation in 1962, 1963 and 1964) and the other by the engineer Godfrey Newbold Hounsfield (who built the first prototype in 1971), for which they received the Nobel Prize for Medicine in 1979.

The conventional CAT provides axial planes of the body by way of sections of a quality that is often higher than anatomical slices. This is achieved by using the simultaneous rotation of the tube producing the ray beam and the corona detectors. A computer calculates the dose absorbed at the different points of the slice during the rotational motion of the whole system, which displays an image on a screen.

Since the first TAC images in 1976, different generations have appeared in the search for ever faster processing speeds and better image quality while attempting to obtain reconstructions on other different axial planes that are of an acceptable quality, with a larger number of detectors and shorter study times.

Thanks to the important advances in hardware during these years a new computerized tomography (CT) has been developed, helical CT (HCT), which uses the continuous rotation of the detector and the X-ray source in combination with the continuous movement of the examination table. With this method of examination 100% of the time is put to use. Moreover, with this system, data capture is not slice by slice as in axial CT, but results in the entire volume being captured so that slices can be reconstructed in all three dimensions of space. Combining this new hardware with the progress in software for processing the images taken enables more efficient diagnoses to be made from the more realistic and exact reconstructions achieved with 3D textures and images. An HCT 64 detector model was used for this work due to its having the precision required for subsequent customized design.

In fact, medical circles are now benefiting from the ability to exchange information from different medical image acquisition systems between centres and researchers. This is due to the "DICOM" (Digital Imaging and Communication in Medicine) standard having been set up and its now generalized use as a working format for a range of three-dimensional image reconstruction software, particularly since the introduction of version DICOM 3.0 in 1993.

As an additional development tool, "Mimics" (Materialise NV) and similar programs have also appeared which not only perform three-dimensional reconstruction from medical images but also carry out simple operations on these reconstructions and convert them to other formats that can be accessed by "CAD-CAE-CAM" computer-aided design, engineering and manufacturing programs. These "CAD-CAE-CAM" programs (Solid Edge, Catia, NX-5, I-DEAS, Rhino, Solid Works and others) form a wide range of computer tools that are at the service of engineers, architects and design professionals, as has previously been explained regarding modern product development methodologies. The power of these software packages together with their ability to manage information from medical images as a basis for design, means that at present, customized designs, specially for the medical device industry, can be designed in a matter of hours, while comparing alternative designs is also made easier (Hieu, 2002, Harryson, 2007).

However, the use of customized designs, products, prostheses or implants has been historically sporadic, practically always the fruit of research projects. This is basically due to problems of cost and timescale which have always prevented these customized products, prostheses and implants from competing with standard mass-produced designs.

Nonetheless, in recent years "rapid prototyping" has also led to reduced timescales and costs by manufacturing parts directly from the information on their geometry stored in the files of "CAD-CAE-CAM" programs or Mimics and to the advent of new capabilities for a customized response in the product development industry, with a social impact that is likely to be highly positive (Schwarz, 2005, Kucklick, 2006).

There are several softwares, for handling the information obtained from medical imaging technologies, and enabling computer-aided design, engineering and prototyping tasks. They are usually referred to as "Mimics-like" programs (due to the relevance of Mimics (Materialise NV). Among such programs, due to their industrial impact and quality of results, it is important to mention at least:

- Mimics (Materialise NV), for general purpose applications.
- Simplant (Materialise NV), especially oriented to Odontology.
- Surgiguide (Materialise NV), especially oriented to Odontology.
- 3D Doctor, for bone modelling from CT scan and soft tissue from MRI.
- Analyze (Mayo Clinic), for handling images from MR, CT and PET.
- MRIcro Software, for converting medical images to SPM friendly Analyze format.
- Biobuild, for converting volumetric imaging data to rapid prototyping file formats.
- Volume Graphics, for general purpose applications.

Listed below are the main applications of computerized tomography, together with software for processing medical images and "CAD-CAE-CAM" tools, for optimizing product design and development activities:

- Personalized and special designs (Bibb, 2000, Chang, 2003, Díaz Lantada, 2010).
- Reverse engineering, modular developments and design optimization (Flisch, 1999, Vasilash, 2009).
- Object reconstruction (Effenberger, 2008, Vasilash, 2009).
- Prototyping and trials (Flisch, 1999, Effenberger, 2008).
- Inspection of inner details and defects during manufacturing processes (Losano, 1999, Effenberger, 2008).
- Inspection of inner details and crack propagation during service life (Losano, 1999, Effenberger, 2008).
- Multipurpose non-destructive evaluations (Losano, 1999, Effenberger, 2008).

These technological combinations provide novel ways of tackling the design process, but also for validating manufacturing processes and verifying service life. It is very important to mention that the whole process is economical and non-destructive. In addition CT allows inner details and defects to be registered, which proves to be a great advantage when compared with other monitoring processes, such as three-dimensional laser reconstructions or surface ultrasound-based examination technologies.

Figure 1 includes a schematic description of the main applications of computerized tomography for product design and development, taking into account the whole lifecycle, from the design stage to the end of product life or replacement by novel products. The different typical formats conventionally used are also included in the diagram, taking into account the related studies and software for design, calculation or manufacturing.

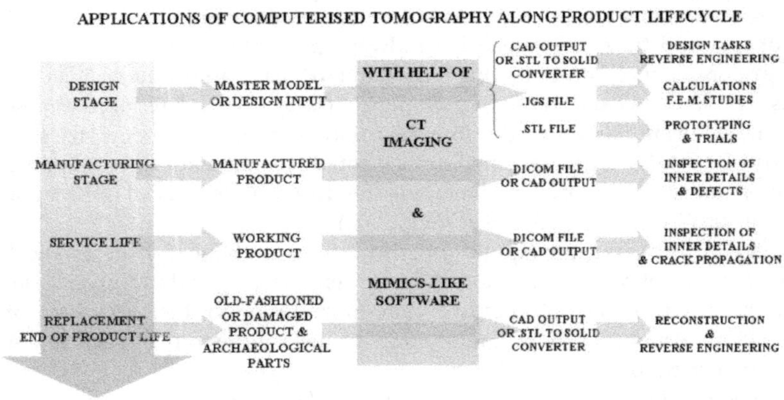

Fig. 1. Schematic review of applications of computerized tomography for product lifecycle.

The combined use of such technologies is of recent appearance; in fact, the main evolution has been registered in the last decade, as Figure 2 shows. The Figure represents the evolution of "ISI Web of Knowledge"-indexed publications related to the use of computed tomography for promoting product development activities, such as design, calculations or engineering and prototyping.

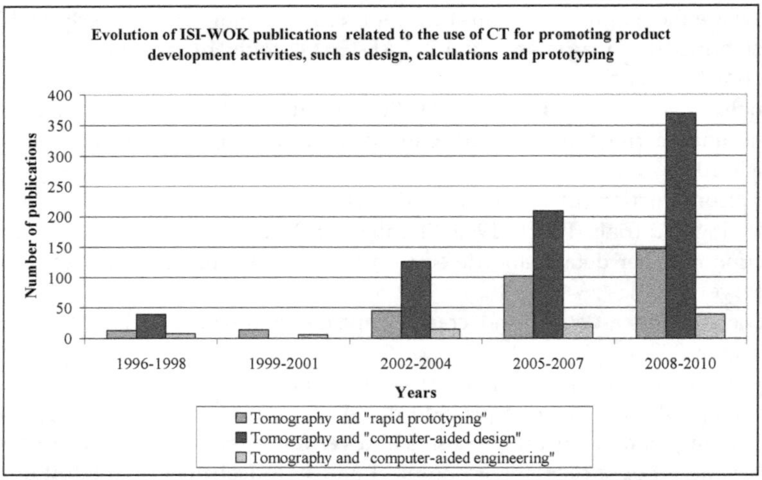

Fig. 2. Evolution of ISI - Web of Knowledge publications including the combination of "tomography" with "rapid prototyping", with "computer-aided design" and with "computer-aided engineering".

All these novel possibilities and applications can be included or described under the terms "CT-aided engineering" or "CT-aided product development". The main application fields of these technological combinations focusing on product development are discussed further on in the following section.

3. Main application fields

The first approximations, around 15 to 20 years ago, linked to using computed tomography as a support tool for product design and development correspond to the industry of personalized medical prosthesis and devices, as well as to some studies linked to the prototyping of human body structures for subsequent surgical planning and training tasks. As the main applications of computed tomography imaging have always been within the medical field, it is normal that the first experiences connected to CT-aided product development would be related to the development of medical devices or surgical support tools. However, during the last decade, the application fields have greatly expanded and there are examples of remarkable CT-aided product design and development case studies in sectors such as the plastics processing industry (Reinhart, Losano, 1999), the automotive sector (Vasilash, 2009), the medical device area (Bibb, 2000, Díaz Lantada, 2010), with especial growth in dentistry and oral surgery (Chang, 2003) and other industries (Filsch, 1999). There are even application experiences related to archaeology and art (Vasilash, 2009), including remarkable teaching consequences and proposals.
For a more detailed analysis regarding the main application fields of CT in product development, searches of the main scientific publications related to ["tomography" and "rapid prototyping"], ["tomography" and "computer-aided design"] and ["tomography" and "computer-aided engineering"] were carried out. Such mentioned searches were done in September 2010 using the capabilities of ISI - Web of Knowledge databases and the main results are shown in Figures 3, 4 and 5. Of course, computed tomography is not the only imaging technology of application for promoting product development activities and we have to mention other possibilities, such as obtaining information from laser digitization or

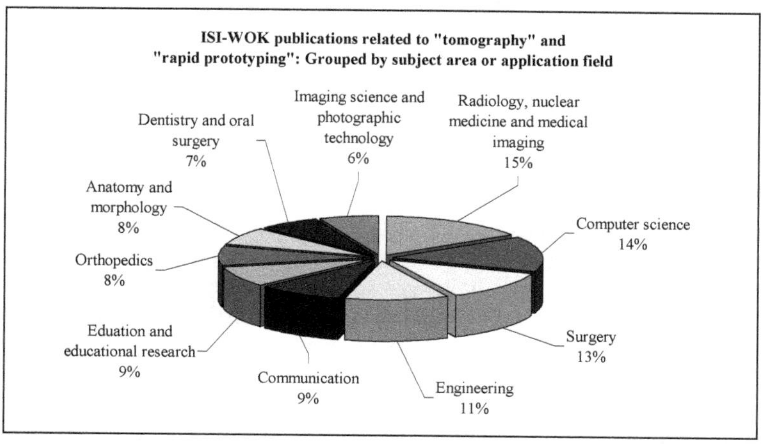

Fig. 3. ISI - Web of Knowledge publications with main topics "tomography" and "rapid prototyping" grouped by subject area or application field.

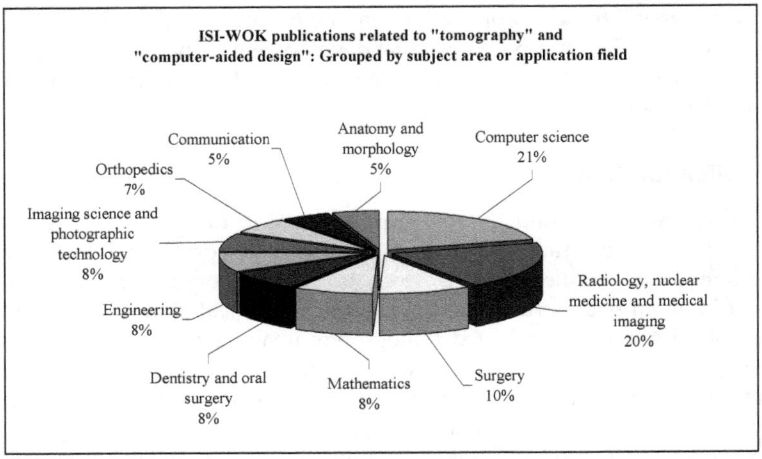

Fig. 4. ISI - Web of Knowledge publications with main topics "tomography" and "computer-aided design" grouped by subject area or application field.

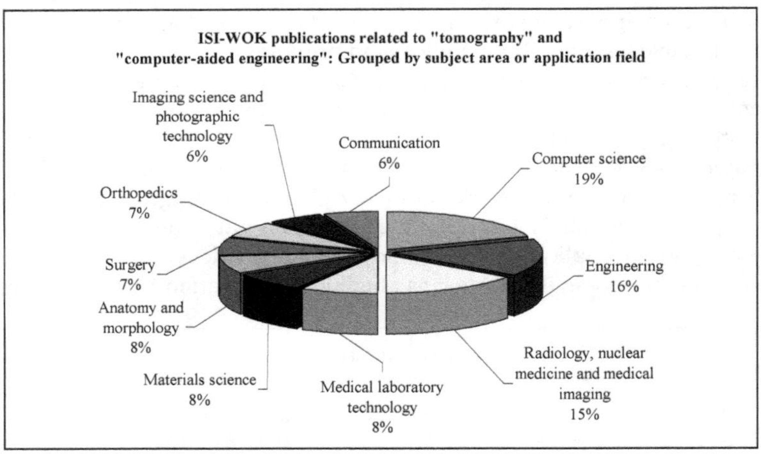

Fig. 5. ISI - Web of Knowledge publications with main topics "tomography" and "computer-aided engineering" grouped by subject area or application field.

using information from nuclear magnetic resonances and even positron emission tomography. A more detailed comparison between the capabilities of these technologies is included in the section regarding "Challenges and Future Trends".

Medical applications are most relevant according to all statistics, covering around 45 to 65% of applications, when considering surgery, orthopaedics, dentistry, radiology and anatomy together. Engineering studies (mainly related with product development, computer science and materials science) cover around 25 to 39% of applications of tomography combined with rapid prototyping, computer-aided design and computer-aided engineering, which is also an important number. Among medical applications there are several examples of publications regarding fields such as surgical training, medical device development,

development of diagnostic models and even development of models for teaching activities. Among engineering applications, the most important advances based on CT-aided processes correspond to the automotive and aeronautic industries.

4. Case studies: CT applications in product development

This section provides a couple of case studies, linked to the development of several prosthetic devices, regarding the use of computed tomography for enhancing personalized product developments. Traditionally, references of CT application to the design of personalized devices have been more linked to source images from hard tissues, but novel advances on quality and precision of the CT equipment also provide remarkable possibilities for designing prostheses adapted to soft tissues. Both approaches are compared further on, showing the design process of a hip prosthesis (including an evaluation of its influence on the patient's femoral structure) and explaining the development of a prosthesis adapted to cardiac tissue.

4.1 Design of personalized prosthesis adapted to hard tissue

The case study set out in this subchapter as an example details the process for producing a customized hip prosthesis design from the information from medical images. The aim was to produce a non-cemented prosthesis where the metal part is pressure-mounted inside the femur and must therefore be made to fit the available space. The design was made in the Machine Engineering Division of Universidad Politécnica de Madrid (www.upm.es) with the aid of the available CAD-CAE-CAM technologies. More detailed information may be found in the references (Osuna, 2008, Ojeda, 2009).
The usual procedure for carrying out a customized examination with a view to using a prosthetic device usually begins either by taking a computerized tomography - CT or a nuclear magnetic resonance - MRI / NMRI of the patient needing the prosthesis. Then, with the aid of .dicom or .dcm (Digital Communications in Medicine) format, the information from the CT or MRI can be transferred to a program such as "Mimics", so that it can be displayed in 3D, as Figure 6 shows. These programs usually include modules that allow selecting part of the patient's bone geometry and storing it in .stl or .igs formats that can be read by other CAD programs after processing the images "slice by slice". Having selected the relevant part of the patient's femur (in this example, the internal cavity to which the metal part of a customized prosthesis must be adapted) this three-dimensional geometry can be transferred to a format that is valid for a design program and this femoral zone can be used as the basis for a customized prosthesis design, as can be seen in Figure 7 (Ojeda, Osuna, Lafont, Díaz Lantada, 2009).

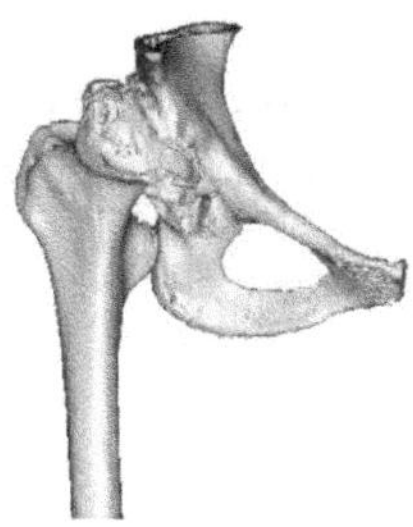

Fig. 6. 3D reconstruction of hip joint based on the information from CT images.

Mimics software for computer-aided designs based on medical images.

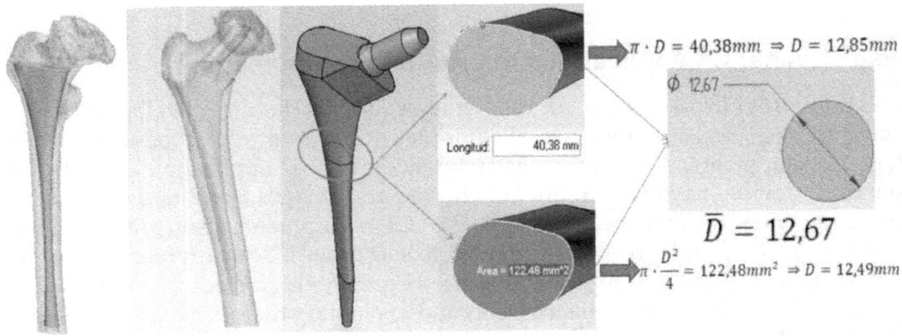

Fig. 7. Example of personalized prosthesis designed from the information of CT images.

4.2 Mechanical studies of body structures regarding the development of prostheses

Taking the designs produced by CAD programs, geometries can be converted into files that are recognized by CAE programs, that is, computer-aided calculation to which the finite elements method can be applied as a simulation tool for verifying that the designs are adequate for the in-service loads to be borne by the final product.

Until just a few years ago, this conversion was not always direct and the use of .igs or .stl formats led to some loss of information. However, the most widely-used CAD design programs are becoming more and more flexible in saving files and using different formats that are compatible with other CAD and CAE programs with FEM capabilities (Catia, NX-6, Solid Works, Rhino, Ansys, Nastran...). In fact, some programs like "Mimics" with the ability to reconstruct the information from medical images in 3D, cannot only transfer files to other design programs (and rapid prototyping machines) through their use of .stl format, but are also beginning to include specific outputs for finite element calculation and simulation programs.

In this study we have taken the relevant part of the patient's femur, from previous case study, and used a ".slt to solid" converter, so as to obtain a .igs file, for subsequent FEM calculations with the help of CAE programs. After introducing the geometry in such programs, material properties can be applied, the part can be meshed for optimizing calculations and loads and boundary conditions can be applied, so as to obtain a systematic study.

Figure 8 shows an example of how a patient's femur behaves, when the attached prosthesis receives a load from the acetabulum (2000 N is the value usually chosen for critical situations) and where the metal part is pressure-mounted inside the femur. The simulations were performed with FEM software taking an initial CAD design and allow us to study the stresses induced to a patient's femur, during loading of the prosthesis in conventional daily-life activities, so as to analyse the convenience of a prosthetic solution.

By using different contact models, the in-service behaviour of the implant and its effects on the surrounding tissue (bone in this case) can be reproduced. Some studies examine the influence of active prostheses on the geometry of soft tissues (Díaz Lantada, 2009). These studies are anyway essential for evaluating any harm that may be caused to the receptor organism by the designed implants.

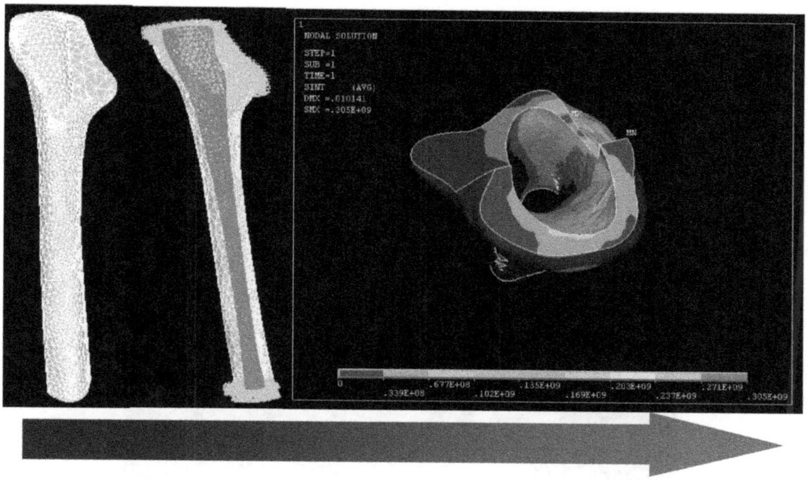

Fig. 8. Example of mechanical FEM study based on the information from CT images.

4.3 Design of a personalized prosthesis adapted to soft tissue

The major advances in customized prosthesis design have traditionally been linked to bone structures, since bone tissue density is easily identifiable, making it easier to produce the associated design more easily than for soft structures and tissue. Bone tissue appears as a very distinct white on the Hounsfield Scale, which is an important advantage when processing information from medical imaging tools, with programs like "Mimics" and those previously mentioned. However, in soft organs the difference in density between tissues is very small and does not let the different structures be identified separately, which is an enormous barrier to customized design work. This is the case with cardiac prostheses and in particular, regarding mitral annuloplasty rings, shown here as an example of application (Díaz Lantada, 2010).

In these cases, due to the similar densities of soft tissue, surrounding cloth and blood, some reference points need to be found in the medical images that will help the three-dimensional reconstruction of the target zone of the organ or soft tissue. In the example shown, cardiac CT images were used to identify in each "slice" the points of insertion of the valve leaflets in the patient's mitral ring (marked in blue in Figure 9). These points were inserted through their Cartesian coordinates in a CAD program, in order to get an idea of the three-dimensional morphology of the patient's mitral ring, to which the prosthetic annuloplasty ring is to be adapted, as well as for design tasks, as can be seen in Figure 10. Such prosthetic rings provide additional stiffness to the structure of a patient's mitral valve and help to reduce the degree of mitral insufficiency. There are several models and sizes in the market, as no design has yet proved to be especially beneficial, so personalization may well be a promising solution. The proposed design was also carried out in the Machine Engineering Division of Universidad Politécnica de Madrid (www.upm.es), with the aid of the available CAD-CAE-CAM technologies.

Further information on the complete design process of prostheses adapted to soft tissue and the customized design methodology proposed may be found in the references cited. Whatever the case, the information from medical imaging technologies combined with rapid prototyping technologies, are not only enormously useful in planning surgical work

(Binder, 2000, Gilon, 2002, Mottl-Link, 2008, Kim, 2008), but also have considerable advantages when rapid customized implants are required.

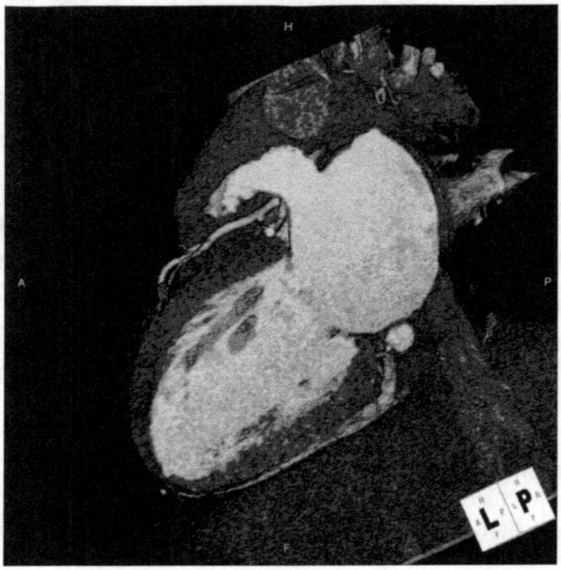

Fig. 9. Cardiac CT reconstruction of left atrium and ventricle, connected via mitral valve (Image courtesy of Raquel del Valle - Lennox Hill Heart and Vascular Institute NY).

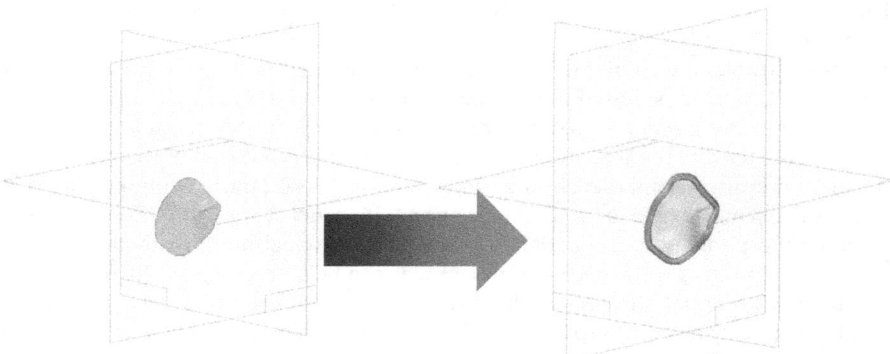

Fig. 10. Reconstruction of mitral valve section of a patient with mitral insufficiency and design of personalized annuloplasty ring, based on the information of cardiac CT images.

From the first solid models manufactured by layer manufacturing technologies, other rapid prototyping technologies denominated as "second stage" can be used to produce moulds by rapid-form copying. These moulds can be manufactured in numerous materials such as, silicones, ceramics, ceramics with a metal load and others, and allow casting stronger materials inside them than the original models. They enable prototypes to be produced for meeting the in-service specifications.

5. Challenges and future trends

5.1 Quality, precision and cost of equipment

A limiting aspect for using computed tomography for promoting product development activities, in different industries not directly linked to the medical sector, has traditionally been the cost of medical imaging equipment and the surrounding installations needed. To overcome such limitations, some enterprises now offer imaging and prototyping services, including the possibility of carrying out CT scans and subsequently providing a CAD file with the geometry of the desired part of the product. Outsourcing such medical imaging and format conversion tasks is a remarkable solution for research teams or small enterprises, that might need the help of computed tomography (or other imaging technologies), without having the possibility of acquiring their own equipment. Regarding the costs of digitization equipment, laser scanners and CCD (charge coupled device) film digitizers are more economic (around 1000 - 60000 €) than CT scanners or NMR equipment (from 150,000 even up to 500,000 €). However, laser and optical systems do not allow the reproduction of inner details, so important not only for personalized design processes, but also for non-invasive in-service verifications. New trends in the medical imaging industry are trying to mount different technologies, for combining their respective advantages, in one machine (CT+PET, CT+SPEC...) and regarding product development enhancement, perhaps it would be very positive to combine in one machine the fastness of laser scans with the capabilities of reproducing inner details of computed tomography. Such advances, together with an increase in precision and more competitive prices will help to spread the industrial applications of these technologies.

5.2 Normalization and standardization of formats

An aspect requiring additional dedication, to simplify the tasks of designers and to promote the information exchange regarding 3D designs, is the development and decision to use a common universal file format for computer-aided design activities and another one for computer-aided manufacturing and rapid prototyping processes (if possible, the same one). Nowadays there are several formats for CAD programs (.par, .prt, .asm, .cat, .obj, .3ds, .iges, .step...), as well as numerous alternatives for information exchange and subsequent rapid prototyping (.stl, .ply, .vrml, .iges, .step...). Format conversions suffered by a part, throughout the design, calculation and manufacturing process, entail information and quality loss. Furthermore, the possibility of using different CAD-CAE-CAM tools, for profiting from their respective advantages, is limited due to incompatibilities. Previous attempts at standardization have been carried out by private and military initiatives (.iges) or have appeared as an answer to proposals from international organisms such as ISO (.step format was a consequence of ISO10303 Standard), although the initial objectives have not yet been achieved. However, in other areas there are remarkable examples of collaboration, as happens in document processing (with the use of .pdf) and in the medical sector (with the DICOM standard for medical imaging). Once these limitations have been tackled, the advantages of the combined use of computed tomography with CAD tools and rapid prototyping will become evident. Such homogenization would also imply a cost reduction for teaching centres, due to the need for fewer software licenses, and the distribution of teaching resources would also be more adequate.

5.3 Promotion tasks: Teaching issues and collaboration between researchers

To promote the industrial expansion of CT-aided product development and CT-aided engineering, and facilitate their use for the development of new devices in several fields, it is very important for universities, research centres and major sector companies to collaborate and exchange information in respect of the scientific-technological progress in these materials and their applications. It is an inherent mission of teachers and researchers to focus attention on these new fields of study and on the importance of examining them together in a coordinated manner and to look on other researchers as companions and never as rivals. Cooperation among technology branch and health branch teachers in the preparation and teaching of courses related to these subjects is also important. It is in this respect that the participation of departments from different universities is very positive as they can make their laboratories and research centres available to students. It is interesting to consider ways to exchange information and enhance teaching, like those listed below:

- It would be highly beneficial to set up a specific forum on medical imaging and its industrial applications, beyond the medical sector, with a specific section devoted to engineering and product design and development, where researchers, universities and companies can get in productive contact.
- Congresses and scientific meetings are very useful instruments for bringing together the main researchers in an area of knowledge, particularly when this is done according to a fixed schedule to discuss specific topics, and it would be very positive to arrange regular international meetings on CT-aided product development and CT-aided engineering, possibly also including topics linked to alternative technologies, such as nuclear magnetic resonance or laser digitization.
- To encourage the use of these technologies in Industry it is important to make known the advantages expected from their use. Therein lies one of the basic benefits of carrying out research work in the University, since the discoveries made encourage changing and gradually updating the syllabuses of the related subjects. This helps to promote and maintain students' interest and to increase the transfer of knowledge arising from research to Society as a whole.

5.4 Reverse Engineering: Related risks

We cannot finish the chapter without warning about the risks derived from the misuse of these combinations of technologies, especially regarding industrial piracy and the usurpation of intellectual property rights. Of course computed tomography, combined with computer-aided design and rapid prototyping, can give new life to old or damaged parts and products no longer available and promote restoration activities (for example for the classic automotive industry), as well as archaeological processes and modular design activities. However, it has also led to the appearance of pirate companies that plainly copy the designs of products from all kinds of industries (automotion, entertainment, household, furniture...) and start up production directly, without having invested in the development process. It is therefore always advisable to protect novel developments by means of patents, not just as a very positive advantage related with marketing activities and negotiation processes, but also as a way of being protected against the risks of reverse engineering. For a powerful protection, patents should provide a description, as detailed as possible, of the novel developments and be written with the help of specialized lawyer's offices.

6. Conclusions

Several technological advances during the last two decades have promoted novel approaches to product design and development. The generalized use of computer-aided design and simulation tools, together with the advances in materials science and manufacturing technologies (especially rapid manufacturing technologies or "layer manufacturing technologies"), has enabled the development of more complex geometries and products. The additional possibility of using the information obtained from CT images as input for computer-aided design and for computer-aided engineering programs has opened up new horizons for carrying out personalized and ergonomic designs, as well as for promoting all kinds of tasks linked to product design and reverse engineering (reconstruction of damaged products, reproduction of delicate parts and studies related to inner non-visible geometries, among others).

This chapter has tried to cover some of the most important applications for such combination of CT imaging, design and manufacturing technologies, including industrial design, automotive engineering, aeronautics, bioengineering, archaeology and even teaching or art. Some case studies related to successful developments have been explained in detail, so as to analyse the most common procedures and in order to provide advice for conventional difficulties. It is important to note that the impact of combining information from medical imaging technologies with the advantages of novel design and manufacturing tools is so remarkable and its applications so widespread, that we can speak of "CT-aided product development" or even "CT-aided engineering". The main present challenges for improving the end-quality and industrial impact of such developments have been also discussed, together with some analytical reflections on the most important risks derived from these novel capabilities, especially concerning the limits between reverse engineering and plagiarism. Current remarkable study and research trends have also been analysed, with the hope of promoting collaboration among universities, research centres and enterprises.

7. References

Bibb, R.; Brown, R. (2000). The application of computer aided product development techniques in medical modelling topic: Rehabilitation and prostheses. *Biomedical Science Instrumentation*, 36, 319-324.

Binder, T. (2005). Stereolithographic biomodeling to create tangible hard copies of cardiac structures from echocardiographic data: In vitro and in vivo validation. *Journal of the American College of Cardiology*, 35, 230-237.

Chang, C.C.; Lee, M.Y.; Ku, Y.C. (2003). Digital custom dentare design with new abrasive computer tomography and rapid prototyping technologies. *Biomedical Engineering Applications, Basis and Communications*, 15(3), 115-119.

Cormack, A.M. (1964). Representation of a function by its line integrals with some radiological applications. *Journal of Applied Physics*, 35, 2908-2913.

Díaz Lantada, A.; Lorenzo Yustos, H.; Lafont, P.; Munoz-Guijosa, J.M.; Echavarri Otero, J.; Muñoz Sanz, J.L. (2007). Teaching applications for rapid prototyping technologies. *International Journal of Engineering Education*, 23(2), 411-418.

Díaz Lantada, A.; P. Lafont, P.; Muñoz-García, J.; Muñoz Sanz, J.L.; Munoz-Guijosa, J.M.; Echavarri, J.; Lorenzo, H. (2009). Stress-strain simulations for optimizing the design of shape-memory polymer based annuloplasty rings. *World Congress on Medical Physics and Biomedical Engineering 2009*. Munich, 7 - 12 September.

Díaz Lantada, A.; Del Valle Fernández, R.; Lafont Morgado, P.; Muñoz García, J.; Muñoz Sanz, J.L.; Munoz-Guijosa, J.M.; Echávarri Otero, J. (2010). Development of Personalized Annuloplasty Rings: Combination of CT Images and CAD-CAM Tools. *Annals of Biomedical Engineering*, 38(2), 280-290.

DICOM Standard - Digital Imaging and Communications in Medicine, Strategic Document available from: http://medical.nema.org

Effenberger, I.; Kroll, J.; Verl, A. (2008). New solutions and applications of 3D computer tomography image processing. *Proceedings of the SPIE*, 6813, 68130A.

Erkens, A. (1928). Beiträge zur Konstruktionserziehung. *VDI-Z Verlag. Integrierte Produktion*, 72, 17-21.

Flisch, A. (1999). Industrial computed tomography in reverse engieering applications. *International Symposium on Computerized Tomography for Industrial Applications and Image Processing in Radiology*. DGZfP Proceedings.

Freitag, D.; Wohlers, T. (2003). Rapid prototyping: State of the Art. *Manufacturing technology information analysis centre*. Chicago Illinois.

Gilon, D. (2002). Effect of three-dimensional valve shape on the hemodynamics of aortic stenosis: Three-dimensional echocardiographic stereolithography and patient studies. *Journal of the American College of Cardiology*, 40(8), 1479-1486.

Harrysson O. (2007). Custom-designed orthopaedic implants evaluated using FEM analysis of patient computed tomography data. *BMC Musculoskeletal Disorders*, 8(91).

Hieu, L.C. (2002). Design and manufacturing of personalized implants and standardized templates for cranioplasty applications. *Industrial Technology*, 2(11-14). 1025-1030. IEEE ICIT '02.

Hounsfield, G.N. (1973). Computerized transverse axial scanning (tomography): Part 1. Description of system. *British Journal of Radiology*. 46, 1016-1022.

Kaiser, W.; König, W. (2006). Geschichte des Ingenieurs. Ein Beruf in sechs Jahrtausenden. *Carl Hanser Verlag*. München.

Kesselring, F. (1954). Technische Kompositionslehre. *Springer*. Berlin.

Kesselring, F. (1951). Bewertung von Konstruktionen. *VDI Verlag*. Düsseldorf.

Kim, M. (2008). Rapid prototyping: A new tool in understanding and treating structural heart disease. *Circulation*, 117, 2388-2394.

Kucklick, T.R. (2006). The Medical Device R&D Handbook. *CRC Press, Taylor & Francis Group* (1st Ed.).

Kuhlenkamp, A. (1971). Konstruktionslehre der Feinwerktechnik. *Hanser*. München.

Lafont Morgado, P.; Lorenzo Yustos, H. (2000). Rapid tooling: Moldes rápidos a partir de estereolitografía. *Revista de plásticos modernos*, 524, 150-157.

Losano, F.; Marinsek, G.; Merlo, A.M.; Ricci, M. (1999). Computed tomography in the automotive field. Development of a new engine head case study. *Computerized Tomography for Industrial Applications and Image Processing in Radiology*. DGZfP Proceedings.

Matousek, R. (1957). Konstruktionslehren des allgemeinen Maschinenbaus. *Springer*. Berlin.

Mottl-Link, S. (2008). Physical models aiding in complex congenital heart surgery. *The Society of Thoracic Surgeons. Annals of Thoracic Surgery* 86, 273-277.

Niemann, G. (1950, 1965, 1975). Maschinenelemente. *Springer*. Berlin.

Ojeda Diaz, C. (2009). Estudio de la influencia de estabilidad primaria en el diseño de vástagos de prótesis de cadera personalizadas. *PhD Thesis. Universidad Politécnica de Madrid.*

Ojeda Díaz, C.; Osuna López, J.; Lafont Morgado, P.; Díaz Lantada, A. (2009). Estudio de la estabilidad primaria, influencia en el diseño de vástagos de prótesis femorales personalizadas: Aplicación a paciente específico. *3º Congresso Nacional de Biomecânica. Sociedade Portuguesa de Biomecânica.* 11 - 12 February in Braganza.

Osuna, J.E. (2008).- Combinación de tecnologías para la optimización del desarrollo de prótesis. *Master Thesis. Universidad Politécnica de Madrid.*

Pahl, G., Beitz, W. (1996). Engineering design: A systematic approach. *Springer Verlag*. London.

Reinhart, C.; Poliwoda, C.; Günther, T. How industrial computer tomography accelerates product development in the light metal casting and moulding industry. *Database and Journal of Non-Destructive Testing (www.ndt.net).*

Reuleaux, F. (1875). Lehrbuch der Kinematik, 1: Theoretische Kinematik. *Vieweg und Sohn*. Braunschweig.

Reuleaux, F. (1875). Lehrbuch der Kinematik, 2: Die praktischen Beziehungen Kinematik zu Geometrie und Mechanik. *Vieweg und Sohn*. Braunschweig.

Roozenburg, N.; Eeckels J. (1995). Product design: Fundamentals and methods. *John Wiley & Sons*. New York.

Saaksvuori, A.; Immonen, A. (2008). Product lifecycle management. 3rd Edition. *Springer Verlag*. Berlin, Heidelberg, London, New York.

Schwarz, M. (2005). New Materials Processes, and Methods Technology. *CRC Press (1st Ed.). Taylor & Francis Group.*

Stark, J. (2004). Product lifecycle management: 21st Century paradigm for product realisation. *Springer Verlag*. Berlin, Heidelberg, New York.

Taddei, M.; Zanon, E. (2006). Atlas ilustrado de las máquinas de Leonardo. *Editorial Susaeta*. Madrid.

Tschochner, H. (1954). Konstruieren und Gestalten. *Girardet*. Essen.

Ulrich, K., Eppinger, S. (2007). Product design and development. 4th Edition. *Mc-Graw Hill / Irwin*. New York.

Vasilash, G. (2009). Ford accelerates product development with additive technology. *Time Comrpession (www.timecompression.com)*.

Wohlers, T. (2008). The Wohlers Report - Additive Manufacturing: State of the industry. *Wohlers Associates*.

www.ingramcontent.com/pod-product-compliance
Lightning Source LLC
LaVergne TN
LVHW080712300625
814993LV00006BA/36